To Cindy & Paul
In case you're
interested —
Love, Al & Beth

Under the Apple Tree

*This shall be written for the
generation to come, and children still
unborn shall praise the Lord!
Psalm 102:18*

Under the Apple Tree

Marrying ~ Birthing ~ Parenting

Helen Wessel

Bookmates International
Fresno, California

Under the Apple Tree • Marrying • Birthing • Parenting

International copyright © 1981 by Helen S. Wessel.

Scripture quotations in this publication are from the King James Version (KJV) or author's paraphrases of the KJV, unless otherwise indicated. Other versions quoted include the Living Bible (LB), New American Bible (NAB), New American Standard Bible (NASB), New English Bible (NEB), Phillips (Ph.) and the Revised Standard Version (RSV).

Published by Bookmates International, Incorporated. All rights reserved. Printed in the Unites States of America. No part of this book may be used or reproduced in any manner whatsoever without written permission except in the case of brief quotations embodied in critical articles and reviews. For information address: Bookmates International, Post Office Box 9883, Fresno, California 93795, United States of America.

Cover art: MIC Innovative Creations, Lakeside, California

Cover photo: William Johnson, Chase City, Virginia

Typesetting: Gloria Walters, San Diego, California

Library of Congress Catalog Card Number: 79-52050

International Standard Book Number: 0-933082-02-9

Contents

Foreword: Dr. Walter W. Wessel vii

Introduction: How to Use This Book ix

Part I   Personhood and Marriage

Who is God?
The nature of God, creation, Adam and Eve, temptation, redemption 3

Who Am I?
Personal identity, body and spirit, relationships, fulfilment 16

Unity in Diversity
One in heart and soul, God first, the single person, husband/wife roles 33

Awakened Desires
The frankness of Scripture, the purity of sex in marriage, overcoming sexual difficulties 50

The Song of Songs
Barriers to sexual happiness, love a commitment, growing intimacy 66

When Two Agree
The need for children, birth control, natural family planning and the sympto-thermal method 80

Part II   Life and Birth

The Gift of Life
Eve, Cain and Abel, the death of Jesus Christ, life in the womb, from generation to generation 99

Garden of the Lord
Balanced nutrition, bread from heaven, breathing patterns for good health and for natural childbirth 114

Great Expectation
Exercises and relaxation for good health and for natural childbirth, stages of growth of the infant in the womb 128

Labor of Love
Signs of labor, stages of labor, birth 144

The Way of Wisdom
    Causes of pain in labor, medical attitudes toward childbirth,
    common medical practices, childbirth alternatives 160
No Place Like Home
    Pros and cons, preparation, examples of home birth 182

Part III   The Circle of Love

Baby Makes Three
    Touching, eye contact, naming, breastfeeding 199
New Identities
    Adjusting to new lifestyles, baby in the parents' bed,
    Daddy is a parent too......................................214
The Way of a Child
    Fair expectations, learning to make choices, discipline
    and responsibility...229
A Time to Lose
    Weaning from the breast, from the home, coping with
    loss, grieving 244
A Time to Remember
    The importance of memory, healing of unhappy memories,
    building good memories.....................................257
The Family of God
    Infant dedication, family-style fellowship groups,
    the perfect Church 270

Appendix

Acknowledgments 289
Permission credits 291
Resources 293
Recommended Reading 295
Index 311
About the Author 315
Childbirth in Emergency 316

Foreword

Under the Apple Tree is the result of many years of experiencing the grace and faithfulness of God in the birthing and rearing of six children. The theology and spiritual insights of this book represent the day-to-day lifestyle of its author. What she says in this book comes straight out of a life dedicated to and lived for Jesus Christ.

As Helen's husband, I have been privileged to share in many of the experiences spoken of in the book. One of the most remarkable was the birth of our oldest son Daniel. I was not only present at the birth, which took place at home, I assisted in it! The miracle of birth, as I witnessed it that day, confirmed to me again the biblical teaching of the wisdom, love and grace of God.

For those who read the pages of this book my prayer is that the same wisdom, love and grace of God which is so evident in all creation, may be revealed and confirmed to you.

Walter W. Wessel

Introduction

Is your interest childbirth? Start reading there. Is it marriage? Read there. Is it raising children? Turn to those portions of the book first. Dip in anywhere that is of current interest.

The book provides a biblical base from which all these diverse experiences of family life can be integrated within the Christian community. We live in a fractured society. Even our family and church lives are fragmented. For information on family planning, a couple must go to one place; for childbirth education, to another; for help with breastfeeding, still another. For help in childrearing, we must trot to this or that seminar. For Bible teaching, we turn to the church or Bible study groups, which may fragment families with age and sex segregation. All of these subjects are addressed in this book.

The title, **Under the Apple Tree,** accurately reflects the theme of this book, which begins with God and His natural creation:

> *Nature to a saint is sacramental. If we are children of God, we have a tremendous treasure in Nature. In every wind that blows, in every night and day of the year, in every sign of the sky, in every blossoming and in every withering of the earth, there is a real coming of God to us if we will simply use our starved imagination to realize it.*[1]

Apple trees remind us of the garden of Eden, the great issues of life and death and the forbidden fruit. We move on into courtship and marriage: *Strengthen me with raisin cakes, refresh me with apples, for I am faint with love.*[2]

As an apple tree among the trees of the wood,
so is my beloved among the sons.
I sat down under his shadow with great delight,
and his fruit is sweet to my taste.
He brought me to his banqueting table
and his banner over me is love.[3]

Trees remind us of a "natural" setting for conception (natural family planning) and birthing (natural childbirth):

Who is this that comes up from the desert
leaning on her lover?
Under the apple tree I roused you;
there your mother conceived you,
there she who was in labor gave you birth.[4]

We are reminded of natural foods (breastfeeding), of children climbing trees (sometimes eating green apples!) and of grandmother's apple pies. It reminds us of nurturing and of growth toward maturity: *As the days of a tree shall the days of my people be.*[5] *They shall still bring forth fruit in old age.*[6] It reminds us of God's promised blessings to children's children,[7] the "family tree" branching out from generation to generation.

We end where we began, in the garden of God, where there flows *a pure river of the water of life. On either side of the river is the tree of life with its twelve kinds of fruit, yielding its fruit each month; and the leaves of the tree were for the healing of the nations.*[8] It is here in the garden of God that the heavenly bridegroom waits for His bride.[9]

A leader's manual accompanies the book. Those interested in forming study groups or in sponsoring seminars to train group leaders may write to: Apple Tree Family Life Teaching Series, P.O. Box 9883, Fresno, California, 93795.

I worked hard, . . . yet not I, but the grace of God was with me.[10] May His grace also be with every reader.

Helen Wessel

NOTES
1. Oswald Chambers. **My Utmost For His Highest.** New York. Dodd, Mead and Company, 1965. P. 41.Reprinted by permission.
2. Song of S. 2:5. NAB. **3.** Song of S. 2:3, 4. **4.** Song of S. 8:5. NIV. **5.** Isa. 65:22 RSV. **6.** Ps. 92:14. **7.** Ps. 103:17, 18. **8.** Rev. 22:1, 2 RSV. **9.** Rev. 19:7-9. **10.** 1 Cor. 15:10.

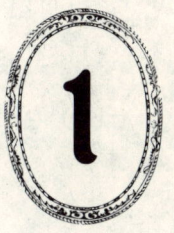

Personhood and Marriage

Who Is God?

And God said, Let us make man in our image, after our likeness. Let them have dominion over the fish of the sea, the birds of the air, the cattle, all animals of the earth and over every thing that crawls on the ground.

So God created man in his own image; in the image of God he created him; male and female he created them.

And God blessed them and said to them, Be fruitful and multiply, fill the earth and subdue it, ruling over the fish in the sea, the birds of heaven, and every living thing that moves upon earth....

And God saw all that he had made, and he found it very good.[1]

The Bible says that people are *made in the image of God*. But who is God? And what is that "image"? How can we understand who we are and in what ways we reflect God unless we have some understanding of who God is?

God is a Person

God is not just an ethereal essence pervading the universe like the atmosphere. He has a specific identity and is called by a name. The God of Moses said His name was **I Am.** The name ***Jehovah*** is from the Hebrew word *to be—yahveh.* When Moses asked God how he could explain to the children of Israel who He was, God said to tell them, **I Am who I Am.**[2]

Centuries later Jesus said, *Before Abraham was,* ***I Am.***[3] When the religious leaders heard Jesus call Himself by God's name,

Jehovah, they were so incensed they tried to stone him to death for blasphemy.

> *Again the high priest asked him, and said unto him, "Are you the Christ, the Son of the Blessed?"*
> *And Jesus said, "**I Am;** and you shall see the Son of man sitting on the right hand of power, and coming in the clouds of heaven."*
> *And the high priest tore his clothes and said, "You have heard the blasphemy! What do you think?" And they all condemned him as guilty of death.*[4]

God is a Person with a specific identity. God has a name: *Jehovah—**I Am.***

Our finite minds cannot comprehend a time in which there was no time, nor space before there was space, for we can only understand the temporal and spatial boundaries which define our own universe. Yet in that time before time, before the worlds were made, there was the great *I Am—Jehovah.* God **was** and **is** and **is to come**[5]—infinite, with no beginning and no end, the eternal *I Am.*

God is a Spirit

Jesus says, *God is a Spirit, and they who worship him must worship in spirit and in truth.*[6] It is hard for us to understand what "spirit" is. It seems unreal, vaporous. The word *ghost* makes us even more uneasy. It is something one cannot see nor touch nor feel and yet is somehow *there.* This is why God one day came to us as a human being, so we could see and touch and hear God in the flesh. Yet Jesus was not only flesh, nor could the body hold Him captive. For when His body was crucified, in those last moments of agony He cried out, *Father, I give back to you my spirit.*[7]

God is a Person—a different kind of Person—a spiritual Person. He has an identity, a name, and is eternal. He is not a static symbol, but is able to make choices, and to enter into relationships.

And in that space before space the universe was not empty, for it was filled with the Presence of the Eternal Spirit, God. Nor was there darkness, for *God is light, and in him is no darkness at all.*[8] Nor was it lonely, for the Bible says, *In the beginning was the Word* (Jesus), *and the Word was **with** God, and the Word **was** God.*[9]

God is a "Family"

This Person who is God, who is Spirit, is really three Persons, a Trinity—a community, a fellowship, a "family." The very first chapter of the Bible makes this plain, for it says *In the beginning God (Elohim).*[10] The Hebrew word **Elohim** is the plural form of another Hebrew word for God, **El.** This "plural" Person could discuss matters, share decision making, and cooperate in creating *(Let **us** make.* . . . [11]).

But **Elohim** is not God's name. His name is **Jehovah.** And we know that He is a Trinity, Three-in-One, rather than several gods because Deuteronomy 6:4 clearly says, **Jehovah, your Elohim** *is* **one Jehovah.** . . . God is manifested in three Persons but is one God, whose name is Jehovah. God the Father, God the Holy Spirit and God the Son are related to each other in perfect unity, three aspects of One Being, the impenetrable mystery of the Triune God.

And the nature of this Being is Love: *God is love.*[12] Love must have an object for its affection. It implies an *other.* God is a "family" of loving relationships, for God the Father loves the Son and the Spirit. God the Son loves the Father and the Spirit. God the Holy Spirit loves the Father and the Son.

What is love? Poets and sages have attempted to describe it, often giving a mother's affection for her child as its highest human example. But is it not from God, who is Love, that this "mother-love" comes into being? Can we speak of the mother-love of God or, dare we, even of God as mother? Some theologians have suggested that the Holy Spirit is the mothering aspect of God,[13] our comforter, guide and protector.

Yes, God is father. The Scriptures affirm this again and again. But God is also mother, and in that knowledge many fearful, lonely ones may safely rest their weary souls. For in this sinful world millions have never experienced love from their earthly fathers. Thus it is difficult for them to think of God as a loving father.

When, in addressing God we use the word "Father," as Jesus told us to, we must not narrow the meaning: we must not put such emphasis on masculinity that we fail to endow God with the tenderness, the affection, the attention characteristic of a mother. . . .

God incorporates into his love for us all the different facets of human love. The love of a father, the love of a mother, the love of a brother, the love of a sister, the love of a husband, the love of a wife—all are present, all are contained in God.[14]

God is Creator
Before the worlds began, heaven and earth were conceived as an idea in the mind of God, who was "pregnant" with the vision of all that could be. Out of nothing but the essence of the One who filled all, heaven and earth burst into physical reality.[15] For this Triune God is also Creator.

*In the beginning God **(Elohim)** created the heaven and the earth.... And the Spirit of God moved upon the face of the waters. And God said, Let there **be...** and there **was.***[16]
*Before the mountains were born **(yalad)** or ever you had given birth **(chul)** to the earth and the world, even from everlasting to everlasting you are God.*[17]

The Spirit of God *moved upon the face of the waters,* hovering, sighing, heaving into life waters, earth and sky. The creative word of God caused light and life to explode into being. Daughter earth was formed in the womb of *the darkness upon the face of the deep,* [18] rocked in the cradle of the sea and bathed in its waters, as is the unborn child in the womb.

The Psalmist describes how God the mother caused the mountains to be born *(yalad)* and "gave birth to" *(chul)* the earth and to the worlds beyond. These Hebrew words which speak of God "giving birth" are the same words used of a mother giving birth to a child.

Earth emerged from the waters, the shoulders of the mountains pushing upward until their peaks pierced the limits of the sky. The Spirit of God wrapped swaddling bands of clouds around the mountain peaks, caressing the valleys with soft gauzes of the breeze. A mist arose to kiss the barren soil until daughter earth herself could bring forth grass and herbs and trees.

Has the rain a father?
  or who has begotten the drops of dew?
Out of whose womb came the ice?
  and who has given birth to the hoar frost
    of heaven?[19]

Although daughter earth emerged into light—for God is light, so that there was no need for sun or stars—yet this penetrating, life-sustaining light of God was invisible to her. So God hung lamps in the ceiling of the sky: a sun to light her day and the moon and stars to light her night.

Daughter earth in turn became the mother, "mother earth," we say. *And God said, Let the earth **(adamah)** bring forth the living creature after his kind, cattle, and creeping things and the animals of the earth after their kinds. And it was so.*[20]

Of course we understand that the term "mother earth" is a figure of speech, for the earth does not really "give birth." Each living creature contains in itself the ability to reproduce its own kind, and earth does not give birth to earth. However, earth is the source from which come all animals, including man.

In the same way, God "gave birth to" and "mothered" the earth only as a figure of speech, for the creation did not share the essential nature of the Creator. After the heavens and the earth had been created, *God saw that it was good,*[21] but was not satisfied.

God longed for beings with the capacity both for intelligent creativity and for loving relationships, including a relationship with Himself. Thus people were created in God's own image.

> *And **Elohim** said, Let **us** make **adam** (mankind—people) in **our** image, after **our** likeness.... So **Elohim** created **adam** (people) in his own image; in the image of God created he him; **male and female** created he them. And God blessed **them,** and God said to **them,** "Be fruitful and multiply, and fill the earth and subdue it; and have dominion....*[22]

The Hebrew word **adam** means "mankind," "men and women," "people." The earth, **adamah**—the feminine form of the word **adam**—is the source from which men and women as well as animals have been made. Both men and women—though they came from earth—are given dominion **over** it. They are to "husband" the earth, to "mother, nurture" it and all its creatures. The words to "husband, mother, nurture" are synonyms describing God's loving care for His creation, a responsibility God shares with men and women.

The Bible says male **and female** are created in the image of God. Woman mirrors God's image equally with man. God has all the finest attributes of everything we call "womanly:" patience, gentleness, sensitivity. He has all the fine qualities we call "manly:" courage, endurance, forthrightness. A man then, to be like God, must reflect the "womanly" as well as the "manly" characteristics of God, just as a woman, made in God's image, is also to reflect His "manly" attributes.

To say that God has the attributes of both man and woman, both father[23] or mother,[24] is not assigning human sex to the persons of the Trinity. God is Spirit, transcending maleness or femaleness. Thus men and women as spiritual beings[25] created in the image of God also transcend the physical limitations of their maleness or femaleness.

The first chapter of Genesis gives us the broad panorama of the creation of people, men and women, the human race, ***adam,*** who come both from the earth and from the Spirit of God. The second chapter of Genesis relates in greater detail the manner in which God brought this to pass.

He began with the man. (In the first three chapters of Genesis whenever it says *"**the** man"* it means Adam only.) The first man, Adam, was named after the earth *(**adamah**)* from which he was made. He was not "brought forth" by the spoken command of God as was the rest of creation.[26]ABather, God personally formed him from the ground with watchful care:

*So the Lord God formed man **(adam)** from the dust of the ground **(adamah)**, and breathed into his nostrils the breath of life, and man became a living soul.*[27]

Did not the other land animals also breathe? Yes, they breathed earth's atmosphere. But it was not only air that entered man: it was also the very breath of God. No other earthly being is "God-breathed," a living ***spirit,*** with the capacity for communion with God. The man was son of God as well as of earth, prefiguring Jesus, who would one day come to earth as Son of God and Son of man. Even the angels of heaven (of whose creation we are not told) do not share our likeness to God.[28]

God planted a beautiful garden and placed the man in it as its "husbandman," to mother, nurture, protect it. God brought to him all the birds and beasts to name and invited him to use every provision in the garden except one:

You may freely eat of every tree of the garden; but of the tree of the knowlege of good and evil you shall not eat, for in the day that you eat of it you shall die.[29]

What does this strange warning of "death" mean? In this exquisite garden of God[30] the lion can lie down with the lamb[31] and there is nothing to hurt nor destroy, for death has not yet entered the world. Adam did not know what death could be. He had no "knowledge" of its evil.

Although the man lived in this perfect environment, he was lonely. He gave names to all the animals and birds of the air, searching among them for companionship. But among all that had been created from the same earth from which he was taken, no companion was found, for in him alone was the breath of God. It is utterly impossible for people, as spiritual beings, to live alone. Just as God's own nature is a fellowship, a "family," so no human being can be fully satisfied without a relationship to some "other" in whom God's Spirit also resides.

Day after day the man searched for the "help" *(ezer)* God had promised him, the one who would be a help *(ezer)* as God was a help *(ezer),* someone who alone was made in God's image. The Hebrew word *ezer* means "to surround, protect, aid, support," and is a word often used of God's relationship to man.[32]

The man looked into the eyes of each of the animals as he named them. A warm, affectionate gaze was often returned, but without comprehension. When he tried to discourse with them they wandered off, uninterested. Although God talked with him, he could not see God, who is Spirit, and his loneliness increased.

One evening when the man lay down God caused him to fall into a deep sleep, the death-like sleep of God's "anesthesia" in which he felt nothing. As he slept God made an incision in his side, took flesh from his side to make a woman and closed the incision. Adam had become a "mother" as if by cesarean section![33]

But there was an essential difference in the woman being "born" from the man than when a man is born of woman.[34] For when a child is born it is fully formed as a human being, though still an infant. Not so with Eve. The Creator fashioned her as Adam had been fashioned, with loving care. Adam sacrificed his own flesh for Eve, but he did not create her. She was not formed **in** his body, but from the flesh taken from his side *(tsela).* (The Hebrew word *tsela* occurs 42 times in the Old Testament and is consistently translated as "side" or "chambers of the side", **except** in the case of Eve, where translators arbitrarily call it "rib"!)

*And the flesh which the Lord God has taken from man's side **made he** into a woman, and brought her to the man.*[35]

Adam stirred in his sleep. When he opened his eyes, it seemed that he had been sleeping for a long time! The sun was high in the heavens and the garden alive with the rustle of creatures and bird song. He tried to sit up, but a stiffness in his side made him wince. Instinctively he put his hand on his side and looked down. Astonished, he noticed a long, faint scar, as if from a fresh wound! As he struggled to his feet a slight movement caught his eye.

What is this! he wondered as he made his way through the foliage toward the strange, lovely creature, the woman. She did not seem to notice him. His heart pounding, he reached out and touched her. Startled, she turned and looked right into his eyes.

How a single look can speak volumes! For the first time a gaze answered his own with understanding. Here was one like himself, with whom he could laugh and cry, talk and pray, plan and wonder. The woman was taken from his side to remain side by side with him, not above him, not below him, but one like himself. She spoke his language—not the language of his lips only—but the language of his heart, of his spirit. Adam exclaimed:

*This at last is bone of my bones and flesh of my flesh; she shall be called (Wo)man **(isshah)** because she was taken out of Man **(ish)**.*[36]

If God had formed the woman out of the ground as he had the man, Adam might have thought her different from himself, as the other earth creatures were different. Instead, she shared both his flesh and spirit. The feminine attributes were all latent in Adam's personality—as they are in every man—before Eve was taken and formed from his flesh. Her creation did not rob him of these attributes. The masculine attributes of Adam were all latent in Eve's personality—as they are in every woman—for man and woman are formed from "one flesh."

The only apparent difference was that she was female and he was male, so that their bodies could mold together in the love-making of sex. This delightful invention of God was given to increase a husband and wife's pleasure in each other in the closest act of physical intimacy and to perpetuate the human race.

And even these sexual differences are not as great as some might think.[37] It is misleading to think that only men have "male hormones," and only women have "female hormones." Rather, it is the **balance** of androgens and estrogens in each person's body which determines the extent of the male or female characteristics of that person.

One's real "self" is not bound by the limitations of flesh or of sex, for each is made in the image of God, a creative personality, a "spirit." Only the body which houses the spirit is in male or female form. The essential "personhood" of man and woman is the same, for each reflects God's spiritual nature.

Thus Eve is a person in her own right, and Adam becomes her head, to husband her, to mother, nurture and protect her. He is to teach her the oracles he has received from God, for she is new to this world. She is the learner, and Adam her priest-husband must teach her God's truth concerning the tree of life which will enable them to live forever. He is also responsible for warning her of God's command not to eat of the tree of the knowledge of good and evil. Although she is like him in potential, the woman so newly formed is still untaught and needs to be brought to maturity.[38]

Does it seem strange that the priestly role of the husband might be described as one of "mothering"? Yet the apostle Paul did not hesitate to call himself a mother, for he once wrote, *My little children, with whom I labor in birth again until Christ be formed in you.*[39] The role of a priest or pastor is that of "mothering" the people. The Church itself is called a "mother."[40]

God is Savior

Adam the priest/husband, from whom Eve was formed and by whom she was taught and nurtured, is an imperfect shadow of the God-man who was to come. For as Adam's bride was taken from his side, even so is the bride of Christ taken from His mangled side, *born of water and of blood,*[41] *born of His Spirit.*[42]

In the Greek translation of the Old Testament by Jewish scholars called the Septuagint, translated 400 years before Christ, the Hebrew word **tsela** (side) from which Eve was formed is translated as **pleura,** from which we get our word "pleurisy"—a pain in the side. This same Greek word occurs in the crucifixion account:

> *One of the soldiers with a spear pierced Jesus' side* ***(pleura),*** *and right away blood and water flowed out.... For these things were done, that the scriptures should be fulfilled, "They shall look on him whom they have pierced."*[43]

Adam is a symbol of Christ, put into a "deep sleep" that Eve might be formed of his own flesh, just as Jesus entered into the utter darkness of real death that we might be born of His Spirit through His pierced side, His life's blood poured out for us.

And as Adam was raised out of sleep to receive his bride, so Jesus was raised from the dead to receive His bride, the Church. Adam said of Eve, *She is bone of my bones and flesh of my flesh.*[44] The bride of Jesus Christ is called *members of his body, of his flesh and of his bones.*[45]

This is the most astonishing fact of all concerning who God is. God is a Person. God is a Spirit. God is a "family," a Trinity of Persons. God is a Creator. Yet this majestic, awesome God humbled Himself to the lowest hell—for you and me. God is Savior!

Adam, the priest/husband to Eve, was not only to love and nurture her with gentleness. As her "priest" he was also responsible to share fully with her the oracles of God that he had received, until they had **both** come to spiritual maturity.[46] He failed miserably in his role! Eve was deceived by the enemy. Perhaps Adam's teaching was inadequate, although we do not know that, for Eve also had direct communication with God and did not have to approach God only through her husband. But she was the learner. She had had less time to experience God, to learn to know Him. Satan always approaches first those most likely to be deceived, those unlearned, new believers who are not yet mature in their faith.

When Eve let doubt enter her heart and was deceived by the enemy of her soul, what did Adam, her priest/husband do? Did he go to God and cry out, "What shall I do for my wife? The enemy got into the Garden that You told me to protect, and has trapped her into disobedience!" Did he make priestly intercession in her behalf, or offer to be sacrificed by the stated penalty of death in her place? Did he cry out to God, "How can I rescue her? I love her! I am willing to die for her! I will take her penalty upon myself, Lord, if only You will restore her!"

No such thing. Adam deliberately, with full knowledge that he was wilfully disobeying God, took of the fruit and ate it with his wife. Adam was **not** deceived.[47] He **knew** he was deliberately disobeying God's express command to him. Then he blamed God—*the woman **you** gave me!*—and he blamed his wife—***she** gave it to me!*[48] The Scriptures repeatedly, say of Adam's sin: *As in **Adam** all die....*[49] Adam's name means "dust," the dust of death. *To Adam God said,... dust **(adamah)** you are, and to dust **(adamah)** you shall return.*[50]

And Eve? Deceived, fallen Eve? To her is given the name "life" from the Hebrew word **havah,** *because she is the mother of all living.*[51] The Scripture says that *she shall be saved through the birth of the Child.*[52] God promised her a *Seed* who would one day destroy the serpent, her enemy.[53] Eve is deceived no longer! She now clearly understands that the beautiful creature to whom she listened was intent on destroying her. The serpent—Satan—becomes her life-long enemy, but a Savior is promised, the Messiah, who will be victorious over Satan.

Eve, forgiven, believed God's promise of a coming Seed who would overcome the power of the enemy. She is the first to voice God's name, *Jehovah.* For when her first child was born she remembered God's promise and joyfully exclaimed, *I have gotten a man from **Jehovah**.*[54]

Alas, Eve, this was not yet the child who would bring deliverance! The promised Messiah awaited another time, centuries later. But He would surely come, born of a woman. It was to Eve, not to Adam, that the Savior was promised. And it is those who follow *her* faith in a Messiah, a Deliverer, who are persecuted by her enemy, Satan.

Eve was the mother of all earth-children, as Adam was the father. She shared his earthly **(adamic)** nature and her body returned to dust. But she is also *the mother of all living,* the first believer, the prefigure of Mary to whom the promised Child was finally born—God in human flesh. Eve is the first of all who believed and who receive eternal life. She is the symbol of God's bride, the Church—deceived, sinning, repentant, redeemed.

God our Savior, our priest/husband, not only intercedes in our behalf, but also took the penalty of our sins upon Himself. The first Adam failed as the priest/husband of his household. The second Adam—Jesus Christ, bore the agony of our sins in His own body on the Cross. For the first time in the history of the universe, the unity of the Trinity was broken, and the Father turned away from the Son. In the total blackness of that separation—that hell without God, Jesus cried out the anguish of **our** guilt, *My God! My God! Why hast thou forsaken me?*[55]

God wants people—you and me—to become members of His family. He wants us to be sons and daughters of the Father, to be the bride of the Son, to be "one" with the Holy Spirit. Through all eternity, we shall never be able to plumb the depths of such an awesome mystery of Divine Love. God is our Savior!

> *Eve, in that blessed period before sin entered, shows us the church fulfilling all God's desire for her in union with His Son. Eve first came forth from Adam, to be then brought back to him as his help-meet. From one there became two; from those two there was again one. This is the mystery of the Church, that in her, what is altogether from Christ returns once more to Him.*[56]

When God first brought Eve to Adam, he put his arm around her and they strolled together in the garden of God until encircling dusk erased the shadows of the day.

Our divine Lover invites us, His bride,[57] to walk with Him through the gardens of the universe. In the light of His presence no darkness ever falls.

> *My lover spoke and said to me,*
> *"Arise, my darling,*
> *my beautiful one, and come with me.*
> *See, the winter is past;*
> *the rains are over and gone.*
> *Flowers appear on the earth;*
> *the season of singing has come....*
> *Arise, come, my darling;*
> *my beautiful one, come with me.*[58]

NOTES
1. Gen. 1:26-31. 2. Ex. 3:13-15. 3. Jn. 3:23. 4. Mk. 14:61-63. 5. Rev. 4:8.
6. Jn. 4:24. 7. Lk. 23:46. 8. 1 Jn. 1:5. 9. Jn. 1:1. 10. Gen. 1:1.
11. Gen. 1:26. Many of the "names" of God in Scripture, such as Almighty, Redeemer, Shepherd, etc., are not names but are anthropomorphic descriptions of His attributes or His actions. The name "Jehovah" appears over 6000 times in the Old Testament.
12. 1 Jn. 5:16.
13. Francis Martin. **Riding the Wind.** Ann Arbor. Servant Publications. 1975. These descriptions cannot be taken literally, for the Holy Spirit as "father" impregnated Mary (Luke 1:35). In Isa. 9:6 Jesus is called not only "prince of peace" but also "the everlasting father." The Holy Spirit is also the Spirit of the Father and of the Son. The Son is the exact essence of the Father and the Spirit. The Trinity is a mystery which we cannot fully comprehend.
14. Leon Joseph Cardinal Suenens. **Your God?** New York. The Seabury Press. 1978. Pp. 36, 37. Reprinted by permission.

15. Job 26:7; Heb. 11:3. **16.** Gen. 1:1ff. **17.** Ps. 90:2. **18.** Gen. 1:2. **19.** Job 38:28, 29. **20.** Gen. 1:24. **21.** Gen. 1:12, 18, 21, 25. **22.** Gen. 1:26-28. **23.** Deut. 32:5, 6. **24.** Deut. 32:11; Isa. 49:20; Num. 11:12; Isa. 46:3, 4. **25.** Mt. 22:23-30. **26.** Gen. 1:20, 24. **27.** Gen. 2:7. **28.** Heb. 1:5-8, 13, 14. **29.** Gen. 2:15-17. **30.** Ez. 31:9-10. **31.** Isa. 11:6-9.
32. *Ezer* is translated as "help" 21 times, as in Ex. 8:4; Deut. 32:7; Ps. 20:1, 2; 33:20, etc. Of the 21 times, 16 times it refers to the Lord as our help—the very same word used to describe Eve's relationship to Adam.
33. Gen. 2:21, 22. **34.** 1 Cor. 11:8-12. **35.** Gen. 2:22. **36.** Gen. 2:23 RSV
37. Helen Wessel. **Natural Childbirth and the Family.** New York. Harper & Row. 1963, 1973. P. 302. Paperback, **The Joy of Natural Childbirth.** 1976, 1979. P. 302.
38. Eph. 4:11-15—"until ALL come to maturity."
39. Gal. 4:19. **40.** Gal. 4:26-31. **41.** 1 Jn. 5:6-8, 11. **42.** Jn. 3:3-6, 16. **43.** Jn. 19:34-36. **44.** Gen. 2:23. **45.** Eph. 5:30. **46.** Eph. 4:13. **47.** 1 Tim. 2:14. **48.** Gen. 3:12; Job 31:33. **49.** Rom. 5:12, 14, 17, 19; 1 Cor. 15:21, 22.
50. Gen. 3:19. **51.** Gen. 3:20. **52.** 1 Tim. 2:15 RSV note; NEB note.
53. Gen. 3:15. **54.** Gen. 4:1. **55.** Mt. 27:48.
56. Watchman Nee. **A Table in the Wilderness.** Fort Washington. Christian Literature Crusade. 1965. Reprinted by permission.
57. Rev. 22:2-5. **58.** Song of S. 2:10 NIV.

Who Am I?

*Those who are led by the Spirit of God are sons of God. For you did not receive a spirit that makes you a slave again to fear, but you received the Spirit of sonship. And by him we cry, **"Abba,** Father." The Spirit himself testifies with our spirit that we are God's children. Now if we are children, then we are heirs—heirs of God and co-heirs with Christ, if indeed we share in his sufferings in order that we may also share in his glory....*[1]

Don't you know that we will judge angels?... The things which have been announced to you by those who preached the good news to you through the Holy Spirit sent from heaven, are things into which even the angels long to look.[2]

A basic misunderstanding of our own identities is the root of many difficulties in relationships. We think of our "selves" as fat or thin, tall or short, young or old, black, brown or white, male or female, smart or not so smart. But who we really are transcends all these differences.

We also confuse our "selves" with the roles we carry out—as husband, wife, father, mother, teacher, student, worker, lay person, prophet, pastor. But who we are is not defined by what we do.

Have we not all at times said, "I've always wished I could.... I've always wanted to be.... Some day I'd really like to...." These wistful longings show that we are not bound to the few feet of earthly space which our physical bodies occupy. Our true selves can cross the continents in thought or explore the vastness of space in imagination. They can rise into the heavenlies to communicate with our Creator/Savior or fall into the depths of discouragement and unbelief. No one looking at us would see any of these things!

I am a person

Others see only our bodies, the temporal houses in which we live and through which we communicate with other human beings. But we are far more than that. Each of us is a person, individual and unique, as God is a Person. Our identity is found in our interior life—in the transcendent inner reflection of God in whose image we were created. Although we are marred, distorted, sinful reflections of God until we repent and receive God as our Savior, we are still precious to Him because He made us in His own image. His love pursues us through all the days of our lives until we turn to Him and receive it.

And like God, we each have a name. God knows our names. The Lord who made us knows every person on earth. He said of Jeremiah what He can say of every one of us, *Before I formed you in the womb **I knew** you....*[3] He said of the heathen king Cyrus, *Thus says the Lord, He who formed you from the womb.... I have called you by your name. I have given you your title, though **you do not know Me**.*[4]

When Jesus first saw Peter He didn't wait for an introduction, but said, *You're Peter.*[5] When He saw Nathaniel coming, He announced what kind of person this was. Nathaniel asked, astonished, *How can you know me?* Jesus said, *Before Philip called you, when you were still under a fig tree, I saw you.*[6] Jesus not only saw him with the eyes of inner vision, but knew all about him, as He knows all about every one of us.

God knows the name of every human being ever conceived, and writes his or her name in the book of Life. For it is not only Christians whose names are written in that wonderful book. Otherwise, how could the names of those who refuse to believe be *blotted out*[7] of that book?

It is the reality of God our Creator, this personal God who is called by a specific Name, that gives meaning and identity to our personal, individual, unique existences. Of all the billions of people who ever lived, God has made no carbon copies. We came *from God,* and we shall one day go *to God,* and be *face to face*[8] with our Creator. He will need no introductions, but will know all about us. *And some will go away into everlasting punishment: but the righteous into life eternal.*[9]

I am spirit

We are "spirit"—as God is Spirit—and that spirit will never die. When our time on earth is completed, *then shall the dust return to the earth as it was: and the spirit shall return to God who gave it.*[10]

As spiritual beings there is *no difference* between male, female, black, brown, white, young or old. *God has no favorites.*[11] Jesus explains that our sexual natures are for earthly purposes only, and that in the spiritual realm there is no distinction between male and female. *In the resurrection they neither marry nor are given in marriage, but are like the angels of God in heaven.*[12] Jesus also made clear that our approach to God is not based on place, position or sex, but upon the right heart attitude. *God is a Spirit, and those who worship Him must worship in **spirit** and in truth.*[13]

Even the apostle Paul, whose teachings have so often been twisted and misconstrued as put-downs for women,[14] said clearly:

> *You are **all** the children of God by faith in Jesus Christ.... There is neither Jew nor Greek, there is neither slave nor freeman, **there is neither male nor female**, for you are all one in Christ Jesus.*[15]

> Jesus said, *You shall know the truth, and the truth shall make you free.... Whoever sins is the servant of sin. The servant does not stay in the household forever, but the Son stays forever. If the Son, therefore, shall make you free, you are **really free**.*[16]

> Paul urges us to *stand fast in the **freedom** with which Christ has made us free, and don't get tangled up again in the yoke of bondage.*[17]

God has created us to be "free spirits." We are free to make choices, a freedom that leads either to our enlargement as persons or to our downfall. For although we are made in God's image, we are not robots who do His bidding automatically. Nor is our behavior just instinctual as is the behavior of animals who have no sense at all of transcendent reality but live only in the present. For example, our instincts for eating and sleeping are strong, yet we can choose to fast at times rather than to eat, choose to stay awake and pray rather than to sleep. God created us with free wills so that we can make choices, and at some time in our lives we are confronted with the most imperative choice: ***choose*** *today whom you will serve....*[18]

The essence of true love is choice—an act of commitment to another. And since God is a Trinity, the Father, Son and Holy Spirit are committed to each other in perfect love for all eternity. But God made another, terribly difficult choice. He **chose** to love us, even though we rejected Him! *For God **so loved** the world that He gave his only begotten Son....*[19] Whether we love Him back or not is of our own choosing. Like Adam and Eve we have the choice of turning to or away from Him.

God longs for intimate relationships with those human beings He created. And it is from our intimacy with Him that we best learn how to enter into right relationships with others. God is not remote, indifferent to us, unfeeling. God has feelings which can be hurt. God loves,[20] laughs,[21] cries,[22] groans,[23] sings,[24] can be angry[25] or grieved.[26] And when God came to earth in His Son Jesus, He experienced all our fleshly frailties. He was weary,[27] tempted,[28] discouraged,[29] wounded.[30]

God experiences all these emotions as the result of our responses to Him. In the same way, when we interact with others we are vulnerable to feeling blessed or hurt by them. And we also bring blessing or pain to those who come into contact with us.

I need "family"

Just as God is not alone, but is Three-in-One—a relationship of perfect, loving unity—so "no man is an island." God said at the outset of human history, *It is not good...to be alone.*[31] We all need an inner circle of loved ones with whom we can share our joys and sorrows. We need a family.

We live in a day when individualism seems all important. But we need to realize that the Bible is a book of "family" covenants. The Lord said to Abraham, *through you all the families of the earth will be blessed.*[32] God repeated this promise to Abraham's grandson, Jacob: *...in you and in your seed shall all the families of the earth be blessed.*[33] Jacob's twelve sons became the nucleus of the nation Israel, each tribe bearing one of the names of Jacob's sons. Before entering the wilderness, the children of Israel were told that each fiftieth year was to be a "homecoming," a Jubilee. *And you shall hallow the fiftieth year, and proclaim liberty throughout the land to all its inhabitants; it* *shall be a jubilee for you, when each of you shall return to his property and each of you shall return to his family.*[34]

When David married into the household of King Saul, his brother-in-law Jonathan became his dearest friend. Later David lamented over Jonathan's death: *I am distressed for you, my brother Jonathan. You have been very pleasant to me. Your love was wonderful, better than the love of women!*[35]

David and Jonathan had a depth of companionship greater than David ever experienced in marriage. And no wonder! David had too many wives,[36] and all kinds of family problems because of the times he disobeyed the Lord. A companionship such as David and Jonathan had **is** possible between a man and wife in marriage. It is more than sexual compatibility, it is an additional level of communion that continues even when many miles lie between them.

Yet in spite of David's family difficulties, the promise to him was a "family" promise. David longed to be creative and do something great for God, building Him a "house" (temple). But the prophet Nathan came to him and said:

> *I declare to you that the Lord will build a house for **you**.... I will raise up your offspring to succeed you, one of your own sons, and.... I will set him over my house and my kingdom forever; his throne will be established forever.*[37]

David was so astonished that *he came and sat before the Lord, and he said: "Who am I, Lord, and what is my family?... And now, Lord,... Do as you promised!"* God kept His promise, and David's son Jesus will reign for eternity. David longed to be creative, but God's idea was far bigger!

I am creative

When we choose each day to walk in God's will, we find ourselves creating. Our minds will be full of new ideas, new plans, new endeavors, our lives full of exciting opportunities. We discover that we are not duplicating anyone else, not displacing them, not in competition with them. We discover who we really are! It becomes a daily delight to discover how "special" we are to the Lord.[38] God will sing over us with love and joy.[39] We will walk among family, neighbors and friends in perfect confidence, unthreatened, gentle, loving, happy to be who we are.

*In your quiet time remember that just as surely as every
snowflake that falls has a perfect design, and no two
designs are the same, so within the folds of your being lies
a design. Ask the Father that this divine inner plan of
your life may stand forth revealed to you as it should be,
unfolding in perfect sequence and perfect order in such a
way as to bring the greatest good to the greatest
number.... Nothing can prevent the fulfillment of your
prayer if it is true to your nature, and a sound reflection
of your inner soul.*[40]

We are free to make choices, free to obey the creative impulses God places within us, free to become that unique individual God planned for us to be.

I need a Savior

But alas, we have made wrong choices and are destined to death. For we are not only spiritual beings. We are also **adam,** dust, whether we are men or women, and our bodies will return to dust. For Adam is the symbol of death.

We are also Eve, **havah,** "life," whether we are men or women, if we have received the Savior. For like Eve, we were all deceived. Paul includes himself when he writes:

*We ourselves were at one time foolish, disobedient,
deceived, living in our own lusts and pleasures. But now
the great kindness and love of God our Savior toward man
has appeared, not by works of righteousness that we have
done, but according to his mercy he saved us.*[41]

Through faith in Eve's promised Seed, the holy child Jesus,[42] we share in her restoration. Deceived, sinning, repentant, forgiven, we are restored to eternal life. The dominion we lost through sin is given back to us. Once again we have authority over the natural world through prayer, and over sin, sickness, Satan and death—in the mighty name of Jesus.

For this Jesus, our Savior God who has all dominion, shares His authority with us!

*The Lord sent them out two by two and said to them,
"The harvest truly is great but the laborers few. Pray that
the Lord of the harvest will send more laborers to help
reap the harvest. And as you go **preach** saying, 'The*

kingdom of heaven is at hand.' Heal the sick, cleanse the lepers, raise the dead, and cast out devils."[43]

After Jesus rose from the dead He repeated this command:

***All power** is given to me in heaven and in earth. Go therefore and teach all nations,... teaching them to observe **all** things that I have commanded you.... Truly I say to you, whoever believes in me—the works I do will they do also, and even greater works than these will they do, because I go to my Father. And whatever you ask in my name, I will do it, that the Father may be glorified in the Son. If you shall ask anything in my name, I will do it.*[44]

I am God's co-worker

Just as God is Savior, so He has called every one of His redeemed children to the work of saving the world. When a field is ready to be harvested, all able-bodied persons, men and women, boys and girls, are needed to help bring in the harvest. Jesus spoke of a ripe harvest on another occasion, when one woman "preacher" brought a whole city to His feet.[45] He said that "whoever"—man or woman—would believe in Him would do the **same** work he did: teaching, preaching, healing, and even greater things. *God was in Christ, reconciling the world to himself, and has given to **us** the word of reconciliation.... We are workers together with God.*[46]

Even as I have been writing these words, I can see little red flags of doubt and disbelief springing up in some readers' minds. "But—but—but. But this is a different dispensation! But the days of miracles are past! But women are not to preach!" But—but—but! The traditions of humanity "butting into" the freedom and authority of the child of God! These human limitations threaten the very things God has given us through the Cross.

One of our sons had such a heart for God as a little boy that he longed to be baptized. He had invited Jesus into his life and wanted to go all the way in obedience to God and be baptized. However, he was refused permission. He was not old enough. Sixth graders could be baptized, but he was only in fifth grade. This was such a serious matter to him that night after night he sobbed into his pillow to receive baptism.

He still has a heart for God. But there was another small boy who was less fortunate. St. Augustine when a small boy requested baptism. No, the church authorities said. He was not old enough. Crushed, St. Augustine turned away from the church and spent long years in sin before he finally returned to make things right with God. The "buts" of tradition hindered the work of God in his life.

A deeply devout person gets ready for church, walks up the street and into the foyer of the sanctuary. "You can't worship here," he is told. Why not? Because his skin is the wrong color. The "buts" of tradition are hindering the work of God in his life, and in the lives of countless others like him.

A gifted, dedicated woman pastors a church of men. She has been accused many times. "Don't you know that women are not allowed to preach? or to teach men? or to be a pastor? You are sinning against the Lord!"

The church she pastors is filled with men she has led to salvation in Christ, prisoners in a wretched prison in a steamy tropical land. The church itself is inside the prison compound, built as a result of her labors. None of her accusers have ever offered to minister in that difficult place for even an hour.

Her answer is, "No one should minister the Gospel without a call from God. I have a call." And she quietly goes on her way obeying God, blessing these desperate people.[47] The "buts" of tradition trying to block the work of God!

Jesus had a sharp warning for legalistic religious leaders like these:

You have made the word of God of no effect by your tradition,... teaching for doctrine the commandments of men.[48] *You shut up the kingdom of heaven against others: for you neither go in yourselves, nor allow those who are entering to go in.*[49]

When I began to hear increasing complaints against women having spiritual ministries to men on the one hand, and complaints against the Bible as a "sexist, patriarchal, chauvinistic book" on the other, I knew it was time to take a closer look. I needed an answer for those who would deny the goodness of our Lord, either way. As I began to search the Scriptures, surprise after surprise began unfolding before my eyes. It was not any "new" truth, but truths I had not fully appreciated before.

For example, the New Testament is full of the word "brethren." If only men are present, it means "brothers." But if women are also present the word means "brothers and sisters." The Greek word ***adelphos,*** translated "brother," really means "from the same womb." The word for sister is in the feminine form, ***adelphe.*** The plural form, ***adelphoi*** means "brothers and sisters" from the same womb. When used of believers, it refers to those born of God, brothers and sisters in the Lord.

*Jesus said, "Behold my mother and my brothers and sisters **(adelphoi).** For whoever will do the will of my Father which is in heaven, the same is my brother and sister and mother.*[50]

Another Greek word translated as "brethren" is ***adelphotes,*** which is a feminine noun. Even the word ***philadelphia,*** which is known as "brotherly love" is a feminine word! Thus one could go all through the New Testament transforming its apparent chauvinistic bias simply by translating the word "brethren" more correctly as "brothers and sisters."

Then I thought back to the patriarch Abraham. Is this not where the patriarchal system seems to begin? But wait a minute. Not all the children of Abraham inherit the promises. Seven sons are named as born to Abraham in addition to Isaac.[51] Only Isaac could lay claim to the promise. Why? Because of his **mother,** Sarah.

But Jerusalem which is above is free, which is the mother of us all. Now we, brothers and sisters, are children of promise, as Isaac was.[52]

In the Old Testament the believing Jews are called God's sons. The word "son" refers to both men and women, for the whole nation was God's "son." *Thus says the Lord, "Israel is my son, even my firstborn."*[53] *When Israel was a child, then I loved him, and called my son out of Egypt.*[54]

But every believing Jew, man or woman, is also "woman" in relationship to Jehovah:

Plead with your mother (Israel), *for she is not my wife, neither am I her husband; let her therefore put away her whoredoms out of her sight.*[55]

Thus says the Lord God to Jerusalem. . . . Behold, your time was the time of love, and I spread my skirt over you and covered your nakedness: I swore to you and entered into a (marriage) covenant with you.[56]

Female symbolism also applies to Christian men, for every believer becomes "woman," that is, a part of Christ's body—His bride. Of course no one would argue that one must become a female physically to become a member of the church, the "bride of Christ." But in spite of this consistent feminine imagery of the Church, it is broadly proclaimed that only males are fit to lead in spiritual or theological matters! This tradition is not consistent with Scripture.

*And the Spirit and the **bride** say, "Come." And let him who hears say, "Come." And let anyone who is thirsty come. And whosoever will, let him take the water of life freely.*[57]

The Lord gives the word: a vast army of women bear the glad tidings. Kings and their hosts are fleeing, fleeing, and the household shall divide the spoils.... Though you have been lying among the pots, yet you shall be as the wings of a dove (f.) covered with silver, and her feathers with yellow gold, when the Almighty scattered kings.[58]

*Speak comfortably to Jerusalem, and cry to her, that **her** warfare is accomplished!... O (daughter) Zion who brings good tidings.... O (daughter) Jerusalem, **lift up your voice with strength. Lift it up, be not afraid, say** unto the cities of Judah, "Behold your God!"*[59]

Awake, awake, put on your strength, O captive daughter.[60]

As the full impact of these glorious truths concerning womanhood burst upon my mind, I could not help but cry out, "Lord—what of my sons? What is there left for them?"

And the answer came swiftly. "Everything! Just as it is all for My daughters, so it is all for My sons. The Church is **one** body, and **all** My children are set free to follow Me wholly."

Jesus prayed, I thank you, O Father, Lord of heaven and earth, because you have hidden these things from the wise and prudent, and have revealed them to babies. Even so, Father, for so it seemed good in your sight.[61] Turning to His followers He added, *Learn from me, for I am meek and lowly in heart.*

And when you pray, you shall not be as the hypocrites are, for they love to pray standing in the synagogues and in the corners of the streets, that they may be seen of men. Truly I say to you, "They already have their reward."[62]

Humble yourselves therefore, under the mighty hand of God, that he may lift you up.[63]

In Old Testament worship, lay persons were not allowed into the inner sanctuary, and only the High Priest could go into the Holy of Holies, once a year. But when Christ died, the veil of the Temple was torn open from the top to the bottom. Now **any** one, man or woman, has direct access to God. If women as well as men now freely enter the presence of God and serve in the Holy of Holies through the torn curtain of Christ's flesh, how can they be forbidden entrance into those church ministries which are only **symbolic** of these deeper realities?

Not long ago I visited a new fellowship of believers. They were deep, loving Christians sincerely attempting to obey God in everything. Every Thursday night the men—and only the men—met for the business of the church, as the elders and deacons. During this time the women met for Bible study and prayer.

How foolish! The women, blessed in the Word and prayer, kept growing and growing spiritually, while the men were hung up on "business" which they thought was too important for women! How the church is robbed of the spiritual maturity of her sons by such foolishness! For Jesus said:

*You are troubled and careful about many things. Only **one** thing is needful. And Mary has chosen that good part, which shall not be taken away from her.*[64]

And in regard to business. Are not women managers of households, stretching income to cover food, clothes, every other need, planning, scrimping, working. The wife in a poverty-stricken home has to have extraordinary management skills if her family is to survive.

In the feminist movement there is a great hue and cry to allow women to fill many of the same roles as men, and receive the same appreciation and pay for the same tasks well done. This is as it should be. But in all the commotion something equally important is in danger of being lost. And that is that men need to be allowed to be like women, that is, to be fully "human." Even God, whom men identify as a male model, does not hesitate to wear the symbolism of the female at times. He even calls Himself a rejected wife! *Judah has been faithless, and has profaned the sanctuary of the Lord by marrying the daughter of a foreign god.*[65] Judah is depicted as the husband of Jehovah, running after harlots rather than being faithful to the heavenly wife.[66]

One of the sound principles of Biblical interpretation is that no doctrine can be safely built on only one or two passages of Scripture, but must take into consideration all the other things said on the same subject. The two "problem" passages concerning women are no problem when looked at in the broad context of Scripture.[67] For example, some people say the Bible does not allow women to teach or to preach. Yet these same people may say that "to prophesy" means "to preach."

And the Bible clearly teaches that women will prophesy. Huldah the prophetess was a counsellor not only to kings, but also to the High Priest![68] The aged Anna who lived in the Temple fasting and praying day and night spoke about Jesus to *all those* (men and women) *who looked for redemption in Jerusalem.*[69] Priscilla and Aquila taught the brilliant Apollos, *expounding the way of faith to him more completely,*[70] and travelled with Paul at times, assisting him in the Gospel. Priscilla is mentioned first in nearly every instance,[71] indicating that she was the teacher and Aquila her "patron." Without the encouragement and support of her husband her gifts would have had less opportunity for expression.

*And I will pour out my Spirit upon **all** flesh. Your sons and your daughters shall prophesy. Your old men shall dream dreams and your young men shall see visions. And also upon the servants and upon the maid servants in those days I will pour out my Spirit.*[72]

Preaching daughters and visionary sons! Wonderful! Free to be whatever God Himself calls each of them to be. Free in spirit! Free to be whole persons! That is my prayer for my own children and for each of you.

Great harm has been done to the cause of Christ by falsely assigning sexual roles to spiritual ministries. To be "religious" is thought to be "feminine." To be an inward, dreaming, praying person is thought to be like "an old woman." But in Scripture it was not so. Joseph the "dreamer" lived to see his dreams come true. Daniel the "visionary" was shown revelations of the end times that still stagger the minds of intellectuals who try to understand them. Paul spoke in tongues, had dreams, visions and revelations. Yet how many assign such experiences to "unstable, emotional women!"

"Women's intuition," we say, and rob our sons of their God-given inner vision. "Your **sons** shall see visions."

"Trying to be a man!" we scoff when a woman stands before others to proclaim God's message. "Your daughters shall prophesy," God declares, "with words for you right from My mouth."

To say that only males can perform certain functions robs God of His freedom of action. It makes men seem indispensable, so that God cannot move freely through whom He will.

In spiritual ministries the Bible clearly teaches that *no flesh,* whether male flesh or female flesh, *should glory in His presence.* God alone receives the glory for all that is accomplished. And He loves to choose those very persons whom we would overlook to fulfill His divine purposes:

> *God has chosen the foolish things of the world to confound the wise; and God has chosen the weak things of the world to confound the things which are mighty; and base things of the world, and things which are despised has God chosen. Yes, and things which are not, to bring to nothing the things which are. That no flesh should glory in his presence.*[73]

How we need to discover who we really are in God so that both men and women can be free to serve the Lord in any way He directs them, totally obedient to the Holy Spirit regardless of our sex.

Who am I? I am Adam. I am Eve. I am a person who reflects in my spirit the image of God, for I have received life through the new Adam, Christ Jesus. If I am totally yielded to the Spirit of God I will be free to enter into every human relationship in the right way, free to do any kind of work. If I am a man, I will be free to follow God in obscure jobs or in public places, to scrub floors or to preach, to make tents or to heal the sick, or perhaps all of these.

If I am a woman, I am free to follow God in whatever He asks me to do, to preach or to keep house, to teach or scrub floors, rock the cradle or be a tramp for the Lord, or perhaps all of these.

> *Now the Lord is the Spirit, and where the Spirit of the Lord is, there is **freedom**. And we all (men and women), with unveiled face, beholding the glory of the Lord, are changed into his likeness from one degree of glory to another; for this comes from the Lord who is Spirit.*[74]

Who am I? I am a son of God, whether I am man or woman. I am a part of His bride, whether I am man or woman. I am a unique creation made by God for God's own purposes. My human spirit is free to be a whole person with all the finest attributes of either sex.

I am the receptacle for that living fountain of waters which is the Spirit of God, who will guide me into what I was created to be, into finding that *good, and acceptable, and perfect will of God* for **me**.[75]

Who am I?

The greatest glory in the universe
is not the evening star—
The sweetest fragrance in the world
is not the rose—
The most exciting treasure God
has gleaned from near and far
is not the diamond.

I am more precious in the eyes of God
than all the Milky Way.
A star can't laugh, or love Him back
or pray to Him each day.
I am a living spark of God
and only He can tell
what galaxies of life await me
*as **his** friend!*[76]

NOTES
1. Rom. 8:14-21 NIV. **2.** 1 Cor. 6:3; 1 Pet. 1:10-12. **3.** Jer. 1:5; Ps. 139:12-16. **4.** Is. 44:24; 45:3, 4. **5.** Jn. 1:42. **6.** Jn. 1:45ff. **7.** Rev. 3:5; 22:19. **8.** 1 Cor. 13:12; 1 Jn. 3:2. **9.** Mt. 24:46. **10.** Eccl. 12:7. **11.** Rom. 2:11. **12.** Mt. 22:23-30. **13.** Jn. 4:24.
14. See Don Williams. **The Apostle Paul and Women in the Church.** Ventura. Gospel Light Press. 1977. See also Gerald Derstine. **Woman's Place in the Church.** Bradenton, Fl. Gospel Crusade Publications (Rt. 2, Box 729). 1977.
15. Gal. 3:28. **16.** Jn. 8:36. **17.** Gal. 5:1. **18.** Josh. 24:15. **19.** Jn. 3:15. **20.** Hos. 3:1; 11:4. **21.** Ps. 2:4; 16:11; 105:43; Jn. 15:11. **22.** Lk. 19:41; Jn. 11:35. **23.** Jn. 11:33; Rom. 3:26. **24.** Zeph. 3:17. **25.** Ps. 79:5. **26.** Ps. 78:40; Eph. 4:30. **27.** Jn. 4:6. **28.** Heb. 2:18. **29.** Mk. 9:19. **30.** Zech. 13:6. **31.** Gen. 2:18; Ps. 68:6. **32.** Gen. 12:3. **33.** Gen. 28:14. **34.** Lev. 25:10 RSV. **35.** 2 Sam. 1:26. **36.** 2 Sam. 2:2, 3; 3:3-5; 5:13. **37.** 1 Chron. 17:7-16 NIV. **38.** Eph. 2:10. **39.** Zeph. 3:17.
40. Glenn Clark. **I Will Lift Up Mine Eyes.** New York. Harper & Row. 1937. P. 57. Reprinted by permission.
41. Tit. 3:3. **42.** Acts 4:30. **43.** Mt. 10; Lk. 10. **44.** Mt. 28:18-20; Jn. 14:12-14. **45.** Jn. 4:27-39. **46.** 2 Cor. 5:19, 20.
47. An article entitled "Women Priests?" in the Minneapolis Tribune. Jan. 27, 1980 made the following points (among many others):
  1. Women often posed as men in the medieval church to fulfill high religious office. For example, Pope John VIII, who reigned from 856 to 859 was a woman. Another woman was a patriarch of Constantinople.
  2. Women also held church office openly through history. Abbesses held jurisdiction in many areas of Europe during the Middle Ages, with the same authority as bishops.
  3. Women were admitted to baptism and membership in the church from the time of Christ's ministry. Not all groups were admitted. For example, non-Jews were denied baptism at first.
  4. An organized priesthood and the traditional figure of the priest did not develop earlier than 100 years after Christ's death.
  5. In Paul's greetings at the end of the book of Romans he names a woman minister of the church at Cenchreae, and also a woman apostle.
  6. The example of Jesus and the apostles providing a norm which excludes women from priestly ministry cannot be sustained on either logical or historical grounds. The only exclusive role Jesus reserved for the 12 was to sit in judgment on the 12 tribes of Israel at the end of the world. As for the other roles of apostles and later priests, "The Twelve were among the followers, or disciples, of Jesus who included both women and men and who, after the resurrection, formed the nucleus of the primitive church and provided its leadership."
  7. To argue that anyone not resembling the 12 apostles is barred from priesthood would automatically exclude people of different races.

48. Mt. 15:6. **49.** Mt. 23:13. **50.** Mt. 12:49, 50. **51.** Gen. 16:15; 25:2. **52.** Gal. 4:26-28. **53.** Ex. 4:22, 23. **54.** Hos. 11:1. **55.** Hos. 2:2. **56.** Ezek. 16:3-8. **57.** Rev. 22:17. **58.** Ps. 68:11 NAB. **59.** Is. 40:2, 9. **60.** Isa. 52:1. **61.** Mt. 11:25, 29. **62.** Mt. 6:5. **63.** 1 Pet. 5:6. **64.** Lk. 11:42. **65.** Mal. 2:10, 11, 14. **66.** Hos. 3:14; 4:1ff.

67. The first of these problem passages is Paul's statements in 1 Cor. 14:34, 35 that women should be silent in the churches and if they have any questions they should ask their husbands at home. The second is 1 Tim. 2:11-14 in which Paul says that he does not permit a woman to teach, and that Eve was deceived.

The Corinthians passage is obviously related to the cultural situation. Paul has already explained that women speaking in the assembly in prophecy or leading the congregation in prayer, are to be appropriately dressed. (1 Cor. 11). Thus the admonition about silence in 1 Cor. 14 is a reference to disturbing conversation. Those who have been in Hindu or Buddhist temples will know what noisy places they are! The confusions of the Corinthian temples for idol worship were being carried over into the churches, so that Paul has been telling them all to learn to speak "one at a time," and not be disruptive (vv. 26-33).

The Timothy passage refers to a woman who is a **learner**, who is not to teach and is easily deceived. The reason she is easily deceived is not because she is a woman, but because, like Eve, she is still a learner. Earlier in the epistle Paul says that there are persons in Ephesus who want to be teachers but "wander away into vain discussions" "having never learned!" (1:5-7). This does not mean they have not heard the Gospel, but that they have not **submitted** to its teaching.

Adam was created first, and received the oracles of God. Eve was created later, and was the learner. She was deceived because she had not yet completely submitted to the teaching. Her understanding was incomplete.

Timothy would clearly perceive that Paul was not talking about all women being forbidden to teach any man, for Timothy himself was well taught in the faith by his own mother and grandmother, as Paul confirms. (2 Tim. 1:5).

In the verses just preceding this restriction on a woman teaching, Paul has been talking in the plural about the men and women in the fellowship of believers, their prayers for the community and public witness. In the next verse he drops to the **singular,** "Let **a woman**" learn. It is the same word as the word "wife."

"**Let** a wife learn." Women were untaught in that culture, so that Paul is moving against the stream of popular opinion in saying she is to be permitted to receive instruction. But this does not reverse God's order for the home, sending her back to act as the authority over her **"husband"**. The word translated "man" is also the word for "husband." The wife who is learning the ways of faith is not to preach to her husband, as Peter agrees (1 Pet. 3:1, 2), but to win him to the obedience of the Word by her changed behavior.

"Permit a wife to learn, in silent submission (to the teaching, and to those teaching her—most likely another woman). *But I do not permit a*

woman to teach or seize authority over a husband. For Adam was formed first.... This is in harmony with Paul's other instruction concerning husbands and wives in Eph. 5:21-33 and Col. 3:18, 19.
68. 2 Kgs. 22:11-15; 2 Chro. 34:19-23ff. **69.** Lk. 2:37, 38. **70.** Acts 18:2. **71.** Acts 18:18, 26; Rom. 16:3; 1 Cor. 16:19;2 Tim. 4:19. **72.** Joel 2:23; Acts 2:16. **73.** 1 Cor. 1:27-29. **74.** 2 Cor. 3:17, 18 RSV. **75.** Rom. 12:1, 2. **76.** Hermon Pettit. **God of the Wilderness.** Fresno, Ca. Bookmates International. 1981. Reprinted by permission.

Unity In Diversity

Submit yourselves to every human institution for the sake of the Lord.... For it is the will of God that by your good conduct you should put ignorance and stupidity to silence.
Live as free men; not however as though your freedom were there to provide a screen for wrongdoing, but as slaves in God's service. Give due honour to everyone....
In the same way you women must accept the authority of your husbands, so that if there are any of them that disbelieve the Gospel they may be won over, without a word being said, by observing the chaste and reverent behavior of their wives.... Do good and show no fear.
In the same way, you husbands must conduct your married life with understanding: pay honour to the wife's body, not only because it is weaker, but also because you share together in the grace of God which gives you life. Then your prayers will not be hindered.[1]

The prayer of Jesus for all believers is that we be one in Him. *Holy Father, keep through your own name those whom you have given me, that they may be one, as we are.... I in them and you in me, that they may be made perfect in one.*[2]
Just as the Trinity is One, so the many and varied members of the body of Christ are to be in unity, com(with)-unity, com(m)unity, one. There ought to be no disharmony, no malfunctioning in the body of Christ. It was so in the early church, for a little while. *And the multitude of those who believed were of one heart and of one soul, and none of them said that any of the things which he possessed was his own. They shared all things in common.*[3]

A Christian man and woman in marriage are to be a concrete example of that larger unity which is Jesus' prayer for the whole church. Unity is not like photo copies. They will have differences in tastes, preferences and abilities, yet they are to be one in mind, heart and purpose, two unique personalities knit together in the closest possible human relationship.

Someone has said that the reason marriage is called a "bond" in Scripture is because God binds a man and woman together in such a way that they can't run away from each other when problems arise. In other adult transactions a way of "escape" can be found, changing contracts, changing locations, starting over. But in marriage it is not so. There can only be a wrenching, a tearing apart of the soul, heartbreak, trauma, for many people—not only the marriage partners—when a marriage is broken. God ordained marriage in a way that is not easy to escape because He wants us to work problems through to unity, wholeness, oneness.

No other gods

Paul said those who marry *will have trouble*.[4] One reason for their difficulties is the temptation to violate the first commandment: *You shall have **no other gods** but Me.*[5] God must remain our first love, even if we choose to marry. Jesus said, *No man can serve two masters, for he will either hate the one and love the other, or else he will hold to the one and despise the other.*[6]

One of the tragedies of many marriages is that young people enter into this most intimate and complex human relationship with false expectations. They expect to "live happily ever after." They expect the marriage partner to give them the sense of wholeness and inner security which only God provides. They expect a little "heaven on earth" to become theirs, through fulfillment from each other.

A young couple in love may have only one consuming interest. The young man dreams of his princess day and night and she of her prince charming. This can carry over into the honeymoon period and eventually become a form of idolatry. The wife or the husband and later the children may hold first place in their hearts. Even when they discover that their "idols" have feet of clay, their primary **attention** is focused on them. God is displaced in both their affection and attention and the first commandment broken. The apostle Paul warns of this danger:

> *I do not want you to be distracted. He who is unmarried cares for the things that belong to the Lord, how he may please the Lord. But he that is married cares for the things that are of the world, how he may please his wife.*
>
> *There is a difference also between a wife and an unmarried woman. The unmarried woman cares for the things of the Lord, that she may be holy both in body and in spirit. She that is married cares for the things of the world, how she may please her husband. I speak this for your own profit, that you may serve the Lord without distraction.*[7]

Paul does not say it is impossible to live wholly for Jesus if we are married, but that it is much more difficult. Thus the first question each young person must ask is: "Lord, is it Your will for me to marry or do You want me to remain single? Do You have a ministry for me which I can best fulfill without the responsibilities of a family?"

It may not be easy to choose to remain single even though we believe it is God's will for us. Some have grabbed a mate anyway and regretted this disobedience in the griefs and problems which followed. Those who are willing to remain unmarried if God so wills receive from Him the grace necessary to live joyfully as a single person.[8]

The single person is to remain chaste, foregoing sexual relationships. *Flee fornication*[9] Scripture warns again and again. Only in the marriage of a man and woman is sexual contact chaste, pure, holy.[10]

Hundreds of thousands of unmarried people today openly proclaim lesbian or homosexual tendencies.[11] This is a cry for help, for understanding, and loud condemnation only compounds the problem.[12] Such people are not necessarily indulging in sexual contact (though many are), but are sexually attracted to those of the same sex rather than to the opposite sex. Other persons struggle with transsexuality. These are suffering, hurting people, with a confusion concerning their own personhood. Before these unnatural feelings can be changed there is need for compassion toward them, for their inner healing, perhaps for deliverance, perhaps for salvation. But we must not assume that only non-Christians wrestle with lesbian, homosexual or transsexual tendencies.

Anyone struggling with such things has access to the same solution as the hetereosexual person who struggles with unclean thoughts.[13] One can be set free from inner bondage to sinful thoughts by turning the problem over to Jesus, *bringing every* **thought** *into captivity to Christ.*[14] Jesus will set us free to think only of those things which are true, honest, just, pure, lovely, leaving no room in our minds for those thoughts which bring only guilt, sin and trouble as their consequences.

If we choose to marry, the Bible clearly teaches that it is for life:

> *You have covered the altar of the Lord with tears, with weeping and crying out, because he does not regard your offering any more, nor receive it with good will at your hand.*
>
> *Yet you say, "Why is this?" It is because the Lord has been witness between you and the wife of your youth against whom you have dealt treacherously. Yet she is your companion, and the wife of your covenant. For the Lord, the God of Israel, says that he hates divorce.*[15]

Jesus restates this truth when He was asked the question about divorce. He said, *What God has joined together, let no one break apart.*[16] The disciples were dismayed at His answer and exclaimed, *If that's the case of a man with his wife, it's better not to get married!*[17]

Some have used the statements of Jesus concerning God's purpose for marriage to impose a harsher law than even the Old Testament law, which permitted divorce.[18] Jesus was not imposing a new "law," but announcing the high standard of God's moral law. He alone could fulfill all the righteousness of God. He came to give us grace, the grace of God which will forgive, restore, and *make all things new.*[19]

In 1 Corinthians 7 Paul says that a person may remarry if their spouse has left, refusing to live with a believer. But he or she may remarry only *in the Lord,*[20] that is, to a believer. But he adds that it is better for those who have been married before not to remarry, whether they were widowed or divorced. Many years later he modifies this by saying *younger* widows should marry again rather than become a burden on the church. Having known the security of marriage before, their commitment to the single state may waver.[21] He does not say that younger women who have chosen virginity from the outset need to marry.

An equal yoke

When a man or woman believes that it is God's will for him or her to marry, it is important to wait until the God-sent person comes. Marrying too young or too quickly, just to be married, is a great danger that cannot be warned against too strongly. Infatuation quickly fades in the hard realities of day-to-day living with another person, for life.

The Bible warns against our being *unequally yoked together*.[22] This is an illustration borrowed from the Old Testament: *You shall not plow with an ox and an ass together.*[23] If one wants to live wholly for God and the other is satisfied with church attendance only, it is an unequal yoke. If one feels a strong call to the mission field and the other to stay at home, it is an unequal yoke. If one values quiet and privacy and the other loves a houseful of constant bustling activity, it is an unequal yoke. The marriage is to **begin** in unity, a unity which is deeper than doctrinal unity. Each may have different tastes and abilities, but their vision should be a single one so that they can move toward it as a team yoked together, each belonging to the other.

> *Let the husband show every kindness to the wife, and the wife to her husband. The wife does not have authority over her own body. It belongs to the husband.*
> *In the **same way**, the husband does not have authority over his own body. It belongs to the wife.*[24]
>
> *Neither is the man without the woman, nor the woman without the man, in the Lord. For as the woman is of the man, even is the man also from the woman. But all things are from God.*[25]

Jesus said that the first great commandment is to love God above all others. *And the second is like the first. You shall love your neighbor as yourself. On these hang all the law and the prophets.*[26] One's husband or wife is first of all one's "neighbor." How easy it is to be polite to others all day long and at the end of the day tear our spouse apart with bitter words! It has been said that we save our courtesies for strangers whom we may never see again, and save our most abusive verbal behavior and discourtesies for the one with whom we will have to live the rest of our lives. It is to be an **equal** yoke, each treating the other as he or she wants to be treated.

C.S. Lewis speaks of his wife, after her tragic death from cancer, as an equal:

> *For a good wife contains so many persons in herself.
> What was H. not to me? She was my daughter and my
> mother, my pupil and my teacher, my subject and my
> sovereign; and always, holding all these in solution, my
> trusty comrade, friend, shipmate, fellow-soldier. My
> mistress; but at the same time all that any man friend
> (and I have good ones) has ever been to me. Perhaps more.
> If we had never fallen in love we should have been none the
> less together, and created a scandal. That's what I meant
> when I once praised her for her "masculine virtues." But
> she soon put a stop to that by asking how I'd like to be
> praised for my feminine ones. It was a good **riposte,** dear.
> Yet there was something of the Amazon, something of Pen-
> thesileia and Camilla. And you, as well as I, were glad it
> should be there. You were glad I should recognize it....*
>
> *It is arrogance in us to call frankness, fairness, and
> chivalry "masculine" when we see them in a woman; it is
> arrogance in them, to describe a man's sensitiveness or
> tact or tenderness as "feminine." But also what poor,
> warped fragments of humanity most mere men and mere
> women must be to make the implications of that arrogance
> plausible. Marriage heals this. Jointly the two become fully
> human. "In the image of God created he **them.**" Thus, by
> a paradox, this carnival of sexuality leads us out beyond
> our sexes.*[27]

Marriage is a relationship in which one's own aspirations and concerns are to be harmonized with those of the husband or wife. Marriage is

> *... neither dependence on authority nor independence,
> nor even interdependence. It calls for life on much higher
> spiritual planes and levels. It calls for a oneness in the
> Body so totally at one with Jesus, and hence with the
> Father and the Holy Spirit, as to become in truth a
> trinitarian body.... It is achieved by intense and constant
> prayer,... becoming lovers and servants of one another,
> people of the towel and the water.*[28]

A man shall leave

God has ordained certain structures for marriage, to provide for harmony in the relationship between husband and wife. Both have certain God-appointed responsibilities toward the other in order to fulfill God's design for a Christian home.

The first responsibility begins with the husband, as he is commanded to *leave his father and mother and be joined to his wife, and they shall become one flesh.*[29] Jesus repeated this principle of the man leaving his home to go to the bride.[30]

Man has reversed God's order down through many centuries throughout most of the world. Man's way is for the **woman** to leave her parental home and come to wherever **he** is! What grief and degradation this has brought to millions of women! Taken away from the protection of her family, the wife has become subordinate not only to her husband, but has often been brought into the husband's family home and made subservient to his family as well.

In the early kinship system brides remained near the parental home, where the parents would be aware of the way in which she was being treated. It was the groom who made the risk of change. The woman's mother was thus available to help in times of childbirth, sickness or other periods of stress. This practice can be seen in the Old Testament custom of often naming cities and towns after women. Most of the names are in the feminine gender, including "Zion," and may reflect a system in which the husband came to the home of the bride.

There are other Biblical examples of this God-ordained pattern. For example, Sarah's name is "Princess," from the word *sar* which means prince, or chief. Her father Terah was an influential man from whom she received her title. When Abraham left Ur of the Chaldees Sarah did not leave her parental home, for her father came too. (Abraham and Sarah had the same father.[31]) And it is for **her** that the new Jerusalem is named[32] in the promised land to which they journeyed.[33]

When the time came for Abraham and Sarah's son Isaac to marry, the practice of the husband going to live near the wife's parents was one of Abraham's great anxieties. He sent his servant to Nahor to find a wife for Isaac among his God-fearing relatives there. But he warned, *If the woman is not willing to follow you back to this land, you are free from this my oath. But be certain that you don't take my son there again.*[34]

When Isaac's marriage proposal was given to Rebecca's family, she was asked, **"Will** you go?" She said yes.[35] A generation later Rebecca's son had to **ask** his two wives, Leah and Rachel, even after twenty years of marriage, if they would be willing to go with him back to his own parental home.[36]

Generations later, when Samson married a Philistine wife, she remained with her family, as was the custom.[37] This is one of the reasons his parents were so upset that he did not marry a daughter of Israel.

In Jesus' parable of the bridegroom, the virgins wait near the home of the bride and then go out to bring the approaching bridegroom to the bride's home.[38]

Jesus is the perfect example in this, for He left His Father in heaven to come win His bride. But wait a minute, some might say. Isn't Jesus going to take His bride back to heaven with Him? Yes, the bride of Christ is caught up to Him, but then the wedding party descends to **her** home, earth renewed!

*And I saw the holy city, new Jerusalem, coming **down from God out of heaven**, prepared as a bride adorned for her husband, and I heard a great voice out of heaven saying, "Behold, the dwelling place of God is with mankind."*[39]

Christ, the model husband

After leaving his father and mother, the new husband sets up his own household with his wife. In this new marriage relationship, God has declared him to be the head of the home. *For the husband is the head of the wife, even as Christ is the head of the church.*[40] The husband is the head, whether he accepts this responsibility or not. Whether he is a good man and husband or a bad or uncaring one makes no difference. His **position** is that of the head of the home. But what does it mean to be the "head"?

A headstone is the secure foundation around which a structure rises. It may be no bigger nor better than any of the other stones in the structure, but its **placement** is important. The security of the whole structure rests upon this stone. When the foundation stone is incorrectly placed the whole structure is in jeopardy. In the same way, when the husband who **is** the head of the house, is not living in the will of God, his whole family suffers the consequences. The headstone is out of place.

The head is also a pacesetter, preceding the others, leading, making the way safe. He is like the prow of the ship piercing through the waters so that the body of the ship may follow in its wake. He is like the guide who leads the way up a mountain or who cuts a swath through the jungle for those who follow.

The head is also the one who carries responsibility for the whole. The husband is responsible for his wife's happiness and welfare. He bears this same responsibility for his children. He is responsible **whether he accepts this responsibility or not.** He is like the head of a nation. The **office** of president is an honorable one, even though a dishonorable person may hold the office. The president is responsible for the welfare of the whole nation and receives the blame when things go wrong, even though it may not be his fault. As head of a family, a man is praised or blamed for whatever transpires, whether or not it was his decision. Are the children rebellious? He bears the shame. Is his wife disrespectful? He is blamed. In the same way Jesus Christ, the perfect head of His bride, the Church, bears the blame or praise for whatever the Church does, even when it is flouting Him as its head.

The head is also a covering. A cover is *a shelter*[41] in the storm, *a shade*[42] from the noonday heat, *a hiding place*[43] from danger, as well as a *love that covers all sin.*[44]

Ruth said to Boaz, *Cover me with your robe.*[45] To cover means that nothing is left **outside.** Boaz' whole estate became Ruth's as well, and she shares with him the honor of being listed in the genealogy of Jesus Christ.[46]

Sometimes the word "lord" is used in the Bible rather than "head" for the husband. We tend to choke on that, because we don't understand what it means! It does not mean "God," but is another word for head. For example, the lord of an estate is the person responsible for the whole estate, answerable for the welfare of all those living on the property. Sarah considered Abraham her "lord," but certainly not her God![47]

Thus when Abraham said to Sarah, "God is calling me to be uprooted," Sarah replied, "All right. Let's obey God." She said goodbye to her friends, packed her belongings and went with him to Haran, to Palestine, even down into Egypt. But though she called Abraham lord, she didn't hesitate to speak her own mind. She insisted that he send away the Egyptian maid Hagar and Ishmael, Abraham's son by the maid. Abraham didn't want to! He grieved over Ishmael. Finally he went to the Lord and complained about what his wife was telling him to do. And the Lord replied, *In all that Sarah has said to you,* **listen** *to her voice; for through Isaac will the Promise come.*[48] And Abraham obeyed Sarah, for she, rather than he, correctly understood the will of the Lord in this matter.

Jesus Christ is not only our God. He is our Lord, the model for every husband to follow as head of the house. He was gentle and kind, saying, *Fear not, daughter, for your king comes to you on a donkey's colt.*[49] He said to his disciples:

> *You know that the princes of the Gentiles lord it over*

*them. But it shall not be so among you! Whoever will be great among you, **let him be your servant.** Whoever wants to be chief, let him serve the others. For the Son of man did not come to **be** served, but to serve others, and to give his life as a ransom for many.*[50]

Scripture never says that a husband is to bring his wife into subjection! He is not to say to his wife, "I'm the head, so you have to do what I want. I'm the spiritual authority and I understand the Bible better than you. I have more theological and spiritual insight and am not as easily deceived as you are."

Beware! Such an attitude breeds arrogance. The sin of loving to be pre-eminent, Jesus rebuked in his disciples over and over again, and it was the cause of Satan's downfall. It is the sin that makes some men prefer a "dumb blonde" to a brilliant girl, no matter how graceful and lovely that girl might be.

Jesus as the model husband shares all His authority with His bride. His disciples were arguing one time about which one was the greatest. Jesus said, *Don't worry about that. Look. I'm assigning to **you** the kingdom assigned to me!*[51] Jesus is not threatened by the success of His followers, then—or now. He shares His authority and dominion with His bride. He says, *Come. Rule by my side. Share my riches, my wisdom, my responsibilities. All I have is yours.*[52] He is not jealous of His bride's attainments.

A husband who is confident of his own personhood under God is not threatened by any successes of his wife. My grandparents were married for 50 years in perfect harmony. My grandfather had only an eighth grade education (although he read widely to make up for it), while my grandmother had been to college and was a teacher. In nearly every church they attended she taught the adult Bible class, and he sat admiringly in her class. At one time she was mayor of their town—the second woman mayor in the entire United States. He was one of the town's citizens under her.

He often said to me, "Your grandmother is a most remarkable woman!" As he said it, the expression on his face softened, and he would look in her direction with love and pride in his eyes. He considered himself enriched and blessed by her achievements, not diminished. Neither of them ever questioned his position as head of the home.

The ultimate test of a man's headship in the eyes of God is not how domineering he is, but rather how he treats his wife. He is the **husband,** an awesome responsibility, not to be undertaken lightly.

A husbandman is one who husbands the earth. He nurtures it, cares for it, coaxes it into luxuriant fruitbearing. In return for his good husbandry he is abundantly blessed. At times my husband and I have driven past midwestern farms with acres of flourishing crops, healthy livestock, large, shiny silos and newly painted barns. In the middle of this would be a little old house with the paint peeling off. Some of these homes had no modern conveniences, although the farmer had every possible piece of up-to-date equipment. He "husbanded" everything but his wife! In this he impoverished himself in ways he never dreamed.

The husband is called *the savior of the **body**,*[53] following Jesus' example. He is to protect his wife's health and energy, bear with her the stress of childbearing and childrearing, help carry the work load in whatever way he can, "husbanding" her strength.

Not only is the husband to leave his father and mother to cling to his wife and become "head" of this new household, "husbanding" it. He is also to be the priest of his household, responsible for each member's standing before God. Adam and Eve both sinned, but when God came He called, *Adam, where are **you**?*[54] Adam had an imperfect wife and blamed his problems on her. Jesus also has an imperfect wife. But unlike the old Adam, this new Adam (Jesus) has taken the imperfections of His bride upon Himself, still interceding for her.[55] The husband/priest is to be like Jesus, the intercessor who lifts his wife to God in prayer, bestows blessings on her in the name of the Lord, forgives her faults and prays for God to forgive her also.

Let every one of you love his wife as much as he loves himself.[56] Whatever the husband enjoys, let him see that his wife has opportunity to enjoy it also. Whatever fulfillment the husband finds, let him make sure his wife has the opportunity to be fulfilled. Whatever ministry he has, let him joy in the prospering of her ministry also. Let him be humble enough to wash her feet,[57] and perhaps even die for her safety. *Husbands, love your wives, even as Christ also loved the church and gave himself for it.*[58]

A godly wife

And what responsibilities must the wife shoulder in the marriage relationship so that the joy of the unity of the Holy Spirit may fill the home? Her first duty is an attitude of **respect** for her husband. This would not seem to be difficult if the husband were fulfilling all his responsibilities as head and husbandman of the home. But, as the new wife soon discovers, her prince charming has many faults.

At first it may be just little things. He doesn't pick up his clothes. He forgets to take out the garbage. He picks his fingernails and drops the sharp pieces on the rug. Sometimes he forgets to pay the bills. He never notices how tired she is at the end of the day but asks, "What do you do around here anyway?" He considers her work of no importance compared to his, a breeze that he could easily dispense with in an hour. She does all the dirtiest work. He would never think of cleaning the toilet or scrubbing the bathtub.

And so, little by little, the enemy of our souls gets a foothold in the wife's heart. Self-pity. Disrespect. Pride. "Me? Respect *him!* No way!" But then the Word of the Lord comes: *Let the wife see to it that she **respects** her husband.*[59]

Many women who consider themselves as model Christians subtly treat their husbands with disrespect. Such a wife may make snide remarks behind her husband's back, or even to his face, or belittle him in public. In this way she is tearing down her own house[60] by undermining the headstone.

Not only is the wife to respect her husband, she is also to honor him above herself. *Therefore as the church is subject to Christ, so let the wives be to their husbands in everything.*[61] Now if the husband were perfect like Jesus, this would not present a problem! But alas, he is full of faults, so how can she yield her own way to what he wants?

Again, Jesus is the model. At twelve years of age he was so brilliant that he confounded the wisest men in the nation with His questions.[62] Yet he returned home with his parents *and was **subject** to them.*[63] Was He subject because they knew better than He? Not at all! They couldn't even understand what He was trying to explain to them about God. Even though He was only twelve, He was far superior to His parents, who were humble peasants, perhaps not even able to read and write. Yet He yielded to them because of their **position** as parents.

In the same way, a godly wife who is secure in her own personhood before God can voluntarily yield her own way when there is a difference of opinion. If she feels the husband is wrong, she can quietly lift the whole matter to God privately. She goes the second mile, giving her cloak as well as her coat,[64] and follows the example of her Savior who submitted to the authorities who put Him to death wrongfully. Jesus had the power to stop them, but he yielded to them in order that a greater good might come. This is the key that makes yielding possible—God's personal blessing follows. *Humble yourselves under the mighty hand of God, that **he may** exalt you in due time.*[65]

This voluntary yielding of one's own will in obedience to God is a powerful spiritual tool to bring about the very thing we desire. When a wife yields to her husband she is following the same instruction as that given to servants:

> *Servants, be subject to your masters with all respect; not only to the good and gentle, but **also to those who are perverse**.... For Christ also suffered for us, leaving us an example, that we should follow in His steps.... He committed himself to him who judges righteously.*[66]

The Christian servant knew he was his master's equal,[67] yet he treated him as he would treat Jesus. A wife is to treat her husband as she would treat Jesus. The husband may be far from being like Jesus, but that makes no difference. She must treat him with respect, believing God for a work of grace in his heart, honoring him as she would honor him if her prayers had already been answered. She is not to threaten him by her piety but to affirm his manhood, his personhood, his headship. Then he is free to grow into his role, becoming more and more like Christ the husband. Even though the wife may be more spiritually mature at a given time in her marriage, she should still encourage the husband's spiritual leadership, giving him breathing space to grow into what God wants him to become. And at **that** time, the husband will gladly welcome her by his side in all his ministries. God will lift her up!

> *If a woman has a husband who does not believe, and if he wants to stay with her, let her not leave him. For the unbelieving husband is made holy by the wife....*[68]

> *Wives, yield to your own husbands so that although they **do not obey the Word**, they may be won without the Word by the manner of life they see in you.... Let your adorning be your inner self, a quiet and gentle spirit which is of great price in the sight of God.*[69]

When a wife believes God's promises and affirms her husband as the head of the home she will be blessed far more quickly than if she preaches at him and *usurps his authority*.[70]

However, there is a warning here, for there are wrong as well as right ways of yielding. Some wives yield like child brides who have no brains. Ask such a wife any question about a difficult Scripture passage and she may say, "Oh, I'll have to ask my husband what he thinks about that." This kind of blind yielding is terribly dangerous. Not only does it leave the wife undeveloped and infantile in her spiritual thinking but it also leaves her open to being misled and deceived by Satan—the very thing she is trying to avoid by letting her husband do her thinking for her.

This kind of yielding cost one woman her life. Her name was Sapphira. She agreed with her husband that they should sell their property and give the money to the church, pretending that they were giving it all but keeping a little for their own needs. They agreed to lie. When Ananias brought the gift to Peter, Peter knew at once through the word of knowledge that he was lying about the proceeds, and Ananias dropped dead at his feet. A short time later Sapphira entered:

> *And Peter said to her, Why is it that you have conspired together against the Spirit of the Lord? Look, the feet of those who buried your husband are at the door, and they will carry you out too. And she fell down at his feet, dead.*[71]

A wife needs all the gifts of the Holy Spirit, including the gift of discernment, in order to know when God is speaking through her husband, when it is his own spirit, or when it is the deceiver speaking through him. If she discerns that what her husband is saying is not of God, and he refuses to listen to her objections, she has direct recourse to Jesus, who will tell her what to do. The Lord may prompt her to wait, to be quiet about it, and He will frustrate the wrong action Himself. Or he may prompt her to speak and promise to put words in her mouth.[72] If it is a serious matter of obedience to God or to the husband, as with Ananias and Sapphira, the wife's first loyalty is to God no matter what the cost, even if it means losing her home.[73] *We ought to obey God rather than men.*[74]

If God is calling her to a public ministry, there is no need to push her own way forward. If the anointing of God is genuine, it cannot be hidden, just as Moses could not keep his face from shining when he came from the presence of the Lord.[75] God Himself will open the door to her at the right time.

A common difficulty which a wife experiences with an overbearing husband is that he threatens her own identity. She has not yet learned the security of her own personhood in Christ. But as she sets her heart to follow God, an inner calm and strength will come to maturity. The more Christlike and mature she becomes, the easier it will be for her to yield peacefully to the wilfulness of another, because she is confident that God in time will make things right.[76]

Too often a Christian husband reads the Bible to see how his wife should act. The Christian wife does the same to see what the Scriptures say about a husband. This leads to the confrontation of finger-pointing: "The Bible says you ought to...!" That's not God's way. It takes all the grace of the Holy Spirit for each of them to fulfill his or her **own** Scriptural role.

Give thanks always for all things unto God and the Father in the name of our Lord Jesus Christ; submitting yourselves to one another out of reverence for Christ; wives to their husbands as to the Lord.[77]

Several years ago I attended a Catholic weekend retreat called a "charity workshop," in which we learned ways to love one another in Christ. A couple in their mid-forties attended the workshop. I asked them jokingly, "Who wins the arguments in your house?"

To my astonishment they replied, "We never argue."

"Which one of you is responsible for that?" I pressed them.

They each pointed to the other and responded simultaneously, "She is." "He is."

Two are better than one, for they have a good reward for their labor. For if they fall, the one will lift up the other. But woe to him who is alone, for he has no one to help him up when he falls.[78]

Again, if two lie together, they can have heat. For how can one be warm alone? And if someone comes against one of them, two will stand against the attacker. And a threefold cord (God, husband, wife) *is not quickly broken.*[79]

NOTES
1. 1 Pet. 2:13-16; 3:1-9. **2.** Jn. 17:11, 23. **3.** Acts 4:34. **4.** 1 Cor. 7:28.
5. Ex. 20:3. **6.** Mt. 6:24. **7.** 1 Cor. 7:32-35. **8.** Mt. 19:12.
9. 1 Cor. 6:15-18; 10:8; 2 Cor. 11:2; Gal. 5:19; Eph. 5:3-5 etc. **10.** Tit. 2:5; Heb. 13:4.
11. The Bible teaches that homosexuality is "unnatural" (Rom. 1:26), and it is forbidden (Lev. 18:22). But we need to remember that heterosexual activity outside of marriage is also condemned. Paul wrote to the Christians in Corinth, *I am afraid that when I come again my God will humble me before you, and I will be grieved over many who have sinned earlier and have not repented of the impurity, sexual sin and debauchery in which they have indulged* (2 Cor. 12:21).

Sympathy for homosexuals is growing because of the false notion that they are "born that way." Although this is not true, the troubled one may not know the roots of his condition. Deliverance is possible for those who want to be set free from this bondage, just as deliverance is possible for anyone else who is in bondage to any other evil. Mercy and forgiveness are the paths to healing rather than condemnation.

12. Mt. 7:1, 2; Rom. 2:1, 9-11; James 4:11, 12. **13.** Mt. 5:28. **14.** 2 Cor. 10:5; Phil. 4:8. **15.** Mal. 2:11-16. **16.** Mt. 5:31, 32; 19:4-11. **17.** Mt. 19:10. **18.** Deut. 24:1-4. **19.** 2 Cor. 5:17; 1 Cor. 5 with 2 Cor. 2:5-11. **20.** 1 Cor. 7:8-16. **21.** 1 Tim. 5:3-14. **22.** 2 Cor. 5:14-18. **23.** Deut. 2:10. **24.** 1 Cor. 7:3, 4. **25.** 1 Cor. 11:11, 12. **26.** Mt. 22:39.
27. C.S. Lewis. **A Grief Observed.** New York. Seabury Press. Copyright © 1961 by N.W. Clerk. Reprinted by permission of The Seabury Press, Inc., pp. 39-42.
28. Catherine de Hueck Doherty. **The Gospel Without Compromise.** Notre Dame. Ave Maria Press. 1976. Pp. 57, 58. Reprinted by permission.
29. Gen. 2:24. **30.** Mt. 19:5. **31.** Gen. 11:27-31; 20:11-13. **32.** Gal. 4:22-31. **33.** Heb. 11:13-6. **34.** Gen. 24:4-8. **35.** Gen. 24:57, 58. **36.** Gen. 31:14-16. **37.** Ju. 14:1-4. **38.** Mt. 25:1-13. **39.** Rev. 21:1-3. **40.** Eph. 5:23; 1 Cor. 11:3. **41.** Ps. 61:2, 3. **42.** Song of S. 2:3. **43.** Deut. 33:12; Ps. 119:14. **44.** Prov. 10:12. **45.** Ruth 3:9-11. **46.** Mt. 1:5. **47.** 1 Pet. 3:6. **48.** Gen. 21:9-12. **49.** Jn. 12:15. **50.** Mt. 20:25-28. **51.** Lk. 22:24-30. **52.** Mt. 11:28-30; Jn. 20:19-23; Rev. 3:21. **53.** Eph. 5:23. **54.** Gen. 3:9. **55.** Heb. 7:25. **56.** Eph. 5:28. **57.** Jn. 13:14-16. **58.** Eph. 5:25. **59.** Eph. 5:33. **60.** Prov. 14:1. **61.** Eph. 5:24. **62.** Lk. 2:40-47. **63.** Lk. 2:49-52. **64.** Mt. 5:40, 41. **65.** 1 Pet. 5:6. **66.** Eph. 6:5-8; 1 Pet. 2:18-23. **67.** Philemon 16, 17. **68.** 1 Cor. 7:14. **69.** 1 Pet. 3:1ff.
70. 1 Tim 2:12. *Let a wife **(gune)** learn quietly in submissiveness. But I do not permit a wife **(gune)** to teach nor to **usurp** authority over a husband **(aner)**. For Adam was formed first, then Eve.* Paul is saying that a wife is not to be held back from any learning, but that her growth in spiritual knowledge does not give her headship over her husband, *for Adam was formed first.* The husband is still head, even though he may be an unbeliever, as he most likely was in this case. See 1 Pet. 3:1ff and also note #67 in "Who Am I"?

71. Acts 5:1ff. **72.** Mt. 10:18-20. **73.** 1 Cor. 7:15. **74.** Acts 4:17-21, 5:27-29. **75.** Ex. 34:29-35. **76.** Rom. 15:1-3.

77. Eph. 5:20-22. In the earliest Greek manuscripts the verb **hupotasso,** translated "submit" or "subject to" does not appear in v. 22. Thus v. 22 must be linked to 21 to make sense: *submitting to one another out of reverence to Christ; wives to their husbands....*

The eminent biblical scholar, Dr. Leon Morris, one of the translators of the NIV, commented on this in an address entitled "The Ministry of Women" at a forum for the Faculty of Fuller Seminary in 1976:

"... while there can be little objection to the translation, 'let wives be in subjection to their own husbands' in Ephesians 5:22, there is no verb there. It has to be supplied from the preceding sentence, 'be subject to one another in the fear of Christ.' In other words, the subjection of wives to husbands is not some great and unusual thing, but a particular example of a universal Christian duty. Christians are not to be self-assertive, but humble. They are to be subject to one another, not domineering over one another. And the main thrust in this passage is not on the subjection of the wives, but on the sacrificial love of the husbands. This brings Paul to the thought that Christ loved the church and gave Himself for it. He is the Savior of the body, but the husband is not said to be the savior of the wife. In this most important matter both depend on Christ. We ought not accordingly to make too much of the differences between them. That is not the thrust of the passage. There is self-denial on both sides. Now if ALL Christians are to be subject this applies to elders as well as to others. On this ground then there may exist no insuperable difficulty in the way of ordination of women. P. 18.

78. Eccl. 4:9, 10. **79.** Eccl. 4:11, 12.

Awakened Desires

*Who is this that comes up from the wilderness
  leaning upon her beloved?
Under the apple tree I awakened your desire.
It was there that your mother conceived you.
  It was there she gave birth to you.*

*Set me as a seal upon your heart,
  As a seal upon your arm.
For love is strong as death,
  Jealousy cruel as the grave.
The coals thereof are coals of fire,
  Which burns with a fiery flame.*

*Many waters cannot quench this love,
  Neither can the floods drown it.
If a man would give all that he possessed
  for love,
  It would be utterly despised as too
  small a price.*[1]

The open Book

The Bible is amazingly frank about sexual matters. Much of this frankness is lost in translation. For example, the word translated to "know" one's wife means to experience sexual relations with her, to "know" her vagina with the penis. In the King James Version we read:

Abimelech, king of the Philistines looked out at a window and saw, and behold, Isaac was sporting with

Rebekah his wife. And Abimelech called Isaac and said, Behold, of a surety she is thy wife. And how saidst thou, "She is my sister?"[2]

This sounds as though King Abimelech looked out of his house window and saw Rebekah and Isaac playing ball or some other "sport." How could he know from this that she was not Isaac's sister? In 1954 I looked up this passage in the **Septuagint.** The **Septuagint** (seventy) is a translation of the Hebrew Old Testament into Greek by seventy Hebrew scholars 400 years before Christ. I discovered that this translation clearly shows that Abimelech looked into the window of the tent and saw Isaac having sexual intercourse with his wife. Of course Abimelech exclaimed, "She's not your sister!"

The frankness of Scripture (at least in the original) makes it clear that it is not wrong to speak candidly about sexual matters. We need to become familiar with our own bodies if we are to be able to share them freely with our husband or wife.

Sexual self-knowledge

A boy can never escape the reality of his sex. His penis and testicles are visible. They are handled when he urinates, when he washes. He sees the genitals of other boys and men in locker rooms and elsewhere. He learns when very young that it "feels good" when he rubs his penis. At some point during his years of puberty he experiences his first nocturnal emission, which is the ejaculation of semen from the erected penis. It feels so good that as a young man it is hard to keep from stimulating himself, and he struggles not to become addicted to self-stimulation. He may know nothing about the genitals of the female. But he knows that his penis is for girls. It is supposed to go in somewhere, somehow!

By contrast, a girl's genitals are largely hidden. Because she does not see them easily, and may have been told that it's naughty "to look," she may grow up unfamiliar with her own body. She doesn't want anyone to see her undressed (even though most of her genitals are not visible). If she accidentally arouses herself while riding a bicycle or in wiping herself on the toilet, she quickly represses the feeling because it's "not nice." She believes that a nice girl doesn't think about, talk about or feel such things, until marriage.

Furthermore, a woman is subjected to the indignity of genital examination in a doctor's office as a matter of necessity. She must carefully draw a mental curtain between herself and the doctor. It is unthinkable to allow the doctor's touch to cause any sexual feeling whatever. Thus women learn to inhibit all sexual responses so that it is not surprising if they think they don't have any!

Then the wedding comes. The honeymoon. And suddenly there are no restrictions at all! She is expected to give her body to her groom freely and experience all the joys of sexual intercourse. But it is not that easy suddenly to reverse a whole lifetime of modesty! And to her unhappy surprise, she may even experience pain rather than pleasure, for the **hymen,** the membrane at the back of the vaginal opening, must be stretched or broken enough to allow the penis to be inserted comfortably. Both bride and groom may be a little disappointed.

One young couple stayed in the minister's home on their wedding night. They were to leave early the next morning for their honeymoon. Thoughtfully the minister's wife had placed a plate full of wedding cake on the dresser for them. The bride spotted it at once as they came into the room. She was famished. She had been too excited to eat before the wedding and too busy at the reception. "Look!" she exclaimed. "Let's have a piece of cake."

Who wanted cake? Certainly not her sweetheart! He was hungry for **her.** He had waited a long time for this moment. Not wanting to displease him, she went to bed with him at once. It was over almost before it began, wetter than she had expected, disappointing. They fumbled around with the towel. Lying in her husband's arms afterward she soon found him snoring. And she was still hungry for cake.

A bride and goom should not expect their first sexual experiences to be perfect, but approach them with a sense of humor and compassion. One does not play a concerto when first touching the piano.

Sexual arousal

Sexual arousal comes quickly for most husbands. A touch on the arm from his wife or a glance at her or the thought of coitus stimulates the nerve centers which control erection of the penis. Its tissues fill with blood so that it becomes firm and erect, pointing upward. But he has much to learn about the intricacies of a jointly fulfilling experience.

Sexual arousal for the wife is more complex. Let every godly woman know that it is all right to learn about her own body, for how can she possibly give to another what is strange to herself?

How can a wife yield to the pleasure of her husband's touch if she is not even willing to touch herself? She cannot give away what she has never discovered.

Let the wife get a mirror and examine herself. The external female organs are called the **vulva.** At the top over the pelvic bone is a mound of flesh called the **mons pubis,** covered with hair. Below the **mons pubis** between the legs are an outer and inner pair of lips, called the **labia majora** (major lips) and **labia minora** (minor lips). Between the **labia minora** just below the **mons pubis** is the **clitoris.** Just below the **clitoris** is the **urethra,** a small opening which leads to the bladder. Below the **urethra** is the **vagina.** Across the lower portion of the vaginal opening is a membrane called the **hymen,** sometimes called the "maiden head," which is usually broken during the first intercourse. The area between the vagina and the anus is called the **perineum.**

A young wife can help dilate (stretch) her own hymen. This is done by inserting a finger into the vagina and gently pressing back toward the anus. It can be streched a little further each day. If the hymen proves resistant to stretching, a physician can correct the problem so that intercourse will not be so uncomfortable. Some women have a fragile hymen that has broken accidentally before marriage. A broken hymen is no proof that a woman is not a virgin.

The **clitoris** is the key to feminine sexual arousal. But because it lies below the surface of the skin except for its **glans** (head), many women are unaware of its existence or function. The clitoris is like a small, hidden penis. It extends upward from its glans under a sheath of skin for an inch or two. Let the wife place her index finger in the upper portion of the channel between the inner labia. As she moves her finger back and forth slowly across the center of this channel, she will feel a ridge under the skin, parallel to her finger. This is her clitoris. If she continues moving her finger back and forth gently across the clitoris, she will discover that it begins to harden and is easier to define with her finger. If she were to continue stroking over the shaft of the clitoris she would begin to feel sexually aroused.

The vagina can also be explored with the fingers, feeling up along the vaginal walls inside the body. If a woman stands with one foot on a chair, she can reach all the way up to the **cervix** with her index finger. The cervix extends down into the vagina from the womb and feels firm to the touch. A slight depression like a dimple can be felt in its center. This depression is the **cer-**

vical os, the "mouth" of the cervix which leads into the **uterus,** or womb. It is through the cervical **os** that the menstrual flow comes each month. In a woman who has never given birth to a child the cervical **os** is so tiny that a thread can barely pass through, yet it has tremendous capacity for stretching, for it is through this opening that a baby is born. It is "the baby door."[3] The cervix is about an inch to an inch and a half long. Think of it as similar to a spool of thread with a tiny hole down the center. The depression the woman feels with her finger is the **external os,** opening into the vagina. The other end of the opening, which leads into the uterus is called the **internal os.**

In both men and woman an interwoven series of muscles provides a firm pelvic floor, shaped something like a hammock. The outer layers of muscle are called the external perineal muscles. The inner muscle layer is the **pubococcygeus** muscle, or **levator ani.** This inner muscle controls the outlets of the urethra, vagina and rectum. Both men and women can contract and release these muscles at will.

The tissues of the vaginal walls have little sensation. Some of the wife's sensations during coitus come from **pressure** exerted on the inserted penis by her tightening this inner muscle layer which is just beneath the surface of the vaginal walls. This pubococcygeus muscle has been named the "Kegel" muscle, after Dr. Kegel who discovered its importance for feminine sexual pleasure. A woman can learn just where this muscle is by inserting her finger into the vagina and trying to tighten the vagina around her finger.

To exercise the Kegel muscle, the wife can sit on the edge of a chair and slowly draw her vulva up, up, until it is no longer touching the chair. Then gradually she can release the pelvic muscles until the vulva is again resting on the chair edge. She can also try to stop the flow of her urine when on the toilet, placing her legs far apart and contracting these muscles so that only about a teaspoonful of urine is released at a time. If she cannot control her urine flow in this way, her Kegel muscle is weak and needs to be strengthened through systematic exercise.

Once the Kegel muscle has been discovered, it should be contracted as tightly as possible many, many times a day, when standing, sitting, walking, lying down. It is an exercise every woman should learn and practice all her life. This exercise will keep the muscles of the pelvic floor firm and strong, and help prevent the involuntary leaking of urine that afflicts many older women. Pediatricians even advise it for children who suffer from bed wetting.

Men who exercise their Kegel muscle so that they learn to control it, will be able to contract it during intercourse, thus preventing premature ejaculation.[4] This voluntary control also increases the pleasure of their own orgasms.

One of the most delightful functions of the Kegel muscle is its role in female orgasm. At a certain point of sexual excitement the muscle may begin to contract rhythmically and automatically of its own accord. It is a most profound, delightful sensation, and even the uterus may be felt contracting as this female orgasm continues. A warmth sweeps over the wife's whole body until even her breathing is caught up into this profound rhythm.

When husband and wife expect to come together in coitus, the wife can begin preparing herself ahead of time by experimenting with the Kegel exercise. She can s-l-o-w-l-y draw up the muscle, release it just as slowly, and do it again and again, enjoying how it pulls down on the clitoris, how the labia tighten, how the contracting and relaxing of the muscle is like a "sucking" of the vagina that longs for a "drink," longs for the penis, longs to draw the sweet fruit of the male, the semen, into her body. She will become aware of each little sensation throughout the whole pelvic area as she continues to contract this important, wonderful sexual muscle, even before her husband has touched her.

The wife can continue contracting the Kegel muscle as her husband holds her, guiding him in caressing her shoulders, breasts, nipples, abdomen, and genitals. As she becomes sexually aroused, the inner lips begin to engorge and the shaft of the clitoris becomes firm. Her husband can stroke her inner thighs, along the shaft of the clitoris or whatever feels comfortable to her. The glans of the clitoris is extremely sensitive, and stroking it directly may not be comfortable. Instead, the husband can gently caress the surrounding tissues, the inner and outer labia. He might hold the whole vulva in his hand and rhythmically press and relax, press and relax his hand, to increase clitoral stimulation indirectly.

As the wife becomes sexually aroused, the lining of the vagina secretes a lubricant which makes the insertion of the penis easier. Either she or her husband can reach up into the vagina and draw some of the lubricant to the mouth of the vagina. If there is not enough natural secretion, a lubricant such as K-Y Jelly will help. A small amount applied to the head of the penis or around the rim of the vagina is enough.

Now the wife is aroused, the clitoris responding, the vaginal walls moist and receptive, the penis enlarged and ready to insert. But another problem may arise, for the husband may be so aroused by trying to prepare his wife that he is ready for ejaculation, too soon! This causes him anxiety and compounds the problem each time they proceed toward coitus. He becomes afraid that he will "come too soon" and a pattern of failure develops. But there is a way in which his ejaculation can be delayed.

Because ejaculation—the release of semen—is controlled by nerve centers **other** than those controlling erection, the husband can learn to maintain an erection for some time without ejaculation. When he feels he is near ejaculation too soon, his wife can take his penis between her thumb and first two fingers. Her thumb should press upon the ridge just below the head of his penis on the side away from his body. Her two fingers on the opposite side help her to hold the penis firmly and maintain pressure on the "ridge" she will feel under her thumb. This is the "squeeze" technique, and must be done to the husband by the wife. It is not effective when a man attempts to do it on himself.

The squeeze technique can be done several times during the period of lovemaking before the insertion of the penis, whenever necessary to delay ejaculation. If the penis has already been inserted into the vagina when the husband's urge comes prematurely, he should quickly withdraw it and let his wife press it between her fingers again. The couple can learn over a period of time how they can jointly control the timing of the husband's ejaculation, so that the penis can be in the vagina for several minutes during each coital act. Men must learn to maintain an erection in the vagina up to 15 or 20 minutes before ejaculation.

These two difficulties—the inability of the wife to achieve orgasm even after several months of marriage, and premature ejaculation by the husband—can be overcome. More thorough discussion is needed than is possible here, for couples with either of these problems. Dr. Ed Wheat, through his excellent book **Intended for Pleasure**[5] and his tapes, has enabled thousands of couples to overcome these problems.

One flesh

Before inserting the penis into the vagina for the first time, the husband should carefully feel the slope of its walls with his fingers, so that he can guide the penis in at a comfortable angle. The insertion of the penis into the vagina does not provide a woman with much sensation. The vaginal walls do not have many sensory receptors, in order to make the passage of a baby downward painless during childbirth. If the husband thrusts his penis rapidly back and forth he will quickly come to ejaculation but his wife will be disappointed.

Only the outer third of the vagina responds pleasurably to pressure, movement and stretching. This is where the Kegel muscle lies just beneath the surface. Deep thrusting of the penis is not necessary. Instead, after inserting the penis, the husband should let it rest quietly in the vagina while the wife begins to contract the Kegel muscle around it. This will heighten her pleasure and will not overstimulate him too soon.

The couple may experiment with a variety of positions for coitus, although the most common is with the wife on her back and the husband above her. Some find this position more stimulating when the wife closes her legs after the insertion of the penis, while the husband's legs are placed outside hers. This gives him more complete contact, and even his testicles may be pressed gently between her inner thighs.

She can continue to contract the Kegel muscle around her husband's penis: tighten, release, tighten, release. She can experiment, doing it now faster, now slower. breathing deeply, enjoying him. If she has learned the Kegel well and has used it to arouse herself before the insertion of the penis, she may have experienced orgasmic sensations already. But that's all right, for unlike the husband, the wife can experience these waves of orgasmic pleasure again and again.

Dr. Ed Wheat explains that, contrary to popular opinion:

> ... *the vagina is not passive but is a very active organ which when sexually stimulated increases in length and widens to twice its diameter. At the beginning of arousal the upper vagina expands, and the uterus lifts up toward the abdomen. When thrusting begins, the vagina constricts to conform to the penis. After orgasm the uterus moves downward, so that the cervix rests in a pool of semen deposited in the upper vagina.*[6]

The husband reaches orgasm at the time of the ejaculation of his semen. He feels a wave of heat over his whole body, then begins to relax and the penis begins to recede in size and firmness. He may break out in a sweat. The feminine orgasm,

> ... *like the male orgasm, consists of thrusting actions of the organism, releasing tension and seeking unity outside itself.... The feminine contractions in orgasm resemble those of childbirth; they are expulsive, and as outer directed as those of the male whose rhythms they match.*[7]

It is not necessary for the husband and wife to experience orgasm at the same time, and it is not likely in the earlier years of marriage before they are well attuned to each other though years of close sexual communion. The wife may experience orgasm before, during or after coitus, or not at all. She may wake up during the night several times after coitus to find the Kegel muscle contracting spasmodically, the uterus rhythmically contracting, and a release of heat flowing all through her body. Or she may never experience orgasm. The more she worries about having a "successful" orgasm, the less successful she may be. This may lower her self esteem, disappoint her husband, and gradually she may seek to avoid sex. She should know that many wives have learned to enjoy the closeness of coitus without ever experiencing orgasm.

The hormone **oxytocin** has been called "the hormone of love" because of the important physiological role it plays in sexual functions. Oxytocin sets off the let-down reflex in breastfeeding, produces vigorous uterine contractions during childbirth, and is the cause of the uterine contractions during female orgasm. Recent evidence suggests that oxytocin also stimulates male ejaculation. "Biochemically there is much reason to suspect that all types of family love are closely related."[8]

It is extremely important to continue physical closeness after orgasm for at least a half hour, with touch and cuddling. If the husband is sleepy, let him doze a few minutes and then wake up again. For if he listens to his wife at **this** time, he will learn more about her than he ever dreamed! Some couples have asked if they should have prayer together at this time. If it seems natural and spontaneous, of course.

"Talking" hands

Many a wife has learned that if she touches her husband or gives him a hug, he always interprets it as a signal that she wants sexual intercourse. He associates any physical contact with a sexual approach. So the wife, longing for human closeness, learns to avoid touching him unless she is willing to go all the way to the marriage act.

A back rub works the same way. A wife's back may be aching after a long day of housework, lifting children, leaning over the stove. After the couple falls into bed her husband begins to rub her back. But at the touch of her skin he is stimulated into wanting coitus. This means that she cannot relax and go to sleep under his gentle massage, but must always rouse herself again to minister to his sexual needs. Why doesn't he rub her back **after** coitus? But he's already snoring.

Whenever I mention these things in a group of women, I see heads nodding, eyes filling with tears. Their husbands may have knowledge of many of the techniques of sexual intercourse, for magazines, newspapers and books are full of it. But "technique" is not enough. Women resent a husband thinking that if he could only "push the right button," she would respond.

Most men have never learned to appreciate the pleasurable sensations of touch apart from sex, combined with eye contact that speaks volumes. From the moment of birth, bonding deprivation, absence of breastfeeding, and inadequate touching have been the rule for most boy babies. And after they become "big boys" of two or three, they receive even less touch stimulation in the way of hugs, kisses and cuddling so they won't become "sissies."

By contrast, although a girl may suffer the earlier bonding and breastfeeding touch deprivation as an infant, she receives much more physical closeness and cuddling, and for a longer period of time. And she receives many warm caresses from her lover's arms during the courtship period. She looks forward to marriage as a time when she will receive even more. But the touching may cease soon after marriage! Now that her husband is sexually satisfied, he may be indifferent to her continuing need for communication through non-sexual touching, and he almost never looks into her eyes to see what she is thinking or feeling. Even if he still enjoys being touched and held close, he may think it is "unmanly." His appreciation for the subleties of touch apart from sex are unawakened. When a woman touches his arm, he thinks she is making a sexual advance. He is unaware that the skin is the most complex and extensive organ of the body,[9] and a marvelous means of communication with others.

Women more often know the power of touch, the many things it can say, the comfort it can bring to a troubled child. In the healing arts, some of the health professionals have learned that when they gently touch a patient where it hurts and say, "Does that feel better now?" the answer is often yes. This compassionate human touch reassures the hurting one, stimulates the healing process and helps him or her begin to get well.

Does the husband know the healing power that is in his hands? Not only is there the gentle human stimulation to healing, but as the head of his household the supernatural power of the Spirit of God can flow through his hands to bring blessing to the sick in his own family.[10] Does the husband know what comfort and peace his loving touch can bring his wife when she is not sick? Does he let her touch him?

Even a warm handshake is a form of communicating through touch, a way of saying "I like you." We shake hands with friends and strangers. But does the husband ever take his wife's hand as a way of saying, "I love you," looking into her eyes? Such a touch asks nothing for itself, but is given only to comfort, heal, give joy and peace.

Communication

But communication through touch alone is not enough. A couple must also verbally express to each other their sexual needs and desires, just as they discuss many things that seem easier to talk about. Sometimes a husband hesitates to tell his wife that he feels a need for much more frequent sexual release than he has been experiencing. He may be wrestling with undesirable dreams or temptations to lustful thoughts because they are having coitus infrequently. A thoughtful wife will recognize her responsibility to minister to his sexual needs, even if she does not feel the need as often. She will respond positively to his lovemaking in word, reassurance, and a willingness for more frequent sex.

Husbands generally desire coitus more often than the wife, or the desire may not strike both at the same time. Women are not immune to sexual hunger and some may crave more frequent coitus than the husband. It helps to know that the sex drive for most men is lowest late at night and strongest on awakening in the morning. A woman need not hesitate to tell her husband of her need for more frequent coitus, and to help him find times in which he is best able to fulfill it.

The husband must give the wife what is due her, and the wife equally must give the husband his due. The wife cannot claim her body as her own; it is her husband's. Equally, the husband cannot claim his body as his own; it is his wife's. Do not deny yourselves to one another, except when you agree upon a temporary abstinence in order to devote yourself to prayer; afterwards you may come together again; otherwise, for lack of self-control, you may be tempted by Satan.[11]

Today's woman feels free to expect that her husband will learn to provide the **quality** of lovemaking she desires, urging him to learn more about feminine response. Yet she must be willing to reciprocate by offering her husband the **quantity** that he needs. Each should be concerned about the sexual needs of the other and do their best to fulfill that need.

Sometimes it is important to talk during the lovemaking, explaining to each other what one does and does not like. For example, it is important to talk about sex acts that are different from the usual routine. One can say, "It would please me if,... would you mind?" Or if a suggestion bothers, one can say, "Why don't we do it this way? Is that okay?" One should never condemn a spouse's suggestion or action, or accuse him or her of wrong desires by saying, "That's not nice!" One must never belittle the other by saying, "You ought," or "You ought not to...." Our bodies are holy. Our marriage is holy. Sexual contact within the marriage is holy.

Occasionally a partner, usually the wife, yields to certain sexual acts which give her a strong sense of revulsion. Her yielding without comment is terribly harmful to the relationship, for it is living a lie, blocking communication, building defensive barriers between the two. Sometimes women complain to me about such things but when I suggest they be honest with their husbands they say, "Oh, I could never tell him that." Why not? Because he wouldn't even try to understand? wouldn't listen? or care? Perhaps. But perhaps he would.

One woman complained that her husband would say in midafternoon, "Shall we have fun tonight?" She thought it unromantic for coitus not to be spontaneous, but to be "planned" for in advance. Another wife is upset by spontaneous sex and has too much on her mind to drop everything abruptly at any time. She would prefer to plan a time to look forward to. All these differences of feelings and expectations need to be talked out in mutual trust in an unthreatening, undemanding way.

As family responsibilities increase it is important to plan ahead for time to enjoy sex together, perhaps even a whole night away from home to avoid the interruptions of phone, doorbell, and other activities.

Privacy

Privacy is extremely important during times of sexual intimacy, making certain that no one will enter the room or overhear any sounds husband or wife might make. The fear of the invasion of privacy greatly inhibits the sexual performance and pleasure of the couple.

But privacy is needed at other times too, a little breathing space within the home. A wife often has more opportunity for moments alone than her husband, even if they have a large family. She can relax and be alone at least a few minutes while the baby sleeps or while the children are at school.

But her husband is with people all day long. When he comes home he is with the family until bed time. Does he have at least a corner to call his own where he can be by himself for a time of prayer or thought without intrusion? Even Jesus left the crowds and His disciples, to go off alone for awhile.[12]

Holy sexual union

One of the most amazing teachings of the Bible is that even the "flesh" of a believer is holy. His or her body is a "church," a "temple" in which God lives. The holy sanctuary of the body is still holy when husband and wife come together in the most intimate physical union. This act of marriage was designed by God for our pleasure and to deepen the commitment of ourselves to one person more than to any other, for this act is to be experienced with no other.

> *Marriage is to be held in honor by all and the marriage bed kept holy, because God will judge fornicators and adulterers.*[13]

Fornication is having sexual relations when both partners are single persons. Adultery is indulging in sex with someone other than the marriage partner, whether one or both are married.

> *Now the physical body **(soma)** is not for fornication, but your physical body **(soma)** is **for the Lord,** and the Lord for your physical body **(soma)**.*
>
> *Don't you know that your bodies are members of Christ's body? Shall I then take a member of Christ and make it part of a prostitute? God forbid! What? Don't you know that he who joins his body to a prostitute is one body with her? "For two," says he, "shall be one flesh."*

> *He that is joined to the Lord is one spirit.*
>
> *Flee fornication! Every sin that a man commits is outside his body, but he that has sexual intercourse outside of marriage sins against **his own body**.*
>
> *What? Don't you know that your physical body **(soma)** is the temple of the Holy Spirit which is in you, which you have been given from God, and that you are not your own? For you are bought with a price. Therefore, glorify God in your **body**, and in your spirit, which are God's.*[14]

Is it not an awesome thought that one of the ways in which we can **give glory to God** is by having sexual intercourse with our husband or wife? It is a great mystery that the genital union in marriage is a symbol for the holy relationship between Jesus and the Church! The comparison breaks down because our physical union with Jesus is even more complete than our physical union with the marriage partner, for the Spirit of Jesus pervades our entire body. Our physical body is actually a part of the body of Christ himself.

> *So ought men to love their wives as their own bodies. He that loves his wife loves himself. For no man ever hated his own flesh, but nourishes and cherishes it, just as the Lord Jesus nourishes and cherishes the church: for we are members of His body **(soma)**, of his flesh, and of his bones.*
>
> *For this reason a man shall leave his father and mother, and shall be joined to his wife and they two shall be one flesh. This is a great mystery. But I speak concerning Christ and the church.*[15]

The Bible carries this mystery even further. It says that if one of the married partners has sexual intimacy with anyone ouside marriage, that one actually **defiles Christ,** because the body of a Christian is a member of His body. But the opposite is also true. It is an awesome thought that an unbelieving husband or wife is "made holy" because he or she becomes "one flesh" with the believing partner! A Christian wife is not made unclean by having sexual relations with her unbelieving husband. Rather, he is "made holy" by coming in contact with **her** body. In the same way, the Christian husband makes his unbelieving wife holy in the love union.

This truth destroys any of our objections to yielding our physical bodies to the closest of intimacies with the other because he or she is "not walking in the Lord." The Bible guides in the opposite way, toward **more** intimacy, not less.

For the unbelieving husband is made holy by the wife, and the unbelieving wife is made holy by the husband. Otherwise your children (born of this sexual union) *would be unclean. But now they are holy.*[16]

When the Bible says that the unbelieving spouse is "made holy" by contact with the believing spouse in intercourse, it does not mean salvation, for he or she is still personally responsible to accept Christ as Savior. But it does bring the unbelieving spouse and the subsequent children into the circle of God's covenant to bring our families to Himself. He or she is "marked," so to speak, to be pursued by God with special fervor.

God the Creator designed every part of our bodies, including every detail of our sexuality. He designed our bodies for our pleasure in each other.

And they were both naked, the man and his wife, and they were not ashamed.[17]

And God saw everything that he had made, and behold, it was very good.[18]

Thus the husband and wife can learn and grow together in their sexual experiences as well as in the other aspects of their marriage, knowing sex is holy and good. They can forget about "technique," forget unrealistic expectations based on something they have heard or read. They can learn, but then relax and enjoy each other in their own way, being themselves, enjoying the spices in their own garden of love.

My lover has come down to his garden,
  To the beds of spices,
To browse in the garden and to gather lilies.
My lover belongs to me and I to him.
  He browses among the lilies.[19].

NOTES
1. Song of S. 8:5-7. **2.** Gen. 26:8, 9.
3. Robert A. Bradley, M.D. **Husband-Coached Childbirth.** New York. Harper & Row. 1965, 1974. P. 113.
4. Ingrid Trobisch. **The Joy of Being a Woman.** New York. Harper & Row. 1975. P. 20.
5. Ed Wheat, M.D. and Gaye Wheat. **Intended for Pleasure.** Old Tappan, NJ. Revell. 1977. Reprinted by permission.

On p. 50 of this book Dr. Wheat suggests that if a wife has not experienced orgasm after several months of marriage, the following can be tried. The husband places himself in a sitting position against the head of the bed while the wife sits between his legs. She is to place her legs over his legs, leaning back against his chest with her head on his shoulder. Dr. Wheat says:

"This position allows him freedom of access for creative exploration of your whole body. You should encourage specific direction for this by slight increases in pressure or by gentle directional movement the 'where and how' of your desires at any particular moment. This will allow both of you to learn precise physical communication without the distraction of verbal request or detailed explanation. At this time you should direct his every movement, and he should absolutely refrain from any of his own ideas as to what may be stimulating you.... Often you will want him to just lightly stroke your neck, your earlobes, your breasts, your upper inner thighs, your buttocks, and then return to those most stimulating areas just above the clitoral area or around the vaginal opening.... These are pleasurable times which may extend over a period of weeks....

"While you are learning with your husband you should have complete freedom to stimulate your own clitoris if you feel it is needed to produce your first few orgasms. This will help to start a pattern of response which will later make it much easier to experience orgasm in sexual intercourse. After you have had several orgasms by manual stimulation, you should begin having sexual intercourse in the female-above position. Then use whatever positions you desire." Reprinted by permission.

For additional valuable help, see Dr. Wheat's latest book, **Love-Life for Every Married Couple.** Grand Rapids. Zondervan. 1980. Dr. Wheat also makes available two cassettes called "Sex Technique and Sex Problems in Marriage," which can be ordered from Bible Believers Cassettes, Inc., Dept. S, 130 N. Spring Street, Springdale, Arkansas 72764.
6. Ibid. P. 90.
7. Sidney Cornelia Callahan. **Beyond Birth Control: The Christian Experience of Sex.** New York. Sheed & Ward. 1968. P. 142.
8. Editorial. **ICEA News** (International Childbirth Education Association). Vol. 3. No. 2. 1964.
9. Ashley Montague. **Touching: The Human Significance of the Skin.** New York. Columbia University Press. 1971.
10. Mt. 8:3; Mk. 16:18; Acts 5:12. **11.** 1 Cor. 7:3-5 NEB. **12.** Mt. 14:23; Jn. 6:16. **13.** Heb. 13:4. **14.** 1 Cor. 6:13-20. **15.** Eph. 5:28-32. **16.** 1 Cor. 7:14. **17.** Gen. 2:25. **18.** Gen. 1:31. **19.** Song of S. 6:2 NAB.

The Song of Songs

Let him kiss me with the kisses of his mouth:
For thy love is better than wine.
A bundle of myrrh is my beloved to me,
He will lie all night between my breasts.

As the apple trees among the trees of the wood,
So is my beloved among the sons.
I sat down under his shadow with great delight
And his fruit was sweet to my taste.

He brought me to the banqueting house
And his banner over me was love.
Satiate my thirst, comfort me with fruit,
For my desire is deeply aroused.
His left hand is under my head
And his right hand is embracing me.

Awake, O north wind, and come, O south.
Blow upon my garden, that its spicy fragrances
may flow out.
Let my beloved come into his garden
And eat of his pleasant fruit.[1]

"The song of songs, which is Solomon's," is all about sexual love. Husbands and wives should occasionally set aside a special time alone to read the book together, enjoying all the analogies and nuances of expressions. The phrases about "feasting, eating, drinking," coming "into the garden," "into the vineyard," etc., all refer to the pleasures of genital union. The book is a description of the joys of that deepest union between man and wife which symbolizes the union between God and man through Jesus Christ.

There is a lot of "foreplay" talk in this love song. It describes the sights, sounds, feel, even the smell of the body of the beloved and the "taste" of the roof of the mouth (which is both literal and also an analogy of the penis in the vagina). It displays great sensitivity to all aspects of marital pleasure, of which coitus is only one small part. The lovers feast upon the sight of each other's hair, face, eyes, nose, lips, mouth, teeth, neck, arms, the breasts of the woman, the shoulders of the man, the "belly," the navel, the legs. Notice also that all this visual, verbal and tactile stimulation and enjoyment of each other does not always end in coitus. It is a pleasure also for its **own** sake! But coitus is meant when the wife says "his fruit is sweet to my taste." His fruit is the semen, and she "tastes" it in her vagina.

It's beautiful to read about, isn't it? But is it possible in our marriages? Someone once said that when God brought Eve to Adam he asked, "Lord, what am I to do with her?" God whispered something in his ear. Adam went to Eve and put his arm around her. But after a while he went back to God and said, "Now what do I do?"

Again God whispered in his ear. Adam returned, kissed Eve on the lips and hugged her for a while. But then he went back to God again and asked, "Now what do I do?" This time God whispered a little longer explanation.

Adam came back to Eve, put his arms around her, kissed her on the lips and shared what God had said. "Oh Adam," she sighed. "Not now. I have a headache."[2]

Fig leaves

What is it that causes the "headache" in our marriages? It is Paradise lost. *And the eyes of them both were opened, and they knew that they were naked. They sewed fig leaves together to make coverings for themselves. And they hid themselves from the voice of God.*[3]

There wasn't another person in the world. They were husband and wife. Why should they be ashamed to be naked before each other? But they were.

The result of our sinful nature is the need to put a little distance between ourselves and every other person, including those dearest to us. We feel afraid, ashamed, vulnerable. We want to "cover" ourselves. From what are we protecting ourselves? From discovery. From hurt. The first uncovering of our body may not be easy, but it is not the hardest part.

The ringing of the wedding bells echoes away. The guests have gone their various ways, the rice grains scattered and forgotten. At last the young bride and groom are alone for their long awaited paradise with each other, their private Eden.

Alone? Not really. Physically naked, genitals touching genitals, they are still robed in fig leaves before each other, strangers. Is it possible to be lonely in bed? in each other's arms? even on the wedding night? Yes.

Growing into wedded love takes a lifetime together. The first disrobing of one's body before the other is only the beginning of a long process. It takes far longer to disrobe the inner self before the other, to say truthfully what one is thinking or feeling, to listen with the heart to what the other is trying to say.

The Old Testament says:

> *When a man is newly wed, he shall not go out to war, neither shall he be charged with any obligations; but he shall be free at home one year to bring joy to the wife he has married.*[4]

Of course it is necessary to earn a living. But wouldn't it be a blessing if our churches would follow the Bible and not impose any obligations on newlywed couples for a year, except perhaps those in which they could work **together** in ministry? No separate committee meetings. No separate spiritual retreats. No evenings home alone for either husband or wife, but the newlyweds *free at home one year*. This would help shorten the long journey into the heart and soul of each other and foster open communication between them.

But more is needed than just time alone together. Each one must be willing to open the door of his or her own heart, to listen, and then to enter compassionately and without judgement into the heart of the other. What makes it such a long journey is partly because we don't even know **ourselves.** We feel too threatened and vulnerable to be able to uncover our true selves even to ourselves, let alone before each other. Like Adam and Eve, we make fig leaves and cover ourselves. We hide.

The long journey inward we each must take before God is not

to "analyze" ourselves, but to discover who we are in Jesus, and to see ourselves as He sees us—perfect! For God has given us a covering, the robe of the slain Lamb of God.[5] We can be transparent before each other about our needs and desires, for God has covered all our imperfections with His forgiveness and righteousness.

This is the crux of the matter in the sexual relationships of a husband and wife. A satisfactory sexual experience is far more than body mechanics, knowing all the right "techniques." Deep in the soul of each other is another need that may lie unfulfilled, the need for spiritual union.

This inner need the marriage partner can never fill, although he or she is often expected to do so. This hunger stays, for it is an inner need for God. The wife cannot be God to her husband, nor the husband to his wife. Only God can fill that greatest void in each of us. And until we let Him, we cannot experience that deep spiritual "oneness" which we long for with each other, the heart of the marriage of which sexual intercourse is only the symbol. We each need God for a happy marriage.

But we also need each other. Husbands especially often fail to understand that when a wife gives herself to him in coitus she is giving her **self,** not just her body. She wants to be more to him than a maid who cleans the house, a governess who cares for his children, a mistress who satisfies his sexual hunger. She wants him to notice **her.** She wants him to look often into her eyes, for with the eyes we speak volumes to each other of needs and interests, joys and sorrows. With strangers, our eyes may be guarded, but a man and wife who look often in each other's eyes can speak in depth across a crowded room without a word. When a wife is able to trust her husband's love for her as a real person, their sexual union takes on new intensity of joy.

There is an African parable about a farmer who caught a young woman from the sky for his bride. She was a beautiful creature and was happy to stay with him. But there was one thing that worried him. She had brought a basket from the sky with her, tightly closed with a sealed lid. "Please don't ever open my basket," she made him promise before agreeing to marry him. She warned him that a great disaster would overtake them both if he did so. He promised. He thought it was a small thing to do to win such a lovely bride.

But as the days went by, the weeks, the months, he became more and more curious about that closed basket, so near, and yet forbidden to him. One day while his wife was out he tiptoed over to it, pried the lid open and looked inside. The minute he did so he began to laugh. What had he worried about all these months? The basket was empty!

Soon his wife returned. When she saw his face she looked shocked, put her hand over her heart and whispered, "You opened the basket!"

"Yes," he said. "You silly woman, worrying me all this time about it. There's nothing in the basket."

"Nothing?" she stammered, grieved. "Nothing—in the basket? You saw nothing?"

"Nothing," he laughed. "It's empty."

At that she turned her back, walked out the door straight into the sunset and vanished into the sky. She was never seen on earth again. For you see, the basket was full of all the beautiful thoughts and dreams that she had carefully woven and stored there for them both. It was the most precious thing they had. Because he could not see them and had only laughed at her dreams, she disappeared. He did not know what had been his until he lost his lovely lady of the sky.[6]

How many wives have hidden, lovely things to share soul to soul, but cannot, because the husband would not appreciate them? He has more rapport with people at work, his friends at church, his sports partners. He is seldom home nights but is busy, busy, busy with his own affairs. Then he comes home late, falls into bed and wants sex. He thinks she is cold, frigid, because she doesn't rush gladly into his arms.

Such a husband may not even know himself, never having gone far enough on his inward journey into his own personhood in Christ. All day he plays a role and is unable to drop his mask before his wife and enter into a bond of the inner spirit with her. He is astonished that she seems dissatisfied with him. Is he not a "good" husband? He goes to church with her, earns a living, provides a home, food, clothes. What more can she want?

When a wife is not free to share the deep things of her heart with her husband it is because she does not **trust** his reaction. She believes he will be disinterested. They will be "nothing" to him. This becomes a block to her ability to enter freely into sexual intimacies. It is difficult for her to give such a personal part of herself when he is not interested in the whole. She feels that he is not giving **himself** totally to her either, but is using her only for his own sexual needs.

Or it may be the wife who makes it difficult for her husband to open his real thoughts to her for fear of her rejection. He becomes hesitant and inhibited in his love making or else hurries through. He dare not expose his dreams and longings to her, for she might criticize or laugh. It has been noted that men are more sentimental than women, but they express this sentimentality less verbally. And in our "macho" society the small boy learns to hide his real feelings to keep from being labeled a "sissy." A little girl falls down, is picked up, hugged and the hurts kissed away. A little boy falls down, picks himself up and is told, "Don't cry. You're a big boy!" But little boys sometimes **need** to cry. And so do big boys, husbands. Will a wife think her husband less manly if he shows how he really feels?

Broken hearts

Perhaps the partner senses deep in his or her spirit that he or she is not really loved. And it may be true! How many couples have fallen "out of love" with each other? Usually it is first one, then the other, though the "mask" of a happy married couple may be in place for a long time, even with each other. But in their spirits they sense what their conscious minds are still unwilling to receive. Doubt replaces trust.

The real problem is that they have never truly been **in** love, for true love is a commitment to another from the heart which does not waver regardless of how one may feel and regardless of circumstances.

> *So David danced before the Lord with all his might, and brought up the ark of the Lord with shouting, and with the sound of the trumpet.*
> *And Michal, Saul's daughter* (David's wife) *looked through a window, and saw king David leaping and dancing before the Lord, and she despised him in her heart.*[7]

Michal was the opposite of the godly wife spoken of in Proverb 31:

> *Who can find a virtuous wife? for her price is far above rubies.*
> *The heart of her husband* **safely trusts** *in her. He has an unfailing prize. She will do him good and not evil all the days of her life.*[8]

Let a wife ask herself, "Can my husband safely trust me in his heart? Or do I secretly despise him as Michal despised David, and wish I had married someone else?" This "someone else" need not be a real person. It might be only a dream husband, a fantasy. But it has no rightful place in her heart.

A friend of mine lived with a sickly wife year after year, for long years of married life. He washed the dishes, cleaned the house, did the laundry, cooked the meals, took care of her and took her with him on journeys, pushing her wheelchair wherever she wanted to go. The difficulty was, he could do nothing right! She was continually complaining about him, criticizing the way he cleaned the house, the way he washed the dishes, etc. One day he complained to the Lord about the heaviness of this burden, how unfair it was. She was not the kind of wife he had wanted. And the Lord answered him: *Whoever finds a wife* **finds a good thing,** *and receives favor from the Lord!*[9] The Lord renewed the commitment of his heart to love his wife, and he has been greatly blessed since that time.

> *Live joyfully with the wife whom you love all the fleeting days of your life, which God has given you under the sun, for that is your portion in this life.*[10]

True love is a commitment to keep on loving no matter what, just as God loves us. The temptations to let the heart wander may be great!

> *My son, attend to my wisdom, and bend your ear to my understanding. For the lips of some other woman drop as honeycomb, and her mouth is smoother than oil.*
>
> *But her end is bitter as wormwood, sharp as a two-edged sword. Her feet go down to death; her steps take hold on hell.*
>
> *Remove your way far from her, . . . lest you mourn in the end, when your flesh and your body are consumed.*
>
> *Drink waters out of your own cistern, and running waters out of your own well. Let your fountain be blessed, and rejoice with the wife of your youth. Let her be as the loving hind and roe. Let her breasts satisfy you at all times, and be ravished always with her love.*
>
> *For the ways of a man are before the eyes of the Lord, and He takes notice of all his actions.*[11]

God not only takes notice of the husband or wife whose heart and feet have turned aside to others. He also takes notice of the wounded one and offers His own love to bind up the wounded, broken heart. Hosea the prophet had an unfaithful wife, but God told Hosea to pursue her with enduring love and receive her back, just as God wins us back to Himself with His love, though we are all like unfaithful wives to Him.

> *"She is not my wife* (says the Lord), *neither am I her husband; let her put away her harlotry, and her adulteries from between her breasts,...*
> *"Then I will allure her, and bring her into the wilderness, and speak comforting words to her. And I will give her back her vineyards, and the valley of weeping for a door of hope."* She will sing there, as in the days of her youth. *"And in that day,"* says the Lord, *"she will say to me, '"My husband."'"*[12]

If it is the husband who mistreats his wife, the Lord himself comforts her:

> *Fear not, for you shall not be ashamed. Don't be distraught, for you will not be put to shame. For you will forget the shame of your youth, and will not remember the reproach of your being abandoned any more.*
> *For your Maker is your husband. The Lord of hosts is his name, your Redeemer, the Holy One of Israel, the God of the whole earth.*
> *For the Lord has called you as a woman forsaken and grieved in spirit, and a wife of youth when you were cast off, says your God.... O afflicted one, tossed with tempest and not comforted! Look, I will lay your stones with fair colors, and lay your foundations with sapphires. And all your children shall be taught of the Lord, and great shall be the peace of your children.*[13]

Broken-hearted husbands as well as wives have found comfort in this magnificent passage in Isaiah. Either of them may have experienced the grief of an unfaithful partner. Sin is an impenetrable obstacle to happiness in marriage until there is repentance, turning away from it—even in thought—and receiving the forgiveness of Jesus and the forgiveness of the husband or wife.

Guilt accompanies sin and is a barrier to soul-to-soul communication, even when the sin has been forgiven. "How could I have ever done such a thing!" we moan. It is because we are all sinners. Such a statement is one of pride, like the statement, "I would never think of doing such a thing!" You and I, every one of us, are capable of committing **any** sin, even gross murder. What keeps us from it is the grace and providence of God which has allowed many of us to be born in homes where we have learned about Jesus. That may have brought us early to salvation. None of us can judge another, for this would mean that the death of Jesus was less necessary for our sins than for "worse" sinners.

Those who have committed sexual sins can thank God that they have not only been forgiven, but that they have no room for spiritual pride. And let those who think they have never sinned in these ways beware of boasting, for Jesus says we have **all** sinned in our thoughts.[14] We all need forgiveness, and are not to judge those who have fallen.[15]

All things new

New beginnings are possible in any marriage.[16] In God's eyes the guilty one can become pure again, just as if he'd never sinned. But it may take time to heal the wounds inflicted on the marriage.

If a bride and groom are both virgins at the time of their wedding, they can learn together without comparing their partner's sexual performance with that of someone else. When a virginal bride marries a man who has had sex with other women before marriage, she is at a great disadvantage. Shy, uncertain of herself, she cannot possibly live up to his expectations of a satisfying sexual partner right away. The same is true of the virginal husband who marries a wife who was sexually active with someone else before marriage.

If the guilty one has found the cleansing, refreshing streams of God's forgiveness, he or she need not "tell all" to his bride or groom. This may compound the difficulty, for although their partner might be able to forgive them intellectually or theologically, their emotional response cannot be predicted. This knowledge might bring shock and a wounding of the spirit that would create new inhibitions between them.

It is enough to say to the other, "I've done some things in the past that I'm ashamed of now, but I thank God they're forgiven because of Jesus. I love you with my whole heart, and I love you only." This is a confession each might make to the other, and then each respond to the other, "I forgive you too." That is enough. If either one tries to pry or probe, he or she reveals an unforgiving, prideful spirit. When a sin is buried in the bottom of the sea, it's **buried**.[17] Let it stay there.

But sometimes things don't seem to stay buried! A sense of shame remains, inhibiting husband or wife, even though the partner may be unaware of this. Something lingers just below the surface of the conscious mind, as troubling as a gnat we can't catch or a mosquito buzzing around us in the night. If conscious sin has been confessed and forgiven, the guilt that is still troubling may be from something else.

Nearly every child has had some experiences that were hidden from the parents. It might be taking one's pants down before the opposite sex, or a little boy flipping his penis up and down behind the garage for the others to giggle at, or playing doctor by "taking temperatures" in the rectum with a toothpick, and so on.

Hidden in the memories of everyone reading these words there may be some such unconfessed, unforgiven child's sin. Let each one sit quietly in the presence of the Lord Jesus and ask Him to bring each such memory to the surface of our attention. Think back, a long, long way. Feel the embarrassment that comes when the incident is recalled. Then pray, "Lord, I now confess that I knew that was a naughty thing to do. I was not 'innocent,' but hid my actions from my parents. Please cleanse my mind and heart of this memory with Your forgiving love." He will!

It may be that there were incidents in which our parents or others made us feel "dirty" about some part of our body. Only a "bad" boy or a "bad" girl is wet or messy. We associate all that "messiness" with our sexual organs and functions. A young girl may feel "messy" because she can't control the menstrual flow. Other unpleasant memories which may surface are feelings of rejection from one of our parents, or from both, filling us with a vague sense of guilt for being a boy, or for being a girl. Let the Spirit of God go back into each of these incidents and set us free from this false shame.

Marital pleasure is greatly inhibited by false shame. The vagina is one of the cleanest, most germ-free orifices of the body, far cleaner than the mouth. The menstrual flow is not "dirty." Think of it like sweat. Can we stop our sweat? Are we embarrassed because saliva is secreted in our mouths? Cleanliness is important during the days of the menstrual flow, just as a shower after playing basketball is a good idea. Nor is semen "dirty." It is wet, yes, but colorless, does not stain, and is easily washed off the body and out of the clothing.

We can rebuke this false shame and say, "You false sense of shame, get away from me in Jesus' name! God made me the way I am, with all the parts of my body, including my sexual parts. Because God created me, every atom of my body is pure, lovely, holy. You wicked, dirty, lying spirit, get away from me! I won't listen to you any more!"

Little foxes

But there are other, smaller things that interfere with our pleasure in each other. The Song of Songs warns us to *catch the foxes, the little foxes, that spoil the grapes* (the grapes of sexual pleasures).[18] What are these "little foxes?"

A husband sees his wife bending over the sink washing dishes. She looks so delectable he slips up behind her, gives her a hug and turns her around, wet hands and all. He wants her to drop what she is doing and come to bed at once. Spontaneous romance is good, but a little fox is lurking here. Its name is **Thoughtlessness.**

He would get a much warmer response if he grabbed a towel and helped her finish the work first. Spontaneous sex in the middle of the day tears the bed apart. Who remakes the bed? Thoughtfulness in such little things goes a long way. One husband said that each morning when he got up he first dropped on his knees and asked God what His will was for him that day. Opening his eyes, the first thing he would see was an unmade bed. He decided God's will was for him to make the bed each morning and not leave this chore to his wife.

Controversy is another little fox waiting to spoil the relationship. The biggest arguments are usually over little things. Over the years a husband/wife controversy sounds like a broken record. Comment—retort—defense—defense—. Even the words may not vary! Stop and listen some time. Doesn't it sound familiar? How long ago did it start? The couple is so used to this "recording" they would deny they were arguing, but to others it sounds terrible! The accusations go on and on, over lateness, slowness, miserliness, compulsive buying, the children's behavior, and a myriad of other things. It destroys the unity of the marriage, infects it with bitterness and alienation, takes away the desire for sex together.

We are always trying to remake our spouse into our **own** image of what he or she should be, not letting them be themselves and growing as God wants them to grow. Unity of heart and purpose does not rule out differences of tastes and temperament. The one who was always late before marriage will probably always tend to be late. The forgetful one will continue to be forgetful. The precise, prompt, orderly person will probably become more so. We are to love and accept the marriage partner **as they are.** Any attempt to change them leads only to frustration and anger.

Anger is one of the most destructive of the little foxes that ruin a marriage. Jesus said that it is not what goes into our bodies that defile them, but *the words that come out of our mouths.*[19] Angry words can never be recalled, even after they have been confessed and forgiven. They are like daggers that enter the heart. The dagger may be pulled out but the hurt remains, the trust wounded, and a protective scar builds up over the hurt place.

There are times when anger is not wrong in itself, but the Bible warns us *not to sin*[20] when we are angry. It also warns us not to go to bed without having resolved the anger. Let's put away any anger before going to sleep and start the next day right. *Do not grieve the Holy Spirit of God, but let all bitterness, wrath, anger, arguing and evil speaking be put away from you.*[21]

Anxiety nibbles away at the tender leaves of the marriage, *spoiling the vines.* Anxiety touches every part of our experiences but focuses on becoming sick, getting hurt, having an accident, not having enough money, not being well thought of, not being loved. Jesus said to a harried housewife, *Martha, Martha, you are anxious and troubled about many things. Only* **one** *thing is needed.*[22] That "one thing" is to live in the peace of the presence of Jesus. A husband is often anxious over money, cross with his wife over necessary expenditures for fear poverty lurks around the corner. Yet God has said, *In* **nothing** *be anxious, but in everything by prayer and petition, with a grateful heart tell God your needs.*[23]

There is probably more anxiety and disagreement over money matters than any other aspect of a marriage. Yet these disagreements are only symptoms of a far greater breakdown in communication. Couples who are really united and close can cope with any material lack without disrupting their relationship, supporting each other in their attempt to find ways to overcome the financial difficulties.

Rejection is another little fox that has no place in a marriage. How many times a husband has put his arm around his wife and invited her to come to bed with him but she has put him off. She "has a headache," or is "too tired." A husband should be sensitive to genuine fatigue in his wife. But sometimes this "tiredness" is just a put-off, and he experiences this as a rejection of himself. Perhaps she will relent and they have coitus after all, but his spirit is hurt, and the door of his heart closes a little, protecting himself. It will be harder for him to reach out to his wife the next time for fear of rejection again, even if she really wants him.

> *I sleep, but my heart awakens. It is the voice of my beloved who knocks, saying, "Open to me my love, my dove, my pure one. My head is filled with dew and my locks with the drops of the night."*
> *"I have taken off my coat. Do I have to put it on again? I've already washed my feet. Do you want me to get them dirty again?" My beloved put his hand on the locked door, and suddenly my heart was stirred with longing for him. I jumped out of bed to open the door for him. My hands dropped with myrrh and my fingers with sweet smelling myrrh as I undid the lock. I opened to my beloved.*
> *But my beloved had withdrawn himself and was gone! I searched for him but could not find him. I called him, but he gave me no answer.*[24]

We are all fallible, imperfect. Let's not let little problems overlap into a basically good sexual relationship and marriage, but face up to the problems one at a time, working them through to understanding. When serious marriage trouble comes, let's examine our own hearts again. Am I really seeking the kingdom of God and His righteousness **first?** Who am I in God? Am I willing to give up "my" goals for our marriage and receive my husband or wife on God's terms?

Let's allow our husband or wife to be imperfect, to pursue things differently than we would, to grow in the Lord at his or her own pace. Let's love them and treat them with compassion and hope, as if they were already what God wants them to become.

> *Let's be kind to each other, tender hearted, forgiving each other, even as God for Christ's sake has forgiven us.*[25]

NOTES
1. Song of S. 1:2, 13; 2:3-6; 4:16. **2.** Source unknown. **3.** Gen. 3:7, 8.
4. Deut. 25:5 KJV and NAB. **5.** Rom. 4:7; Rev. 7:14.
6. Laurens van der Post. **The Heart of the Hunter.** New York. Morrow. 1961. Pp. 142-146.
7. 2 Sam 6:14-16. **8.** Prov. 31:10-12. **9.** Prov. 18:22. **10.** Eccl. 9:9.
11. Prov. 5:15-23. **12.** Hos. 2:2, 14-16. **13.** Isa. 54:4-13. **14.** Mt. 5:27, 28.
15. Mt. 7:1; Gal. 6:1-3.
16. Walter Trobisch. **I Married You.** New York. Harper & Row. 1971. See also the other excellent books on marriage by Ingrid or Walter Trobisch.
17. Mic. 7:18, 19. **18.** Song of S. 2:15. **19.** Mk. 7:18-23. **20.** Eph. 4:26.
21. Eph. 4:29-31. **22.** Lk. 10:41, 42. **23.** Phil. 4:6. **24.** Song of S. 5:2-6.
25. Eph. 4:32.

When Two Agree

You shall be called Hephzibah (my delight) and your land Beulah (married). For as a young man marries a virgin, and as the bridegroom rejoices over the bride, so shall your God rejoice over you.[1]

Can two walk together unless they are in agreement?[2]

Again I say to you, If two of you agree on anything they ask, it will be done for them by my Father in heaven.[3]

Two young people walk hand in hand, absorbed in each other. Lovers. We smile at their happiness and look away. The walk leads through courtship and on to the altar where they become husband and wife before God. The beaming couple move as one back down the aisle as if on wings and on out the sanctuary, while we all smile and surreptitiously wipe away a tear. The long walk through life together has begun for them. Will it fulfill the promise of the high hopes of this moment?

Ten years go by. The husband is burdened with heavy responsibilities, the wife absorbed in the children's needs. Are husband and wife still walking together? Still in love? Twenty years pass. The children have grown. Husband and wife face each other alone over the table. What is there to talk about? Are they strangers to each other? Or do they still walk together in the garden in the cool of the day, listening to the voice of Jehovah, blessed in their companionship?[4]

Marriage is of far greater significance than multiplying the human race. It is far more than the legalization of the sex act between a man and a woman. It is to be a companionship, a communion that deepens as the years pass, a growing oneness. Look around at some of the middle-aged couples in your own congregations. How many activities do these couples participate in **together** in the church and community? Do you ever see them look in each other's eyes? Smile across the room at each other? There are many clues which show which couples are still walking together, still finding marriage "sweeter as the years go by...."

The fruit of marriage

It may seem strange at the outset of marriage to look down the years, but it is tremendously important. For the kind of relationship a couple will have then is being built **now.** The added responsibility of children places great stress on the marriage relationship. The trend today is to avoid having children so the couple can enjoy each other without distraction and fulfill themselves. But one glance twenty or thirty years down the road quickly shows this is not the answer either, for all we see are two self-centered, immature older people whose house is full of expensive objects. But who cares what happens to them? What happens when one of them dies?

Children and grandchildren are the best "old age" investment there is, enriching our lives as we see them grow, still loving and caring for us when our lover is gone. Children enhance and deepen the marriage relationship, while the stresses they add hasten the maturity of their parents. The question is not "Should we have children?" but "When does God want us to have each child?" For God does intend that we have children.

> *This you have done again, covering the altar of the Lord with tears, with weeping, and with crying out, but even so he does not regard the offering any more, nor receive it with good will from your hand.*
>
> *Yet you say, "Why is this?" It is because the Lord has been witness between you and the wife of your youth, against whom you have dealt treacherously. For she is your companion, and the wife of your covenant.*
>
> *Did not he make you one? And why one? that he might seek a **godly offspring**. Therefore take heed to your spirit, and let none of you deal treacherously with the wife of your covenant.*[5]

God's desire is for the deep companionship of the marriage to be maintained through the years in order that the children born to this union may be "godly children," added grains of salt[6] for this trouble world, spreading more love, more grace, more healing in each succeeding generation.

May our sons be like plants well-nurtured in their youth, our daughters like wrought columns such as stand at the corners of the temple. May our garners be full, affording every kind of store.... Happy the people for whom things are thus; happy the people whose God is the Lord.[7]

The "population explosion" need be no problem for those who are trusting God, for the Psalmist says, *I have been young and now am old; yet I have not seen the righteous forsaken, nor his children begging bread. He* (the righteous) *is always kind and generous, and his children are blessed.*[8]

When husband and wife seek the will of the Lord and agree about the coming of each child, they can claim God's promises to provide, regardless of the rate of inflation or the standard of living. And God will not only meet their daily needs, but will use these children to help provide answers for the world's needs.

Lo, children are the heritage of the Lord, and the fruit of the womb is his reward. As arrows in the hand of a mighty man, so are children of the youth. Happy is the man who has his quiver full of them![9]

If husband and wife are to agree together through prayer concerning the coming of each child, they need to understand about conception, how it takes place and how it can be avoided. In the centuries past men too often carried little or no responsibility for the consequences of sexual intercourse—even in marriage. It was a means of satisfying his sexual appetite whether or not children resulted. In some cultures this sexual dominance of the male resulted in whole harems of women belonging to one man. And far too often marriages in monogamous cultures became economic arrangements only, while men sought mistresses outside the marriage with whom they indulged their sexual appetites.

Husband and wife who truly walked with God overcame some of these difficulties during the long centuries when knowledge concerning conception was inadequate. Some godly men abstained from coitus for long periods of time, even years, to protect the health of a frail wife. Godly women accepted as many children as God gave them, loving each child, even though the hard work of a big family sometimes affected their health. Fortunately, women often nursed their babies for two, three and even four years, which helped to space the births, as breastfeeding tends to inhibit ovulation.

The miracle of conception

A man might have some rise and fall of sexual desire but his cycle is less obvious than that of the female. The production of his semen is fairly constant. Semen is composed of two types of secretion, the first of which is produced in the testicles and called **spermatazoa** (sperm—the "seed" of the male). The second is the seminal fluid produced by the seminal vesicles and prostate gland. (The **vas deferens** are the tubes which lead from the prostate gland to the testicles.)

When the penis is sexually stimulated its tissues fill with blood so that it becomes firm and points upward, able to penetrate the vagina of the female. Ejaculation is the "climax" for the male, in which his semen is forcefully ejected from the penis. One teaspoonful of semen, which is the amount usually ejaculated, contains 200-500 million sperm. And only **one** sperm is necessary for conception although many thousands are needed to make fertilization possible. Thousands of sperm surround the ovum and release an enzyme to dissolve the ovum outer layer and once this is done the "chosen" sperm enters. This sperm joined to the egg becomes "a living soul." A child is conceived.

In order for that phenomenon to take place, the female must have a ripe ovum for the sperm. But the sperm can survive after coitus for three to five days in the female milieu (tubes, uterus, cervix), awaiting the release of a ripe ovum. Thus a woman might "conceive" up to five days after sexual relations have taken place.

In contrast to the rather constant production of sperm by the male, the ovum of the female is released only once each month. The female sexual cycle is obvious, because the soft lining of the uterus (womb) which has built up during the month to possibly receive the fertilized ovum is cast off when conception has not taken place. This menstrual flow has been called the "weeping of a disappointed uterus." The old lining is discarded and a new one immediately begins to build up on the walls of the uterus.

Another less obvious event is taking place in her body. On each side of the uterus a Fallopian tube branches off, with a small gland suspended below each tube. These glands are the ovaries. (Think of the tubes as like flower stems four or five inches long, one leaning to the right and one to the left of the uterus with a "blossom" below the stem similar to a fuchsia flower or daffodil. This "blossom" is the ovary.) Each ovary contains the complete number of immature ova (eggs) from the time of the tenth week of conception of the female, so that she is born with about 400,000 ova. After she reaches puberty, one ovum matures and is released each month for about thirty years, except when she is pregnant or breastfeeding. None are released after menopause, that is, after menstruations have stopped for a year.

When the ovary on one side or the other releases a ripe ovum, it is drawn into the Fallopian tube and moves slowly along the four or five inch tube toward the uterus. The journey takes about twenty-four hours. If the ovum has not been fertilized by a sperm by the time it reaches the uterus it moves on and is discarded from the body. From the time that it is gone until another ovum is released the following month, conception of a child is not possible.

A child is conceived when the sperm of the male reaches the ripe ovum of the female in the Fallopian tube, penetrates the ovum and merges with it. This living organism then travels through the tube to become attached to the lining of the uterus, its "nest," where it will draw nourishment from the mother until ready to be born nine months later.

Preventing conception

There is a great difference between **preventing** conception and destroying a human life **after** conception. There are methods called "birth control" which may not prevent conception, but literally control births and abort the newly conceived child. Abortion at any time from conception on is the killing of a human being, which is forbidden in Scripture.[10] One of the greatest miracles of all creation is that from the microscopic fusion of two human cells all the potential of a human being is present, awaiting development. Even the potentials of our greatest geniuses of music, art, literature or our greatest saints are present in that tiny union.

One of the possible abortafacients causing abortion, although it is called "birth control," is the IUD (intra-uterine device). The IUD is a plastic or metal piece which is placed in the woman's uterus by a physician and remains in place until a physician removes it. The cervix is dilated (stretched) enough to put the

IUD in or to withdraw it, when the woman wants to have a baby.

It is now thought that the IUD does not prevent the sperm from reaching the ovum, but that it irritates the lining of the uterus so that the fertilized ovum is not able to attach to the lining or to remain attached very long. The sperm may still reach the ovum and the fertilized ovum move down the Fallopian tube to the uterus, but the presence of the irritant IUD causes the child so conceived to be expelled, and no pregnancy develops.

Another possible abortifacient is the mini-pill, a smaller dose of hormones than the regular pill, and now more commonly prescribed. There is less risk to the mother of thrombosis and other health complications with the mini-pill. Unfortunately, the smaller amount of hormones does not always keep the woman from ovulating (as the higher estrogen pill does). Conception may occur, but the woman's altered hormones block the implantation of the ovum in the womb, and the conceptus may be aborted.

The "morning after" pill, taken the morning after coitus, is definitely an abortifacient. If conception took place, the fertilized egg is eliminated and no pregnancy occurs.[11]

Some people may be appalled at the thought that unknowingly they may have been aborting through methods wrongly called "birth control" which they had chosen to prevent conception. The Bible has an answer for them:

If a soul shall sin through ignorance against any of the commandments of the Lord concerning things which ought not to be done, ... let him bring a sin offering. And the priest shall dip his finger in the blood, and sprinkle the blood seven times before the Lord, before the veil of the sanctuary, and the sin shall be forgiven.[12]

Jesus has paid that blood sacrifice for our sin with His death on the cross for us. His sacrifice was necessary for the many sins of which we have not been aware as much as for those which we know. When we become aware of a possible sin, we know what to do. *If we confess our sins, He is faithful and just to forgive our sins, and to cleanse us from all unrighteousness.*[13]

True "birth control" means **preventing** conception, keeping the sperm from meeting the ovum in the first place. The most obvious means of preventing conception is abstinence. If a couple abstains from intercourse during the wife's period of ovulation, no conception will occur. In times past it was not known how to determine this fertile time, so calendar days were counted (the rhythm method). The couple abstained from intercourse for certain days of the month in hopes that the fertile period would be over when they came together in coitus again. Unfortunately, the fertile period varies from month to month, so that this method was often ineffective in preventing conception.

Other couples abstained from sexual intercourse for months and years at a time to avoid conceiving children, but this is unnatural and places great stress on the marriage. After the turn of the century when more became known about how conception actually takes place, some artificial (mechanical or chemical) means of preventing conception were developed.

The most permanent form of mechanical blockage is "tying the tubes." In the female, the Fallopian tubes are closed off so that the ovum cannot reach the uterus. The tubes are tied in two places and then severed between the ties. This is a surgical procedure, and like any surgical procedure is not without some risk to the mother.

In men, "tying the tubes" involves closing off the **vas deferens** (canals) which lead from the prostate gland to the testicles. It is being discovered that this "simple" operation may have some long-term risks. About 25 per cent of vasectomized men develop sperm antibodies, and some say that as many as two-thirds of the men are so affected. These sperm antibodies lower the body's immunological resistance to certain diseases.

Recent reports show that post-vasectomized males with sperm antibodies have developed significant arthritis, and it is believed that susceptibility to such diseases as lymphoma, leukemia and Hodgkins Disease are all theoretical potentials of this sequence of immune events.[14]

Sterilization is mutilation of the human body for social reasons. It is a defeatist attitude, as if one could not trust our human resources, or trust the spouse's ability to practice some periodic abstinence. It is a loss of openness to God's plans for them, as if they were saying, "No matter what Your plans are for us, we have decided to say **no** to any plan but our own." The "openness to life" is lost.

This does not mean that sterilization is not sometimes justified for serious medical reasons. This is not the same as the case when sterilization is done automatically after a couple has one or two children.

A temporary form of mechanical blockage is the use of a rubber condom over the penis, or a cap-shaped rubber device called a diaphragm which is inserted by the woman inside her body over the mouth (cervix) of the uterus. Condoms can be purchased in any drug store. Since the erected penis is approximately the same size in all men, regardless of how large or small the relaxed penis may be, condoms come in only one size. However, the diaphragm or cervical cap for the woman must be fitted to her cervix. Measurement is done by a physician, and she can then purchase the right size for herself.

The cervix extends slightly down into the vagina. At its center is the **os** (mouth), the passageway from the vagina through the cervix into the uterus itself. The diaphragm or cervical cap fits onto the cervix completely covering the **os** or mouth of the uterus.

However, because sperm are so microscopically small and there are so many millions of them, there is always the possibility, of some of them escaping around the condom or diaphragm into the uterus. In order to prevent this possibility a spermicide cream is also used which not only hastens the death of the sperm, but also lubricates the vagina so that its tissues are more comfortable during coitus. The difficulty with spermicide creams and jellies is that some have wondered about the possibility of a damaged sperm (damaged by the spermicide) getting past the barriers and resulting in a damaged conceptus. So far there is no evidence that this has happened, but neither has there been research to disprove the possibility.

A new chemical means of preventing conception has come into favor with the general public in the last twenty years known as "the pill." This involves taking hormones into the body by mouth (occasionally by injection) in order to alter the hormonal balance of the body and prevent fertility. For women, this is intended to prevent ovulation from occurring. The pill is discontinued for five days in each month during which breakthrough bleeding occurs. A new pill is being tested for men which suppresses the production of sperm.

Unfortunately, the widespread use of anything which alters the natural hormonal balance can have harmful consequences over a period of time. Permanent sterility can occur in very rare cases. How distressing it is for a young woman in her late twenties to discover, after discontinuing the pill in order to become pregnant, that ovulation does not return! The menses may return after several months, but ovulation may never return.

Although this is not a frequent problem, it is a real tragedy to the young couples to whom it does occur.

Other unfortunate consequences of the pill have been an increase in the tendency toward high blood pressure, a greater danger of blood clots and strokes, and mental problems such as depression or extreme mood fluctuations. These are far more serious consequences than the unpleasant side effects many women experience from the pill such as nausea and swelling of the tissues.

Experiments on a pill for men involve the same questions. Any artificial altering of the body's natural hormone balance for nonmedical reasons is tampering with God's creation in ways that may have unforeseen long range drastic consequences.

Some couples have decided that they will use no means of birth control but just "trust the Lord." But in order to "trust the Lord," one must also learn to **receive** His guidance and **obey** it. God cannot be blamed if such couples have more pregnancies than they wanted. The spiritually immature are more likely to depend on their impulse for coitus than upon hearing God, mistaking that "impulse" for His guidance. God's guidance would be "no" during a woman's fertile period if another pregnancy was unwise at that time, but how many of us take "no" from God on anything?

Some primitive cultures seem to have knowledge of how to prevent conception.[15] But in many of these cultures coitus is considered taboo until after the child is weaned at about two years of age. This kind of abstinence prevents conception, but it may ruin a marriage!

Natural family planning

Fortunately, our good Lord has made a way in which husband and wife can enjoy genital intimacies without conceiving a child, by learning to recognize the woman's physical symptoms of fertility and infertility. These symptoms have been there from the beginning of creation. It is time we learned God's "built-in" plan.

In the previous chapters we discussed the need for a woman to be comfortable with all aspects of her physical body. There are physical clues, nature's secrets, by which a woman can know when she is fertile and when she is not. These physical clues mean that husband and wife can agree when to have coitus and when to refrain. They will need to talk together about their sexual needs and desires much more openly. This new knowledge is called "natural family planning," because it is based on natural symptoms.

Each woman's fertility cycle extends from the onset of menstruation in one month to the onset of menstruation the following month. But because each woman's fertility cycle is different from that of any other woman and may change from month to month in the same woman, counting calendar days is ineffective for determining fertility.

The fertility cycle is regulated by natural hormones and divided into three periods. The first is the pre-ovulation period, including menstruation, during which no ovum is present. The time length **preceding** ovulation may vary from month to month. Second is the fertile period during which conception of a child can occur. This is the ovulatory period, which lasts about five days. (Ovulation takes place on only one of these days—all others are really pre-ovulatory.) The third period of the fertility cycle is the time after the ovulation period, and this period remains fairly stable (12-14 days) from cycle to cycle. At this time the hormone progesterone is present in greater quantity in the woman's body, preventing the release of another ovum from the ovary until the following month.

The five days of the ovulation period during the central portion of this cycle is the time in which conception may occur. There are physical signs which signal the approach of ovulation (release of an ovum). Although an ovum lives only 24 hours, male sperm can live in a woman's body much longer than that. Thus coitus in the days just preceding ovulation could result in conception. The most reliable sign of the approach of ovulation is the mucus sign. After menstruations the opening (**os**) of the cervix which leads from the vagina into the uterus is closed by a plug of mucus. As ovulation approaches, this mucus thins out and begins to come away. A woman can recognize the changes in moisture at the entrance to her vagina. There is always some moisture in this area, just as the membranes of the mouth are always wet, but now the moisture begins to increase.

During the time in which the ripe ovum is in the Fallopian tubes the mucus plug begins to come away from the cervical opening, and consequently the moisture of the vagina and vulva will increase. At first the mucus is thick but gradually takes on the consistency of raw egg white, and when rubbed between one's fingers slips around (like an egg white between the fingers) and forms threads. It is thus possible to try and tell the difference between cervical mucus and ordinary vaginal secretions or the husband's semen, though it is not easy to tell. Semen or vaginal secretions break apart when rubbed between the fingers so that the fingers become dry. The cervical mucus slides around on the fingers and does not break apart. After two or three days the thready mucus reverts to thicker mucus which leaves a sticky residue on the underwear, eventually drying up totally.

Once the mucus plug to the cervix has begun to come away the sperm has easy access through the uterus into the Fallopian tubes to the ripe ovum. After the ovulation period and time allowed to let the ovum die, there is no possibility of conception for the remainder of the cycle (the monthly cycle ends with the onset of the next menstruation). To be sure the ovum has passed, four "dry" days should be observed before genital contact between husband and wife again takes place. At this time the hormone progesterone is present in greater quantity in the woman's body, preventing the release of another ovum from the ovary until the following month.

Although the mucus sign is the most reliable sign of ovulation, there are other body signs which help to confirm the ovulation period. One is that some women have a crampy pain low in the abdomen on one side or the other each month when the ovum is released from the ovary. In some women this signal is easily recognized. Others may not feel it at all. Because other symptoms can also cause abdominal pain, this is not a reliable symptom by itself.

The presence of fertility can also be monitored by examining the cervical changes with one's finger. The woman uses her index or middle finger, reaching up into the vagina while in a semi-squatting position or with one foot on a stool or chair so that the cervix can be reached by the finger. The examination should take place at the same time each day, using the same position, so that other changes which make the cervix seem higher or lower do not confuse her observation.

Before ovulation takes place the cervix will be firm and thick to the touch. It is about an inch from side to side and extends slightly down into the vagina. The dimple, or depression in the center one feels with the finger is the **os**, which opens into the uterus. Before ovulation, the **os** is tightly closed and relatively dry.

As ovulation approaches, the cervix feels softer to the touch, more open and also moist and slippery because the mucus plug is coming away. And it will be harder to reach because the cervix is being drawn further up into the body.

Once ovulation has passed, the cervix again lowers into the vagina and is drier, closed, and firmer to the touch.

After fertility has passed the woman experiences a rise in basal temperature. The hormone progesterone which suppresses the release of another ovum is also responsible for this rise in basal body temperature (temperature of the body at rest). This higher temperature is maintained until the onset of the next menstruation. A woman can determine this temperature change by taking it each morning before getting out of bed. When her temperature rises and **stays** elevated, fertility has passed.

There are two methods of natural family planning. The first is called the "Billings method" or the "mucus method" in which mucus changes alone are monitored. The second is called the "sympto-thermal" method because temperature and other body signs (pain in the abdomen, temperature change, cervical changes) are noted in addition to the mucus signs. The mucus sign is **essential**, and the additional signs are for confirmation. For example, temperature changes alone would not be reliable because other factors can also cause temperature fluctuation. And during breastfeeding or pre-menopause the mucus sign may be the only reliable symptom of the fertility period.

Natural family planning, when correctly learned and applied, is an ideal way for a couple to "plan" their family. It increases a woman's awareness of and harmony with her own body and increases her confidence in her sexuality. It makes verbal communication between husband and wife necessary about sexual matters, for the husband and wife must discuss and agree on when to come together in coitus, what precautious behavior to adopt if the wife is fertile,[16] and whether or not a child is desired at that time. When they feel the Lord's prompting to have a child, they will have coitus during the wife's ovulation period. Often the wife conceives within the second or third month, and sometimes during the very first try.[17]

Ideally a woman should learn to recognize her fertility cycles before marriage. Perhaps some day this will be part of the premarital guidance in every church and a normal part of all marriage counseling. This brief chapter is only an introduction, and I would encourage the readers to pursue further information in order to use this God-given method in their own marriages.[18]

Keeping love alive

Couples who choose to modify their sexual activity during the wife's ovulatory period find that this periodic cycle of genital activity and restraint can help strengthen the marriage. It is a balance that is in harmony with the biblical teaching for moderation in all things.

> *To every thing there is a season,*
>   *And a time to every purpose under the heaven:*
> *A time to be born, and a time to die;*
>   *A time to plant, and a time to pluck up*
>   *that which is planted;...*
> *A time to weep, and a time to laugh;*
>   *A time to mourn and a time to dance.*
> *A time to embrace,*
>   *and a time to refrain from embracing.*[19]

Abstaining from coitus is a part of every marriage during times of illness, the days surrounding childbirth, separation by distance or other reasons. Most couples abstain during the menstrual period without considering this a problem. John and Sheila Kippley, in their most helpful book on natural family planning, suggest that times of abstinence can be used to foster a return to courtship, followed by a honeymoon.

> *When a husband and wife are in a period of refraining from coitus, they do not simply forget or ignore each other. Rather, it can be compared with the period of courtship that preceded the marriage and honeymoon. There are very significant differences between a chaste and loving premarital courtship and the regular "courtship" phase of natural family planning, for the married couple may morally engage in nongenital behavior that would be highly inappropriate for the unmarried. However, the comparison we would want to make still has validity....*
>
> *During the period before marriage the couple with a commitment to premarital purity looked for and found nongenital and nonpassionate ways of expressing their love and affection. The fact that they did not have intercourse provided no deterrent to their love; on the contrary, the other little niceties of courtship helped to develop their relationship. Tenderness and gentleness instead of passion, conversation rather than coitus, helped to broaden and deepen their friendship.*[20]

During brief periods of abstinence each couple will find their own creative ways of learning things about the other they never knew in this unfolding of an added dimension of the gift of marriage. Each can learn to listen to the other more with the heart, to become more aware of "body language," to observe what the other is saying without words. Physical closeness can be developed in new ways, cuddling at bedtime and talking, perhaps long into the night.

One of the greatest blessings that can come from this period of rest from sexual intercourse is the closeness that can deepen the prayer times together while fasting from sex. If the couple decides to abstain during the wife's ovulation periods they can make this a time of drawing closer to God and to each other in prayer. But fasting from sex should be for short periods only, for long abstentions are not Scriptural.

> *The husband should fulfill his conjugal obligations toward his wife, the wife hers toward her husband. A wife does not belong to herself but to her husband; equally, a husband does not belong to himself but to his wife.*
>
> *Do not deprive one another* (of sexual intercourse) *unless by mutual consent for a time, to devote youselves to prayer. Then resume marital relations. In this way you will be kept from giving in to Satan's temptations....*[21]

When a period of abstinence ends for any reason,[22] the "honeymoon" is all the more joyous. And now the couple is more in tune with each other, more open to receiving God's guidance together. When they believe it is God's will for them to try to conceive, He will bless them with conception. They can keep on walking in agreement together through the pregnancy, through childbearing, through the many changes, stresses and blessings of the long years that follow.

NOTES
1. Isa. 62:45. **2.** Amos 3:3. **3.** Mt. 18:19. **4.** Gen. 3:8a. **5.** Mal. 2:13-15.
6. Mt. 5:16. **7.** Ps. 144:12ff. **8.** Ps. 37:25, 26. **9.** Ps. 127:3-5.
10. Ex. 20:13: *You shall not kill.* Ex. 21:22-25NIV: *If men who are fighting hit a pregnant woman and she gives birth prematurely but there is no serious injury, the offender must be fined whatever the woman's*

husband demands and the court allows. But if there is serious injury, you are to take life for life, eye for eye, tooth for tooth, hand for hand, foot for foot, burn for burn, wound for wound, bruise for bruise. See also Num. 35:30-34.

11. One common medication used for the "morning after" pill is DES (diethylstilbestrol) DES was used in the 1940's and early 1950's to try to prevent miscarriages, but has now been linked to vaginal cancers in the daughters and genital malformation in the sons of women who were given the medication. It's also one of the medications sometimes given to dry up milk in the non-breastfeeding new mother. It's safety for any purpose is not proven. See "The People's Doctor," ed. Dr. Robert Mendelssohn, Vol. 2, No. 2 and Vol. 3, No. 10. For the Pill issue, see Vol. 4, No. 1. Available from 644 No. Michigan Ave., Suite 720, Chicago, Illinois, 60611.

According to a survey by the Alan Guttmacher Institute, about three out of every ten pregnancies ended in abortions during 1977 and 1978. Teenagers had one out of every three abortions, while 75% of the abortions were obtained by married women. These figures of medically induced abortions of course do not include the results of abortifacients.

12. Lev. 4:2-6, 20

14. A study by Dr. Arthur Sackler, research professor at New York Medical College reported that the effects of vasectomy on rats included enlarged cysts in the epididymis, reduction in size of the testes and a drop in certain hormone levels. A 1974 study at the University of Missouri School of Medicine reported that vasectomy in rats produced long-term biochemical effects, including a decrease in blood testosterone (male sex hormone) levels and a 50% increase in body fat. The rats also showed marked increases in blood lipids, one of the substances believed responsible for coronary artery disease. "The People's Doctor," **op. cit.** Vol. 3, No. 12.

15. In ancient times the Bible records a long period before some first children were born. Seth was 105 years old before Enos was born (Gen. 5:6). Enos was 90 before Cainan was born, Cainan 70 before Mahaleel was born (Gen. 5:18). Noah was 500 years old before his three sons were born (Gen. 5:32) and so on. Although the way in which "years" were calculated may have been different, it is possible that marriage often took place much later than the custom today, so that childbirth recorded in the earliest chapters of Genesis would not occur until couples were more mature. Abraham's son Isaac was 40 before he married Rebekah (Gen. 25:20). Long breast-feeding helped to space the children after the first child was born.

16. The Catholic church does not approve of any artificial method of birth control, including the condom or diaphragm. Thus the Catholic couple using natural family planning would be required to abstain during the wife's fertile period if a child is not desired. Protestant couples are free to make their own decision about whether or not to use a condom or diaphragm during the ovulatory period, but should understand that the **possibility** of conception exists because the woman is highly fertile, although it is not likely. Biblical teaching and Orthodox Jewish practice is for abstinence during the menstrual period and for about a week afterward. See Lev. 15:16-24. (The elementary instructions for cleanliness in this passage applies not only to the menstrual flow but also to the seminal fluid of the male.)

17. The ability to identify the ovulatory period accurately can be a help in some cases of apparent infertility.

18. The best method is for a couple to learn from other couples who have learned and are applying natural family planning. This help is especially necessary when learning the method after having been on the pill, after childbirth, during breastfeeding, or when approaching menopause, as the symptoms are more difficult to discern during these times. Sources are listed in the bibliography at the back of this book.

19. Eccl. 3:1-5.

20. John & Sheila Kippley. **The Art of Natural Family Planning.** 1975. Ref. ed., 1979. P. 62. The Couple to Couple League International, P.O. Box 11084, Cincinnati, Ohio 45211. Reprinted by permission.

21. 1 Cor. 7:3-5. NAB.

2

Life and Birth

The Gift of Life

Just as you know not how the breath of life fashions the human frame in the mother's womb, so you know not the work of God which he is accomplishing in the universe.[1]

Truly you have formed my inmost being; you knit me together in my mother's womb. I give you thanks that I am fearfully, wonderfully made; wonderful are your works.

My soul also you know full well; nor was my frame unknown to you when I was made in secret, when I was fashioned in the depths of the earth. Your eyes have seen my actions; in your book they are all written; my days were limited before one of them existed.

How weighty are your designs, O God! how vast are the sum of them! Were I to recount them, they would outnumber the sands.[2]

When we go back to the dawn of history we discover that at the birth of the first child, Cain, his mother Eve joyfully exclaimed, *I have gotten a man from the Lord!*[3] Eve remembered God's promise of a Seed who would crush the head of the serpent, and now she thought the promised Seed had been born! The pregnancy and birth to her were profoundly significant spiritual events, for she remembered God's words to the serpent:

*I will put **enmity** between you and the woman, and between your seed and her seed. He shall bruise your head, and you shall bruise his heel.*[4]

The serpent was cursed and the ground was cursed,[5] but there was no curse on Eve! A Rescuer, a Messiah, was promised instead, who would come through her. It would not be just a Jewish Messiah, for the promise was given long before a Jewish race came into existence. The promised Messiah would be for every one who, like Eve, would receive Him. *For as in Adam all die, so in Christ* (Eve's promised Seed) *shall all be made alive.*[6]

Weep, Eve! This child Cain is not yet the promised Deliverer, the Messiah, the Christ! And you, like Adam, have become subject to the consequences of sin in this earthly life: labor, toil and sorrow all your days until your bodies return to the dust of the earth.[7] *People (adam) are born to trouble, toil and sorrow as the sparks fly upward.*[8]

A sword of anguish will pierce your heart,[9] Eve, for the day will come when your godly younger son Abel will sprawl dying upon the earth. He will be the first person in history to return to the dust of death, a man slain by his own brother, *his blood crying to God from the ground.*[10] Your firstborn son Cain is not the promised Seed but a murderer, the first of many anti-Christs. For it is your second son, Abel, not Cain, who is the symbol of the coming Seed, Jesus Christ, who will pay the penalty of death for sin in order to open the way again to the Tree of Life. *The wages of sin is death.*[11]

Satan defeated

Eve was the symbol of the virgin through whom the promised Seed, Jesus, would one day come in the flesh and win the victory over Satan. For this reason Adam *called his wife's name Eve* (life), *because she was the mother of all living.*[12] This gives tremendous significance not only to the birth of the Savior Child, but to all who believe in Him. It indicates a warfare of cosmic proportions between the offspring of the believing woman and the hosts of Satan, a warfare which began in Eden and will be consummated at the end of the world.

> *There appeared a great wonder in heaven; a woman clothed with the sun, and the moon under her feet, and upon her head a crown of twelve stars: and she being with child groaned, laboring in birth, and strained to be delivered.*
>
> *And there appeared another wonder in heaven, and behold, a great red dragon having seven heads and ten horns, and seven crowns upon his heads, . . . and the dragon stood before the woman which was ready to give birth, in order to devour the child as soon as it was born.*

And she brought forth a man child, who was to rule the nations with a rod of iron. But her child was caught up to God, and to his throne. And the woman fled into the wilderness, where she has a place prepared by God....

And there was war in heaven: Michael and his angels fought against the dragon; and the dragon fought and his angels (demons—fallen angels), *and prevailed not. Neither was their place any more found in heaven. And the great dragon was cast out, that old serpent, called the Devil and Satan, which deceives the whole world. He was cast out into the earth, and his angels were cast out with him.*

And I heard a loud voice saying in heaven, "Now is come salvation, and strength, and the kingdom of our God, and the power of his Christ: for the accuser of our brethren is cast down,... and they overcame him by the blood of the Lamb, and by the word of their testimony. Love for life did not keep them from martyrdom.

And the dragon was furious with the woman, and went to make war with the rest of her offspring, who have the commandments of God and give witness to Jesus.[13]

And I saw an angel come down from heaven,... and he laid hold on the dragon, that old serpent, which is the Devil and Satan,... and the devil was cast into the lake of fire and brimstone... and shall be tormented for ever and ever.[14]

New life in Jesus

The thief does not come except to steal, and to kill and to destroy. I (Jesus) *have come that you might have life, abundant life!*[15] The Seed of the woman, Jesus Christ, born of the virgin Mary, won the cosmic conflict once for all on the cross when He gave up His life for the world. He came to life again and was *caught up to God, to rule the nations with a rod of iron,... that at the name of Jesus every knee should bow, of things in heaven, and things in earth, and things under the earth.*[16]

Every person born into the world needs to come for shelter under the safety of the salvation offered by Jesus Christ and be equipped by Him to share in the "mopping up" of the enemy's forces. *Jesus said to them, I saw Satan as lightning fall from heaven. Look, I give you power to tread on serpents and scorpions, and over **all** the power of the enemy, and nothing shall by any means hurt you.*[17]

Sin, sickness, pain and death come from the thief, Satan. When he brought sickness to the children of Israel in the wilderness, God told Moses to make a serpent out of brass, put it on a pole and place it where all could see it. Every person who looked up at the powerless brass serpent would be healed of his or her sickness.[18]

"What a silly thing," some people thought and refused to look. "How can looking at a piece of wood and brass make anybody well?" They died. But some, in an act of faith, obeyed and looked at the symbol of the dead serpent. They were healed.

For as Moses lifted up the serpent in the wilderness, even so must the Son of man be lifted up, that whoever believes in him should not perish but have eternal life.[19]

When we look at the Seed of the woman hanging on the Cross, what do we see? We see the serpent destroyed, as powerless as the brass serpent on the pole! For Jesus Christ took all our sins and all the serpent's sting upon Himself.[20] He "became" all the ugly things which had to be put to death. Satan thought he had won when Jesus died, but he had lost! The greatest part of the suffering of Jesus was not the dying of the body but the spiritual death, the withdrawal of the Spirit of God because of our wickedness which covered Him. In the blackness of that terrible separation from God, Jesus cried out in agony, *My God! My God! Why have you forsaken me!*[21]

Jesus took away the curse, all of it, for those who accept Him as the promised Seed. He opens paths of blessings for us as promised in Scripture, setting us free from the curse of sin, sickness, pain, death. *Christ has redeemed us from the curse of the law, becoming the curse for us.*[22]

Surely he has borne our sicknesses and carried our pains, yet we considered him smitten by God, and afflicted. But he was bruised for our iniquities; upon him was the chastisement that made us whole, and with his bruises we are healed.[23]

When evening fell, they brought to him many who were possessed by devils; and he drove the spirits out with a word and healed all who were sick, to fulfill the prophecy of Isaiah: "He took away our illnesses and lifted our diseases from us."[24]

The blood sacrifice of Jesus has opened the way for us to live joyfully in this world of trouble, free from anxiety,[25] heaven in our hearts as well as our future hope. Jesus explained to His disciples, *Unless you become like little children you cannot enter the kingdom of God.*[26] He points the way back to the simplicity, lack of worry and absolute trust of a little child in the goodness of his father. In John 3 He carries the analogy back still further, to the unborn child in the womb. He explained to the Jewish ruler Nicodemus:

> *"A man cannot even see the kingdom of God without being born again."*
> *"And how can a man who's getting old possibly be born?" replied Nicodemus. "How can he go back into his mother's womb and be born a second time?"*
> *"I assure you," said Jesus, "that unless a man is born from water and from spirit he cannot enter the kingdom of God. Flesh gives birth to flesh and spirit gives birth to spirit: you must not be surprised that I told you that all of you must be born again. The wind blows where it likes, you can hear the sound of it but you have no idea where it comes from and where it goes. Nor can you tell how a man is born by the wind of the Spirit."*
> *"How on earth can things like this happen?" replied Nicodemus.*[27]

It is not enough to believe that Jesus is the Christ, the Son of the living God. *Even the devils believe, and tremble.*[28] A person must **receive** Jesus, invite Him into his or her life, in order to be born again. *As many as **received** him, to them he gave power to become the sons of God, ... who were born not of blood, nor of the will of the flesh, nor of the will of man, but of God.*[29]

A living spirit

In order to be reborn by the Spirit of God, it is first necessary to be born in the flesh, for the promise of salvation and of reigning with God forever is not made to angels, but to human beings.[30] Even as I write these words my heart is rejoicing, singing a hymn of praise to God in thanksgiving. For I have just learned that our third daughter is pregnant with her first baby. What an awesome thing **life** is! Something exists which did not exist before—a person! Though still only a tiny spark of life, all the potential of what that little person will become is there, not only for this life but also for the life to come.

My daughter and her husband used natural family planning and conceived the child on the first try (during the ovulation period). Their baby is wanted, blessed in its conception by their faith in God, *a godly seed.*[31] This child already has a complete identity before God, though we earthlings have yet to discover who he or she is.

The gift of life is a mystery which we only dimly perceive, *as through a dark glass,*[32] although the Holy Spirit reveals little hints to us of what shall be.

For example, one time another of our daughters called, not knowing if she were pregnant or not, although she and her husband had been trying to conceive during her ovulation period. She was very concerned because of a severe pain in one side and feared the pain might indicate an ectopic pregnancy (the conceived fetus growing in the Fallopian tube without proceeding on down into the womb).

After she called, I sat quietly for awhile before the Lord Jesus praying. Then I asked the Lord to reveal to me more clearly how I ought to pray and turned to my Bible. It fell open to Proverb 31 with verse 2 before my eyes: *What? my son? and what? the son of my womb? and what? the son of my vows?* I praised the Lord, all heaviness lifted, for I perceived three things in my spirit. First, our daughter was indeed pregnant. Second, it would not be a tubal pregnancy, but in the womb. And third, the conceived child would be a son. (It was.)

I cannot explain how the Holy Spirit reveals things to us, but I have known the sex of almost all our grandchildren early in the prenatal period (though I don't tell the parents). It didn't matter to me if each one was a boy or a girl, nor did I ask to know. This experience of a little word of knowledge from the Holy Spirit is not uncommon with Christians who are walking closely with the Lord Jesus, open to His inner voice.

The child conceived is a living spirit, and there are spiritual bonds which link us together through the Lord Jesus Christ. One time our oldest daughter was threatened with a miscarriage during her second pregnancy. I asked Jesus about it, and this time the word came that God would take this little one Home:

> *Then was fulfilled that which was spoken by Jeremy the prophet saying, In Ramah was there a voice heard, lamentation, and weeping, and great mourning; Rachel weeping for her children, and would not be comforted, because they are not.*[33]

Of course I did not tell my daughter! I encouraged her to do everything possible to save the baby, hoping I had misunderstood the Lord. But He confirmed the loss to me again concerning her:

*The children you shall have **after you have lost the other** shall say in your ears, "This house is too small for us. We need more room to live in." Then you will say in your heart, "Who has begotten these, since I have lost my children, and am desolate?*[34]

She lost the child during the eleventh week of pregnancy. Later she told me, "Mother, I knew when the baby died even before the miscarriage. During that difficult time I came to the point of crisis where I said inwardly to my baby, 'If Jesus is calling you, you are free to go.' At that time I experienced a sense of release and knew his spirit was gone, even though the medical pregnancy tests were still positive."

My daughter also knew in her spirit that this lost child was a boy and called him Jeremy. God did not leave her desolate but gave her an unexpected promise: *This time next year you will bear a son.*[35] Exactly twelve months later Jeremy's healthy brother was born.

To have conceived a child and lost it during pregnancy is not the same as though that one had never existed, for it has an eternal spirit, even though its body did not live until birth. Job in his suffering cried out,

*Why then have you brought me forth out of the womb? Oh that I had **given up the ghost** (spirit), and no eye had seen me. . . . I should have gone from the womb to the grave.*[36]

These same words were spoken of Jesus when He died on the cross. *Jesus said, "It is finished!" and he bowed his head and **gave up the ghost** (spirit).*[37]

Elijah prayed, after a little boy had died, *O Lord my God, let this child's soul come into him again.*[38] God answered his prayer. The child's soul came back into his body and the child returned to life.

At death, whether before or after birth, *the spirit returns to God who gave it.*[39] This fact is a great comfort when miscarriage occurs, and should cause grave concern to those who condone deliberate abortion.

The "life-line"

As Christians we need to be more deeply aware of the spiritual reality of the unborn child and its importance in the ongoing plan of God. The aged Jacob in Genesis 49 *called his sons and said, "Gather yourselves together so that I may tell you what will befall you in the last days."*[40] The spirit of prophecy came upon him, and he told what would happen through the offspring of his twelve sons for centuries to come, including a prophecy of the coming Messiah. He even foretold through which of the twelve the Messiah would come.[41]

This "life line" of spiritual descent is pictured in Hebrews 7. *Levi also, who received tithes, paid tithes in Abraham. For he was yet in the loins of his father, when Melchisadec met him.*[42] (Abraham gave one tenth of his spoil from war to the priest Melchisadec.) Abraham was not Levi's father. He was his great-great-grandfather! And the "Levi" mentioned here was not just the great-great-grandson himself, but the entire tribe of Levites who were descended from him, who ministered in the tabernacle and the temple and whose names can still be seen in every phone book. God had a plan for the future of the world hidden in the human bodies of two old people, Abraham and Sarah.

God knows each person long before he or she is ever conceived, but this does not mean we had a "pre-existence." It means that we were first created in the mind of God. He sees the unborn child being *knit together in his mother's womb,*[43] and He sees ahead down the long years of that life to its end and beyond. Thus when Rebekah conceived after Isaac pleaded with the Lord to heal her infertility, she knew to Whom to go with her questions. When her hugely expanding abdomen heaved about like the inside of a butter churn she asked the Lord, *Why am I like this?*[44] The Lord explained to this pregnant young woman that she was carrying twins, and told her that each twin would become the founder of a great nation. *Two nations are in your womb, two peoples are quarreling while still within you. But one shall surpass the other, and the older shall serve the younger.* When the twins were born Esau came out first, followed by Jacob, who became Israel, after whom the Jewish nation is named.[45]

Not only does God know all about the child in the womb, but the unborn child is also responsive to spiritual realities. The Bible says of John the Baptist that he would be *filled with the Holy Spirit even while still in his mother's womb.*[46] When Mary became pregnant with Jesus—even though she had never had sexual relations with a man—the angel told her to go visit her cousin Elizabeth for encouragement. By this time elderly Elizabeth was six months pregnant with John. Mary obeyed the angel, hurried across the hill country to a city in Judah, entered the house and greeted Elizabeth. At once Elizabeth joyfully cried out,

Blessed are you among women! Blessed is the fruit of your womb! And how could it possibly be that the mother of my Lord should come to me?
For as soon as I heard the voice of your greeting, the baby in my womb leaped for joy![47]

We can understand how the Holy Spirit could inspire Elizabeth with words of prophecy, but how could an unborn child sense anything? He could neither see, nor understand language, nor know anything at all. Yet the child in the womb sensed the presence of the unborn Messiah and reacted with excitement. The truth was *spiritually discerned,*[48] that is, perceived in the spirit of the child though not in his conscious mind, which could not yet form rational thoughts.

The apostle Paul says to Timothy, his dearly loved helper,

I thank God and remember you in my prayers night and day. I remember the pure faith that is in you, which dwelt first in your grandmother Lois, and your mother Eunice, and I am persuaded in you also.[49]

Paul does not say Timothy's mother and grandmother **taught** him faith (although they surely did), but that this faith was **in** them. A bit later he adds that *from the time you were a child* **(brephos)** *you have known the Holy Scriptures, which are able to lead you to salvation through faith in Jesus Christ.*[50] The Greek word **brephos** means "newly born" or even "unborn babe." Timothy learned faith not only with his head when he was old enough to understand, but his spirit was receptive to God even before his birth because of the faith of his godly mother and grandmother.

This gives new meaning to the continuity of faith from one generation to the next. Although a child must make his own personal decision to accept Christ as his Savior when he or she is old enough to understand, the child's spirit is being made receptive even before birth when he has believing parents and grandparents.

> *As for me, this is my covenant with them, says the Lord: my Spirit that is upon you, and my words which I have put in your mouth shall not depart out of your mouth, nor out of the mouth of your seed, nor out of the mouth of your seed's seed, says the Lord, from this time and for ever.*[51]

> *Understand then, that the Lord your God is God indeed, the faithful God who keeps his merciful covenant down to the thousandth generation toward those who love him.*[52]

The father/priest

As soon as a child is conceived the husband takes on a new role, that of a father/priest. He now becomes responsible before God to intercede not only for his wife but also for the spiritual and physical well-being of his child. He can place his hand on his wife's abdomen as the baby grows and pray the peace of Jesus over that little spirit, saying, "We bless you in the name of Jesus! We are so glad God has sent you to us. We look forward to the day when we can see you, but we love you already." In this way the father/priest is already laying hands of blessing on his unborn child.

This sensitive concern of a father for his child, even before birth, is a sign of revival, of spiritual renewal:

> *Unto you who fear my name shall the Sun of righteousness arise with healing in his wings.... He shall turn the heart of the fathers to the children, and the heart of the children to their fathers, lest I come and smite the earth with a curse.*[53]

It is awesome to realize that the spiritual condition of a **father** is of utmost importance to the unborn child! While it might seem that the spiritual condition of the mother is of primary significance—because she is the one carrying the baby—in the Bible the "special" children all had God-fearing fathers as well as mothers: Isaac, Samuel, Samson, John the Baptist, even Jesus. For although Joseph was not Jesus' real father, God placed Joseph in the priestly role of protector/provider for Mary and Jesus. God spoke to him in visions and dreams both before and after the child's birth, instructing him how to care for them.[54] God did not have a virgin conceive a child without providing a man to give both physical and spiritual protection to mother and child.

It is because the unborn child is subject to spiritual realities that he or she is vulnerable to evil spirits as well as to God's Spirit.

> *You shall have no other gods besides me. You shall not make any graven image, nor any likeness of anything that is in heaven above, or that is in the earth beneath, or that is in the waters beneath the earth.*
>
> *You shall not bow down to them nor worship them, for I the Lord your God am a jealous God, visiting the iniquity of the fathers upon the children until the third and fourth generation of those who hate Me.*[55]

It doesn't seem fair that children should suffer for the sins of their fathers, does it? But notice that this enslavement of the offspring is linked to the denial of God. The spiritual sin of the father brings the succeeding generations into demonic bondage.

Part of the "visitation of iniquity" is the result of the example of sin set by the parents, which may take generations to break. But children not only learn to be evil from the example of their parents. Often they even seem **predisposed** to wrong doing. How can this be? We know that God's angelic spirits are not bound by time. The fallen angelic spirits also continue working generation after generation. When these wicked spirits capture a man through his disobedience and unbelief, they are still present to infect his offspring for generations after he is gone.

But how good the Lord is! He promises to bless those who love Him for a **thousand** generations! If each generation continues to love Him, that promise to their offspring continues while the world lasts! But those who deny Him bring their offspring under spiritual bondage only for three or four generations, so there is hope for the offspring of the unbeliever. The bondage can be broken! Praise God! Any person who receives Jesus as personal Savior breaks the chain of God's judgment and turns it to blessing for the generations that follow.

Freedom from bondage

No evil spirit can possess a child of God, but it can harrass, tempt and afflict him. When we disobey God, we open a door to the harassment of these spirits. And our unborn child is affected by our negative, sinful thoughts toward them in ways we do not understand.

On a number of occasions I have prayed with people for the

healing of painful memories, but sometimes we could not find the root of the problem, for there was no conscious recall of any cause for the hurt. At a women's conference one time I met a most attractive young woman, the only daughter and youngest of five children, the darling of her older brothers and her parents. She was married to a loving Christian husband, had three beautiful children and was active in an evangelical church.

I was in my room at the close of the day when she knocked on my door, weeping. "I just have to talk to you," she sobbed. "Something is wrong, but I don't know what it is!" Together we went down to a prayer room, while inwardly I pleaded with the Lord to reveal the source of the trouble. As we talked together she said that she had never liked herself and always felt that no one else liked her either. Yet she had been the "darling" of the family!

The Lord put a thought into my mind. "Is it possible," I suggested, "that when your parents discovered your mother was pregnant again, their **first** thought was, 'Oh no! not **another** baby! We thought we had had our last child!"

The words were barely out of my mouth before she began to cry as if her heart would break. It was like touching a raw nerve! A spirit of rejection had attached itself to that tiny fetus and afflicted her for her whole life, even though the parents had quickly adjusted to the reality of another pregnancy. That night Jesus set her free.

Another time I prayed with a seventy year old woman who had been afflicted with the same problem of rejection her whole life, though she had always been an active Christian and had ministered to many people. The spirit of rejection left her. It had apparently been present ever since her parents had reacted against the discovery of the mother's pregnancy. It is astonishing to see the transformation in people when Jesus cuts that link of bondage to the past generation and heals the inner person. I cannot explain how God does it. I do not understand it, though I have seen it happen. I can only exclaim, "Lord, how can these things be!"[56]

If anyone reading these words is concerned for their children or for their unborn child because they were unhappy over the fact of the pregnancy, the remedy is simple. Say to Jesus, "I repent of my wrong attitude toward this child whom You have given to me. I ask in Your name that you remove from him or her any sense of rejection because of my sin. Thank You, Lord, for doing so. Amen."

A prayer-hearing God

A husband and wife who have been born into new life by the Spirit of God are heirs to a wealth of promises in the Bible which they can claim by faith. If they have difficulty conceiving a child they can pray for healing from infertility, and trust God to answer as He did for Rebecca,[57] Rachel [58] and Hannah.[59]

During pregnancy they can pray for the health and safety of the little one in the womb, claiming God's promise: *None shall cast her young* (miscarry) *or be barren in your land. I will fulfill the number of your days.*[60] The couple can pray also for the wife's safety throughout the pregnancy and birth, claiming God's promise: *She will come safely through childbirth if they* (husband and wife) *continue in faith and love and holiness with wisdom.*[61]

And they can pray for the future of the unborn child and all the generations to follow as did the Psalmist:

> *This shall be written for the generation to come, and the people who shall be created shall praise the Lord. The children of your servants shall continue, and their seed shall be established before you....*
>
> *Just as a father's tender concern for his children, so the Lord shows tender concern for those who fear him. For he knows our frame. He remembers that we are dust....*
>
> *The mercy of the Lord is from everlasting to everlasting upon them that fear him, and his righteousness unto children's children.*[62]

NOTES
1. Eccl. 11:5 NAB. 2. Ps. 139:13-18 NAB. 3. Gen. 4:1. According to the Hebrew text Eve says, *I have gotten a man—Jehovah!* The word "Jehovah" has the sign of the direct object! The words "from the" or "of the" Lord are insertions of the translators. Eve named the child Cain, which means "gotten." Her unusual exclamation shows that she believed God was fulfilling His promise of an offspring who would defeat the serpent. Eve is the first person in history to speak God's name, "Jehovah."
4. Gen. 3:15. 5. Gen. 3:14, 17. 6. 1 Cor. 15:22.

7. Gen. 3:16-19. The word translated "sorrow" in the KJV for the woman in v. 16 and for the man in v. 17 is from the **same** Hebrew word, *etzev*. In more recent translations, *etzev* is translated as "pain" when it refers to the woman and "toil" when it refers to the man. This violates the accuracy of the Hebrew text.

The Hebrew word *etzev* refers to labor, toil, with emotional overtones. The same word is used of Noah in Gen. 5:19, where it is correctly translated: *This same* (Noah) *shall comfort us concerning our work and toil* **(etzev)** *of our hands.*

Other Hebrew and Greek words related to childbirth are extensively discussed in my book on natural childbirth, **op. cit.**

8. Job. 5:7. Heb.: ***amal***, which means trouble, toil, sorrow.

9. Lk. 2:35. **10.** Gen. 4:2-11; Heb. 11:4. **11.** Rom. 6:23. **12.** Gen. 3:20. **13.** Rev. 12. This passage is the grand finale of the battle begun at the beginning of the Bible between the woman and her "seed." In v. 5 this "seed" is the Christ-child. In v. 17, "the **rest** of her seed" is defined as those who give witness to Jesus.

The "woman" here is a multiple symbol, Eve, Sarah, Mary, Israel, the church and can be interpreted in various ways eschatologically.

14. Rev. 20. **15.** Jn. 10:10. **16.** Phil. 2:10. **17.** Lk. 10:13, 19. **18.** Num. 21:6-9. **19.** Jn. 3:14, 15. **20.** 2 Cor. 5:21. **21.** Mk. 15:34. **22.** Gal. 3:13. **23.** Isa 53:3-5, RSV margin. **24.** Mt. 8:16, 17 NEB. **25.** Phil. 4:6, 7. **26.** Mt. 18:2-6. **27.** Jn. 3:1-9 Phillips. **28.** Jas. 2:19. **29.** Jn. 1:12, 13. **30.** Heb. 1:14, 2:7-17. **31.** Mal. 2:15. **32.** 1 Cor. 13:12. **33.** Mt. 2:17, 18. **34.** Isa. 49:20, 21. **35.** Gen. 17:21. **36.** Job 10:18, 19. **37.** Jn. 19:30. **38.** 1 Kgs. 17:21, 22. **39.** Eccl. 12:7. **40.** Gen. 29:1ff. **41.** Gen. 49:10. **42.** Heb. 7:1-10. **43.** Ps. 139:12-16. **44.** Gen. 25:21-24. **45.** Gen. 32:28-30. **46.** Lk. 1:15. **47.** Lk. 1:41. **48.** 1 Cor. 2:14. **49.** 2 Tim. 1:2-5. **50.** 2 Tim. 3:15. **51.** Isa. 59:21. **52.** Deut. 7:9-13 NAB. **53.** Mal. 4:2, 6. **54.** Mt. 1:20-24; 2:13-15, 19-21. **55.** Deut. 5:7-9.

56. Recent research by a Christian psychiatrist in England, Dr. Frank Lake, confirms the receptivity of the fetus in the womb:

"We are finding with increasing clarity, evidence that the embryo, which becomes a foetus and then a baby in the womb, is susceptible to all the emotions that are circulating around the mother's body, including her womb and whatever it contains. It thrives on the good feelings and recoils from the bad. Even in the first three months after conception, the foetus experiences either a sense of pervasive pleasure, an infiltration of fine feelings, or a transfusion of terror. If the mother is grieving, the suffusion of sorrow reaches her womb too. No part of the foetal organism is closed to penetration by the distillate of a mother's own despair."

Quoted from "Report from the Research Department," 1979. Dr. Frank Lake, Director, CTA. See also his booklet, **Studies in Constrictive Confusion,** and his book, **Clinical Theology.** London. Dartman, Longman & Todd, LTD. 1966.

57. Gen. 25:21. **58.** Gen. 30:22-24. **59.** 1 Sam. 1:5, 10, 20. **60.** Ex. 23:26.

61. 1 Tim. 2:15. When verses 11 to 15 are correctly translated as a unit, the meaning of "she" and "they" in v. 15 is obvious. *Let the wife (gune) learn.... But I don't permit a wife (gune) to seize authority over her husband (aner).... And she* (the wife) *will come safely through childbirth if they* (husband and wife) *continue in faith and love and holiness with humble wisdom.*

The phrase about "salvation" in childbirth has a double application. It refers both to Eve and her promised Seed, and to the childbearing wife, a promise Christian couples can claim by faith. For a discussion of the rest of this passage, see Note 67 in the chapter "Who Am I?"

62. Ps. 102:18-28; 103:13-17.

Garden of The Lord

Listen, all you who are thirsty, come to the waters!
And you who have no money, come, buy and eat.
Yes, come! Buy wine and milk without money and
  without price.

Why do you spend money for that which is not bread?
  and your labor for that which does not satisfy?
Listen carefully to Me, and eat that which is good,
  and let your soul delight itself in abundance....

For as the rain and the snow come down from heaven
  and do not return without watering the earth,
making it bud and flourish so that it yields
  seed to the sower and bread to the eater,
so is My word that goes from My mouth.
  It shall not return to me empty
but will accomplish that which I please,
  and prosper in that for which I sent it.[1]

God had an idea. "I will make a Garden," He thought, "and put in it everything necessary to sustain life. I will cause trees to grow, their foliage heavy with fruits and nuts. I will plant flowers and herbs, fragrant and beautiful to see. I will carpet the soil with lush vegetation for food which will continually reproduce itself for thousands upon thousands of years. I will put rivers of water in My Garden to keep it flourishing and will fill all the empty spaces with atmosphere. Then I will put people in My Garden. They will have food to eat, water to drink, air to breathe, and lovely things to touch, smell, taste, see and hear. I will come down and walk and talk with them in My Garden." Then through the vastness of outer space tiny Earth spun into its place, a sparkling emerald and sapphire sphere.

Bread and water
God is aware of our need for balanced nutrition, for He has created the earth and the seas to provide everything necessary for our good health. A tremendous variety of flora and fauna all over the earth provide all of the essential nutrients the body needs. Only a few areas, such as the north and south poles and the deserts, lack this great variety of foods.

If today's people are not well fed and are subject to famine and malnutrition it is because we have failed to accept our God-given responsibility to nurture the earth.[2] Deserts expand as the soil is depleted and eroded so that it will no longer sustain crops. Concrete cities send bony, lifeless arms across fertile farmland. Land and water become increasingly polluted by careless use until even the rain brings toxic fallout. Yet even with all this abuse, God has built into the earth ways for it to cleanse and restore itself. When we discover and apply these natural laws, once again *the desert shall rejoice, and blossom as the rose.*[3]

The Bible says that from the time of creation, each species has carried the "seed" of its own kind within itself. This is true of men and women also, so that even future generations are affected by the way in which we nurture our bodies. Thus it is important that both husband and wife learn the laws of nutrition, God's natural law, for both should be in optimum health at the time a child is conceived. Building toward optimum health should have begun in infancy, with special attention during the teen years when the body is under tremendous stress due to its rapid maturation. Since it is not possible to go back, let husband and wife at least learn at the time of marriage how best to eat for good health.

Many families experience undue emotional stress because there are not enough minerals in their diet to maintain energy and keep nerves calm. Urea levels rise, poisoning the body and causing tempers to mount. Blood sugars drop, causing numerous problems. In order to make certain that everyone receives enough vitamins and minerals from the food we eat, a medical doctor has suggested the following basic diet:

> *The diet should contain as much as possible of the following foods: whole grains and whole grain bread, fresh or*

dried fruits, wheat germ, sprouted seeds, legumes (such as lentils, peas and beans), nuts, cheese, eggs, milk, brewer's yeast, skimmed milk powder, sea food, poultry, organ meats and lean meats. In addition, safflower oil should be taken at the level of at least 1 tablespoon daily. The oil can be mixed with wheat germ and used as the morning cereal with milk and fruit.[4]

Both husband and wife should be free of any medication at the time they conceive a child. And during the first three months of pregnancy the expectant mother should not take **any** drugs, not sleeping pills, not "cold" tablets, not weight-reduction pills, not nausea pills, not even aspirin.[5] Birth defects may be caused by a number of substances, especially during the first six weeks of life in the womb when a woman may not yet know she is pregnant. So it is wise for all of us to learn to live without these "crutches" that do not build health.

After a child is conceived the expectant mother must begin to eat for two, not in quantity but in quality, for a healthy pregnancy and a normal, healthy baby. Inadequate nutrition can lead to low birth weight babies with numerous problems, even cerebral palsy. The pregnant woman ought to gain between 25 and 30 pounds from nutritious food which does not include items full of additives and "empty" calories, such as refined flours and sugars. Each day the expectant mother should have the following.[6]

One quart of milk (nonfat or 2% fat if
  she is overweight)
Two eggs
A serving of lean meat, fish or chicken
Nuts and legumes
Fruits and vegetables (as many fresh as possible)
Whole grain breads and cereals

The milk and eggs can be used in cooking. Since eggs grow baby chicks, they contain many of the nutrients a growing embryo needs. If a couple is on a low income and cannot afford much meat, fish or chicken, then the wife should have what there is.[7] The husband can go without them more readily than the growing baby.

Plenty of water is also needed. The fluid (blood and plasma) in the pregnant woman's body increases about 30 per cent during the pregnancy. An ample intake of water also helps flush the wastes from the kidneys of two people, mother and baby.

If nausea is a problem in early pregnancy, the expectant mother should eat a little something every couple of hours such as a piece of cheese, a bit of fruit, a cracker.[8] Since the baby is drawing nutrients continually from the mother's body, small, frequent meals are easier to digest.

Insufficient B vitamins contribute to nausea. A lack of potassium (found in fruits and vegetables) or magnesium (milk is the best supply) can cause feelings of weakness or frequent leg cramps. A craving for starchy foods may be a sign of other mineral deficiencies. If the couple has already developed good nutritional habits, and the expectant mother follows the guidelines above, these problems are less likely to develop. There is ample literature today explaining how to correct these minor problems through the right foods.[9]

The Old Testament provides some helpful insights into good nutrition. I made a study one time of the "clean" and "unclean" animals, birds and sea foods listed. I discovered that one basic distinction[10] was that "clean" ones feed on vegetation only, while the "unclean" are scavengers and are thus potential disease carriers. These "unclean" creatures perform a valuable service, keeping our world free of decay, cleansing the surface of the land and the sea bottoms of refuse. God laid down simple rules for the Israelite people for their own protection, even though they kept the rules only as a religious exercise. If our 20th century wisdom had known such things, the hepatitis outbreaks on the east coast, caused by eating contaminated shell fish,[11] might have been avoided. Seventh Day Adventists (who follow the Old Testament food laws) and Jews who follow these dietary food laws live longer and are less prone to certain diseases (heart attacks, cancer, high blood pressure, etc.) than other segments of the American population.

Although we might observe some of these Old Testament guidelines for good health, the New Testament reminds us not to make food a **religious** issue, for God does not.

> *As for the man who is weak in faith, welcome him, but not for arguments over opinions. One believes he may eat anything, while the weak person is vegetarian. Let not him who eats anything despise the vegetarian, and let not him who abstains from meat pass judgment on the one who eats meat, for God has welcomed him. Who are you to judge each other?*[12]

It is up to each of us to do the best we know in eating only nutritious, wholesome food. We have less control, however, over the additives in our food and the polluting substances that seep into our water supplies. But even in this instance, Christians have an added resource, for we can "say grace." God says:

I will bless your bread and your water; and I will take sickness away from the midst of you. None shall miscarry her young or be barren in your land. I will fulfill the number of your days.[13]

It is amazing that God revealed through His prophets thousands of years ago that there is a relationship between "bread and water" and infertility, miscarriage and birth defects!

What kinds of food can we ask God to bless? **All** kinds! One time the apostle Peter had a vision of a sheet being lowered from heaven full of all kinds of animals. By Old Testament law some were "clean" and some were "unclean."[14] Peter heard a voice which said, *Rise, Peter, kill and eat!* Peter protested vigorously, *Not so, Lord, for I have never eaten anything common or unclean.* The same vision appeared three times, and each time Peter protested. But then the voice said to him *What God **has cleansed**, don't call unclean!*

We need to learn to pray with far more sincerity, "Lord, please bless this food and water for our use, and purify it from anything that might make us sick." I take this prayer very seriously when I am traveling in parts of the world where sanitation is not always the best and travelers often get sick. Jesus said to His disciples before sending them out to minister to people, *I am sending you out as lambs among wolves.... And whatever city you enter and they receive you, eat whatever they set before you.*[15]

I do this, but I also remind the Lord of His promise that He will purify those things I must eat and drink over which I have no choice. *These signs shall follow those who believe,... and if they drink any deadly thing, it shall not hurt them.*[16]

God knows we all need food to live. Jesus taught us to pray, *Father,... give us today the bread we need,*[17] that is, the food sufficient for the needs of our bodies. Centuries earlier, when the children of Israel lived in the Sinai desert where crops could not be grown, the Lord said to them, *I will send you bread from heaven.*[18] The next morning when the people saw the ground covered with white stuff they asked, ***me na?*** which means in

Hebrew, "What's this?" It was a complete nutritional food which could be used as flour for baking, frying, boiling. This perfectly balanced food kept them so strong and vigorous the forty years in the wilderness that the Psalmist later said, *There was not one weak person among all their tribes.*[19]

We are to learn and follow the laws of good nutrition. We can ask God to purify what we eat and use it to keep us healthy. And we need never worry about having enough to eat if we are living in God's will:

> *Look at the birds of the air. They do not plant, nor reap, nor gather into barns, and your heavenly Father takes care of them. Are you not worth much more than they are?...*
>
> *Therefore do not worry, saying, "What shall we eat?" or "What shall we drink?" or "Where can we find something to wear?"... for your heavenly Father knows you need all these things.*
>
> *Seek first the kingdom of God, and all these things will be yours as well.*[20]

But food for the body is not enough. The Bible says, *Man shall not live by bread alone, but by every word that comes from the mouth of God.*[21] The best preparation for parenthood is for a young husband and wife to feed their own souls, *tasting the good word of God.*[22] Let them read the Bible daily, alone and together, meditate on it, memorize it, obey it. May their child not be born into a family where famine rules, *not a famine of bread, nor a thirst for water, but of hearing the words of the Lord.*[23]

Let them feed not only on the Bible, but on Jesus Christ Himself, and *taste the heavenly gift, receiving the Holy Spirit.*[24] Jesus says:

> *I am the living bread which came down from heaven. If any one eat this bread, he will live for ever.*[25]
>
> *Whoever drinks of the water that I shall give him shall never thirst, for the water that I shall give him shall be in him a well of water springing up into everlasting life.... And this he said of the Holy Spirit, which those who believe on him would receive.*[26]

The breath of life

Our little planet earth may be only an insignificant dot in the vast expanse of the heavens, but it contains a precious gift from God that has not yet been found on any other planet. This gift is an atmosphere which sustains life. The air we breathe into our lungs contains exactly the right amount of oxygen. This is carried to every cell of our bodies by the blood stream, which then takes up the waste products from the cells. The blood carries these wastes back to the lungs and it is expelled in the form of carbon dioxide when we exhale.

When God created the earth, He planted a garden. *And out of the ground the Lord caused every tree to grow that is pleasant to the sight and good for food.*[27] But not only are trees pleasing to look at and a source of food. They also draw in carbon dioxide from the atmosphere, and give off oxygen. People were created to live among plant life where the air is freshened by these growing things. It was man's idea to live in concrete cities where pollution hangs heavy in the air.

Oxygen is one of the most important "foods" the child in the womb needs. Without sufficient oxygen he will fail to grow properly and may be deformed or have mental problems. Each of us, but especially the pregnant wife—who is breathing for two—needs a "garden" where the air is fresh. She might find it in a walk down a street where trees are growing or in a little park. Those who live in crowded cities should try to keep growing things in their apartments or homes. And people might be less likely to fall asleep in church if there were more plants growing in the sanctuary. After all, the first "church" was a garden, where husband and wife walked and talked with God.

Fortunately, breathing is automatic and goes on continuously even while we sleep, so that we don't "forget" to breathe. However, people can be taught to make more effective use of breathing for good health.

Cleansing breaths. We seldom use more than a third or half of our total lung capacity. We should learn to take cleansing breaths each day in order to empty the lungs of stale air completely and provide a maximum of oxygen for our bodies' needs. The best time to take these cleansing breaths is when first waking up in the morning. Husband and wife can remind each other to do it.

Inhale slowly, drawing in the air until the lower chest expands, continuing until one can feel the lungs filling up under the armpits and collarbones. When the lungs seem completely full, inhale a little more! Then slowly, slowly exhale, allowing the upper chest to drop and the lower chest to collapse until the lungs seem completely empty. Then, give a little "puff" and blow out even more air.

Begin to inhale again in the same way, slowly, completely, and then exhale slowly, blowing out at the end. Repeat this at least five successive times. This is the best "waking up" exercise there is! I am a sleepy-head in the morning, but when I remember to take these cleansing breaths I begin to perk up by the time I get to the third one. Sometimes by the fifth breath I find that I am already sitting on the side of the bed! Oxygen has reached every part of my body, especially the brain, and cleared away the fog of sleep.

During the day when feeling drowsy, try taking five cleansing breaths rather than a nap, near growing plants if possible. This "quickens" us, makes us feel more alive. It is symbolic of the Holy Spirit, the "breath of God," who quickens us into spiritual life.

Then he said to me, "Prophesy to the wind. Prophesy, son of man, and say to the wind, 'Thus says the Lord God: Come from the four winds, O breath, and breathe upon these dead bodies, that they may live.' "
So I prophesied as he commanded me, and the breath came into them, and they lived and stood on their feet, an exceedingly great army.[28]

Jesus answered, "Truly, truly, I tell you, unless a person is born of water and of the Spirit, he cannot enter the kingdom of God.... The wind blows where it will, and you hear the sound of it. But you cannot tell where it came from or where it is going. So is every one who is born of the Spirit.[29]

It is the spirit which quickens (makes alive). *The flesh is of no avail. The words that I speak to you, they are spirit, and they are life.*[30]

How blessed each day would be if husband and wife not only took cleansing breaths each morning, but from time to time throughout the day revived their spirits with a little "breath from heaven," *times of refreshing from the presence of the Lord.*[31]

Work breathing. This is the normal breathing each person does throughout the day without thinking about it. The harder we work, the faster and deeper we breathe. When we are occupied with quieter work or are resting, our breathing quiets down, responding in a remarkable way to the body's greater or lesser need for oxygen.

When a woman is in labor, this same automatic regulation of breathing takes place if there is no emotional interference to upset the normal pattern of her breathing. If she is at peace with herself, with God, with her labor and with her surroundings, her breathing will exactly meet the oxygen needs of both herself and her baby. As the muscles of the uterus work harder toward the end of the first stage of labor, her breathing quickens automatically.

In order to become aware of the way in which this marvelous mechanism adapts to our activities, both husband and wife can observe their own breathing several times during the course of a day. Most of us breathe more rapidly than we need to because we are too lazy. We take such shallow breaths that we force the breathing mechanism to work faster in order to supply adequate oxygen. If we practice breathing a little more slowly and deeply, making this a habit, it will improve both the quality of our breathing and our health.

Sleep breathing. The need of our bodies for oxygen lowers when we are at rest. Not only does breathing slow down, but as the body relaxes air is drawn deeper into the lungs and the shoulders and upper chest become quiet. This slower deep chest breathing can be observed in sleeping babies or animals, as their tummies go up and down, up and down, with each breath. The air drawn deeper into the chest causes the abdomen to rise and fall in complete relaxation.

This slow, deep chest breathing was first taught by Dr. Grantly Dick-Read for labor and became known as "abdominal breathing." I have heard people say that abdominal breathing is "too hard to learn." Nonsense! It is the most natural breathing in the world and we all do it when we are completely relaxed and sleeping soundly. But because we have never observed our own sleep, we are not aware of this pattern of breathing and have to learn to do it while awake.

In 1972 I had the great privilege of revising the fourth edition of Dr. Dick-Read's classic work on natural childbirth, **Childbirth Without Fear,** which was first published in 1933 under the title **Natural Childbirth.**[32] In this fourth edition I coined the phrases "work breathing" and "sleep breathing," to help people understand that these are natural breathing patterns which our Lord designed for activity and rest.

The natural, slow deep breathing we use in sleep aids the relaxation of the entire body: muscles relax more fully, the heart beat slows down, blood pressure lowers, and all internal body processes work more smoothly and efficiently. This is the natural breathing pattern for the first stage of labor.

An animal in labor instinctively adapts its breathing pattern to the different stages of labor unless its instincts have been disrupted by the tensions of captivity or anxiety. But because we are less in tune with our instincts we need to rediscover these natural breathing patterns in order to apply them during labor and birth.

A simple way to learn sleep breathing is to sit in a lounge chair with one's feet propped up, leaning back (but not reclining). Relax the neck and shoulders so that the shoulders drop slightly and the head tilts forward a bit. Now lay both arms across the abdomen, and sit quietly for a few moments, breathing slowly. Notice how the abdomen begins to rise and fall under the arms, and the upper chest remains quiet. This breathing deeper in the chest is "sleep breathing." Once it is well learned in the chair, practice it in a variety of positions in bed, lying on the back, on the side, even lying face down.

Husbands as well as wives will benefit from spending 10 to 20 minutes each day in "sleep" breathing, learning consciously to **start** and **continue** it for a period of time while awake. During the day brief periods of sleep breathing and the relaxation it induces whenever one feels tired or tense is an aid to better health, calming nerves, aiding digestion, lowering blood pressure. Any position can be used that is most comfortable. It might be with one's arms folded on a desk and the head on the arms, in a chair or even on the office floor. This breathing at bedtime will hasten the relaxation that quickly leads to a sound sleep, and one will awaken more rested.

"Shelf" breathing. This breathing technique is useful for labor. As the first stage of labor advances, the deep, slow sleep breathing tends to quicken slightly toward work breathing because the uterus is working harder. The contractions become stronger and closer together and the need for oxygen to both uterus and baby increases. Shelf breathing is a combination of work and sleep breathing.

Inhale deep in the chest as for sleep breathing, but breathe in a little more air and hold the breath so that the abdomen remains elevated above the uterus. Now, breathe in and out with small breaths in the upper chest **on top of** the air remaining in the lower lungs. This keeps the abdomen lifted off the uterus for comfort during labor contractions, and still meets the body's need for slightly faster breathing. It is very important to take one or two deep cleansing breaths at the end of the contraction and then continue the normal deep sleep breathing until the next contraction. (If one's lips begin to tingle during labor it is a sign of hyper-ventilating, that is, breathing too rapidly and shallowly. If the lips begin to tingle or muscles begin cramping, the mother should breathe into her hands for the rest of the contraction, or until the unpleasant tingling and cramping sensations have disappeared.)

As another contraction begins, inhale until the abdomen rises, exhale only slightly so that the abdomen does not drop, and again breathe in and out in the upper chest, in and out, in and out, until a minute or so has passed (the length of a labor contraction). Then exhale completely. Take two cleansing breaths. The muscles of the abdominal wall must remain completely relaxed, the "shelf" of the abdomen held up over the contracting uterus **only** by the air in the lower lungs. Tightening the abdominal muscles lowers rather than raises them, and this may cause pain.

This shelf breathing should be practiced for a few moments every day during the last weeks of pregnancy, in any position suitable for labor, until it can be maintained for a minute or two with no sense of fatigue. The breathing in the upper chest should not be too fast or it will seem difficult to maintain. It can be learned well enough that one could go on breathing in this way for some time with no sense of effort.

"Pausing breaths." At any time during labor when a woman feels an urge to push too soon, either during the transition between first and second stage or as the baby's head is being born, she must not push! She can keep from bearing down by blowing **out** little puffs of air, "a-**whew!** a-**whew!** a-**whew!**" Emphasis is on the "whew"—the blowing **out**—so that one **seems** to be blowing out more air than one is taking in.

When I was being taught to swim as a teenager I was told to inhale when my face was turned out of the water, and blow the air out when my face was in the water. I could breathe in all right but not out—a -, A-, AH —, AHH — but by this time my lungs felt ready to burst! I was not exhaling as completely as I was inhaling. So at this point in labor the emphasis is on breathing **out.** The breathing in will take care of itself.

But this blowing out is to be gently done, for if one goes

WHEW! a big push will go right along with it! Just little puffs are needed. Elisabeth Bing calls it the "blow the candle" breathing, and has the mothers practice it using the forefinger as the candle. Just a tiny puff is needed to blow out the candle close to the lips.

During one of my trips to the Philippines I had the privilege of teaching an expectant mother how to give birth easily. I had only one short session with her, but she was an apt pupil and quickly caught on to the comfort techniques of breathing, relaxation, and rounded back position for labor and birth. She wrote me later to tell me her baby had come and that she had had a gentle, comfortable labor with no medication. "I paused the baby out," she wrote. I read it twice. Did she mean "push?" But then I realized she was referring to the gentle blowing out I had taught her to use as the baby's head was being born. What a lovely way to say it! She had literally breathed her baby out so gently that there was no damage to her perineum.

The expectant couple can look forward to that beautiful moment when their own baby arrives. What a good, healthy cleansing breath he or she takes in that first moment! Although natural childbirth babies seldom cry at birth, they often make some little sound. How we listen for that first sound of the little voice to show that baby is breathing.

What rejoicing there is now! And watch—see how the breathing patterns of the new mommy and daddy have automatically changed now too!

> *Praise the Lord! Praise Him, heaven of heavens. Let them praise the name of the Lord, for he commanded and they were created.*
>
> *Praise the Lord from the earth, you sea monsters and all deeps; fire and hail; snow and fog; stormy wind fulfilling his word; mountains and all hills; fruitful trees and all cedars; beasts and all cattle; creeping things and flying birds;*
>
> *Kings of the earth, and all people, princes and all judges of the earth, both young men and maidens, old men and children.*
>
> *Let everything that has breath praise the Lord!*[33]

NOTES
1. Isa. 55:1-3, 10, 11. **2.** Gen. 1:26-29. **3.** Isa. 35:1.
4. Carl C. Pfeiffer, M.D., Ph.D. **Zinc and Other Micro-Nutrients.** New Canaan, CT. Keats Publishing, Inc. $2.25. Copyright by Carl Pfeiffer. P. 233. Reprinted by permission.

Safflower is the oil suggested in the quote because it is the lowest in polyunsaturated fatty acids and a good source of linoleic acid which helps lower blood cholesterol (a factor in high blood pressure and heart disease).

5. Even aspirin has been implicated as a possible contributor to birth defects during the first few weeks of pregnancy. Questions are also being raised about the safety of commonly prescribed nausea medications for pregnancy like Benedictin. The rule is: not **any** medication, not **any** time during pregnancy except for diabetic and other ill women under special medical care. Nausea can be lessened by B-vitamins and other dietary means. Learning muscular relaxation in early pregnancy aids digestion and lessens nausea.

Alcohol and tobacco are known to cause low birth weight and other health problems in infants. Research on caffeine shows it may also be a contributing factor in birth defects. (Caffeine is found in coffee, tea, cola, chocolate.)

6. Gail Sforza Brewer with Tom Brewer, M.D. **What Every Pregnant Woman Should Know: The Truth About Diets and Drugs in Pregnancy.** New York. Random House. 1977.

7. Knowledgeable vegetarians such as Seventh Day Adventists learn how to meet all the nutrient requirements, including the various proteins, in meat substitutes.

Christians need to be alert to the fact that at the present time many people have become vegetarian because they have adopted the pagan Hindu prohibitions against meat. After all, if one believes in reincarnation as the Hindus do, one might be eating one's own grandmother! One can be alert to spiritistic non-biblical vegetarian attitudes if the word "carrion" is used for meat, or the statement made that one should only eat "living" things, but meat is "dead." But if a plant is cut off from its roots, is it "living?" Even seeds die. (Jn. 12:24.)

8. Salt is an important element in the pregnant woman's diet, but since most of our diets are too high in salt, sea salt and other natural salts are preferable. Salt-**free** diets for pregnant women are extremely dangerous, Dr. Tom Brewer has proven, and are a common cause of toxemia of later pregnancy. See his research book, **Metabolic Toxemia of Late Pregnancy: A Disease of Malnutrition.** Springfield, IL. Charles C. Thomas. 1966.

9. Pfeiffer. **Op. cit.**

10. Lev. 11. Some "unclean" animals are vegetarian but may cause other problems. The hare, for example, is a rodent. Rodents are carriers of rabies, bubonic plague, etc.

11. The Biblical criteria for clean sea food is that it must have fins and scales. Shell fish are "unclean," as they are scavengers of the bottoms

of the seas, cleansing the waters, and thus potential disease-carriers.
12. Rom. 14:1-4. **13.** Ex. 23:25, 26 RSV. **14.** Acts 10:9-16. **15.** Lk. 10:7. **16.** Mk. 16:18. **17.** Mt. 6:11. **18.** Ex. 16:4. **19.** Ps. 105:37. **20.** Mt. 6:26-33. **21.** Mt. 4:4; Deut. 28:3. **22.** Heb. 6:5. **23.** Amos 8:11. **24.** Heb. 6:4. **25.** Jn. 6:35. **26.** Jn. 4:14; 7:38, 39. **27.** Gen. 2:9. **28.** Ex. 37:9, 10. **29.** Jn. 3:5, 8. **30.** Jn. 6:63. **31.** Acts 3:19.
32. Grantly Dick-Read. **Childbirth Without Fear.** 4th Ed. edited by Helen Wessel and Harlan Ellis, M.D. New York. Harper & Row. 1972. Paper back, 1978.

Dr. Dick-Read's first paper on natural childbirth was in 1919. This fourth edition of **Childbirth Without Fear** is a compilation of the best of all Dick-Read's writings on childbirth, including his first book, **Natural Childbirth,** written in 1933 for the medical profession. He had no idea he was coining a household word! The medical profession strongly resisted his proven research, so in 1943, at the urging of his wife Jessica, he rewrote the book in more readable style, for women. The first American edition was published in 1944 under the title **Childbirth Without Fear.**
33. Ps. 148:1, 4-12, 150:6.

Great Expectation

Have you not known? Have you not heard? that the everlasting God, the Lord, the Creator of the ends of the earth does not faint nor grow weary? His knowledge is far beyond being searched out.
He gives power to the faint, and adds strength to those who are exhausted. Even the youths shall faint and be weary and the young men shall fall utterly exhausted.
But those who wait upon the Lord will renew their strength. They will rise up as if on eagles' wings. They will run and not be weary. They will walk and not faint.[1]

It takes two to make a baby. When a child is conceived the husband's responsibilities as head of the home increase tremendously. Pregnancy and birth are not just "woman's concerns," for at no time in their lives together is a wife more dependent upon her husband than when she is becoming *great with child.*[2] His loving care provides a spiritual and emotional covering both for his wife and for his unborn child. Together husband and wife can learn and plan and practice everything necessary in great expectation, as they wait for the day when their child will appear.

Their preparation for the coming birth of their child should include exercise, sleep and rest, a deepening communion with God, and vision—seeing with the eyes of faith the child still hidden in the womb.

Exercise

Movement is necessary to life. The smooth muscles of our internal organs are continually contracting and relaxing. Our skeletal muscles "exercise" all day long, every time we move and when we shift around in our sleep. Even a baby moves his body muscles continuously, long before he has any motor skills. But certain forms of exercise have special benefits for the expectant woman. If her husband practices these with her he will receive unexpected health dividends himself. Walking, pelvic rocking, tailor sitting, and exercising the muscles of the pelvic floor are four simple activities which require no athletic ability.

Walking. The husband and wife who take a good walk every day are performing the most valuable exercise for any age (not to mention the companionship of being together). A brisk walk stimulates good breathing and good circulation, exercising the heart and lungs. It helps to keep all the body muscles in good tone, giving a sense of physical well-being.

The unborn baby benefits also, for the movement of the mother helps shift the baby into a good position for the birth. During labor, the mother will want to walk as much as possible, as this shortens labor. If she has learned to take long walks without getting tired, she will be in much better physical condition for walking during labor without becoming weary.

No pregnant woman should jog or "run in place"[3] warns obstetrician Dr. Robert Bradley. The uterus hangs suspended in the abdomen on slender ligaments. As the uterus grows heavier, jogging or jumping places undue stress on these ligaments, stretching them past their normal elasticity. This can create problems later on of uterine prolapse (uterus dropping down into the vagina).

The pelvic rock. This is also an important exercise for men as well as women, as it aids good posture and helps prevent or correct backache. The pelvic rock may be performed in a variety of ways. One of the simplest is to stand leaning one's back and head against a wall, with the heels about six inches away. Now, touch the wall with the small of the back. Notice how the pelvis in front tips inward as the back pushes against the wall. The pelvis "rocks" back and forth as one's back moves back and forth touching the wall. Another way is to lie on the floor, bending the knees and placing the feet flat on the floor. Then try to touch the floor with the small of the back. Release and repeat, five or six times.

Still another way to rock the pelvis is to get on hands and knees and release tension by relaxing the muscles all across the small of the back. Now slowly arch the back upward, at the same time pulling the buttocks inward and tightening their muscles. Repeat several times, at least once a day and any time the back feels tired. This hands and knees position does several things: rocks the pelvis, helps relax the back muscles to relieve backache, and builds firmness in the hips and upper thighs.

The pelvic rock can be performed any time. Simply push with the small of the back **as if** there were something to lean against, whether sitting or standing. Then straighten up. Repeat. Notice how this improves posture, lifts the shoulders, and if one is standing it also pulls the tummy in so that the baby fits nicely down into the pelvic basin.

Tailor sitting. Sit on the floor with the knees bent outward and ankles crossed or the soles of the feet together. This stretches the muscles on the inside of the thigh and helps widen the bony pelvic outlet. With a finger, feel the center of the pubic bone. The slight depression in the center is connective tissue called the *symphysis pubis,* which must stretch and move as the baby is being born. Tailor sitting helps both the symphysis pubis and the hip joints to become more flexible and able to move apart readily as the baby's head descends for the birth.

During the second stage of labor the mother will need to be in a position similar to this tailor sitting or squatting position, heels together and knees falling widely apart. The longer she can maintain this position without discomfort, the easier it will be to use this position for labor and birth.

Strengthening the pelvic floor. The muscles of the pelvic floor are like a firm sling or hammock, in the shape of a figure 8 around the anus, vagina and urethra, keeping them firmly closed. These muscles are subject to conscious control. We relax them to open the bowel or bladder at will and then close them again. During the birth of a baby it is important for the mother to be able to relax these perineal muscles fully, to allow the baby passage through without injuring them. This "Kegel" exercise has been described in detail in the chapter called "Awakened Desires." The expectant mother should practice it many times a day. Dr. Robert Bradley calls the Kegel muscle the "baby door muscle," and suggests that husbands can help the wife learn to exercise it correctly.

You can check on your wife's progress in learning control of the muscle of the vaginal opening through which the baby actually passes by having her alternately tighten and loosen this muscle after intercourse prior to withdrawal. ... Your wife should deliberately become consciously aware of the difference between tightness and looseness of

*this muscle so that she can welcome the baby with an open
door policy during the act of pushing the baby out. Like
any other muscle it will become more flexible and more
functional with exercise.*[4]

The parallel between feminine sexual response during coitus
and during childbirth has already been noted.[5] Childbirth is a
deeply moving sexual experience in which the wife opens the
door of her vagina to give back to her husband the baby which
has grown from their love union nine months earlier, when he
placed his sperm in her body.

*In coitus a man bestows his most precious gift of love
upon his beloved. Her opportunity to be the donor of love's
gift occurs during the birth experience when man and wife
exchange roles and he becomes the receiver of love's gift
through the organ of his cupped hands.*

*Therefore, highly-refined communication between man
and wife is the very best preparation for birth. This requires much patience, care and thoughtful preparation.
During the nine months of pregnancy both should take advantage of their opportunities to communicate marital love
and to really get to know each other.... A woman's
response to her man comes during the birth embrace when
her body yields into his eager hands her gift of love, communicating, "This is how much I love you."*[6]

Sexual intercourse may be freely engaged in during pregnancy as long as everything seems to be normal.[7] It can take place in
any position. The baby can't be hurt if the husband is above, as
the baby is cushioned in the amniotic sac. As the baby grows
larger however, this position will not be comfortable and a side
position may be preferred or the wife can sit across the
husband's thighs. If the wife prefers not to have coitus as the
pregnancy advances, the couple can practice love-making
through touch and caresses.

Sleep and rest
Sleep. Although sleep has been researched, it remains an
enigma and it is not yet known just what causes it. Sleep rests
the muscles of the body, but that is not its only important function. One of its primary functions is to renew the mind. A person
deprived of sleep for long periods of time becomes disoriented

and confused and shows personality changes. Some forms of insanity have been traced to sleep-deprivation of the dreaming level (one of the four levels of sleep which have been identified).

Sleeping pills may put people to sleep, but they interfere with the normal dreaming periods. On awaking, the user often feels tired rather than refreshed, because it was not a natural sleep. And of course, pregnant women should never take sleeping pills because of the risk to the baby.

Dr. Carl C. Pfeiffer suggests that those who "never dream" may have a zinc deficiency[8] which prevents dream recall on awakening. The purpose of dreams seems to be like a complex computer sorting out all the data fed into it during the waking hours, arranging it in an orderly pattern before storing it away in the memory bank. We wake refreshed.

The Bible says that we are to *bring every thought into captivity to Christ.*[9] But how can we do this when we are asleep? Many ugly, sinful things that we ignored have passed by our eyes and ears during the waking hours. Sometimes these surface in our dreams, haunting us with fears or nightmares or illicit sexual desires. We need not feel guilty over such dreams, but neither do we need to suffer from them. God promises to **keep** *our hearts and minds through Christ Jesus.*[10]

We need to go to sleep with Jesus on our minds. Each night we can ask the Holy Spirit to keep active control of our minds while we sleep, to pray through our minds and spirits even though we are not aware of it, and to keep them pure. One's first thought then on awakening is—Jesus! If one has difficulty relaxing and falling asleep, try memorizing Scripture. It is a marvellous soporific! I've memorized many Psalms in that way. It flows along for awhile, familiar,—and then it's morning. *The Lord is my shepherd. I shall not want. He makes me....to lie down.... He ....*[11] "Good morning, Lord!"

Keep (God's words). *Bind them continually upon your heart, and tie them around your neck. When you go, it will lead you. When you sleep, it will keep you. And when you wake, it will talk with you.*[12]

He who loves silver shall not be satisfied with silver; nor he who loves abundance with increase. And what good is there to the owners, except to look at it with their eyes? The sleep of a laboring man is sweet, whether he has little or much to eat. But the abundance of the rich man does not allow him to sleep.[13]

It is in vain that you rise up early and sit up late, to earn a living through worry. For God gives sleep to his loved one.[14]

Lord, you have put gladness in my heart, greater than the gladness of those who spend their time eating, and drinking wine. I will lie down in peace, and sleep. For you, Lord, are the only one who keeps me safe.[15]

Rest. Rest and sleep are not synonymous, for one can sleep without resting either body or mind, tossing all night, plagued with worries and frustrating dreams, or drugged in an unnatural sleep which does not refresh. However, we can learn to rest without sleep, and learning this will increase our ability to fall asleep easily and sleep well. This "rest" is the release of muscle tension, combined with the deep "sleep" breathing discussed in the previous chapter. Although we have no conscious control over the internal, smooth muscles of our organs—lungs, stomach, intestines, blood vessels, glands, uterus, etc.—we do have conscious control over the skeletal muscles of our body, and over our breathing.

The skeletal muscles (the long, striated muscles that build the muscle "frame" of our body) respond to our commands. These commands are channeled through the brain, and the right muscles are activated. When I want to walk, the command goes out and my legs begin to move. This command-response becomes so highly refined that I may not be aware of the fact that I do it. A desire comes to do something, and without conscious thought I am already moving in that direction. But it is **me** commanding, for I can stop at will, turn around and go the other way. This response of the muscles to the brain's commands can be refined to such an acute degree that a concert pianist or violinist puts on a muscular performance that astonishes us all. His or her muscles have learned the desired responses so well that they almost seem to be performing by themselves. Yet the performer could stop in the middle of the most complicated cadenza if he or she wanted to. The muscles have "learned" the musical responses, but are still under the performer's control.

Negative emotions disrupt this intricate interchange of

command-response, and also disrupt the normal functioning of the internal organs. A nervous pianist hits many wrong notes because of muscle tension, though his private performances were perfect. An angry driver is a menace, though normally he has good control of his car. Negative emotions can actually make us sick if they are indulged in over a period of time. They cause high blood pressure, ulcers, asthma, migraine headaches, arthritis, etc., and lower resistance to all diseases. They interfere with the normal processes of pregnancy and cause unnatural, severe pain in childbirth. Our emotions have far more to do with our health than any other factor. The Bible is clear in this regard:

A soft answer turns away wrath, but a harsh word stirs up anger. A gentle tongue is a tree of life, but perverseness in it breaks the bones.
A glad heart makes a cheerful face, but by sorrows of heart the spirit is broken. All the days of the afflicted are evil, but a cheerful heart has a continual feast.
A cheerful heart is good medicine, but a downcast spirit dries up the bones. He who restrains his words has knowledge, and he who has a cool spirit is a man of understanding.[16]

The husband who is aware of this will keep a *cool spirit* when his pregnant wife is cross or discouraged. He will remember that *a cheerful heart is good medicine* and try to lift her spirits.

One's emotions seem to have a will of their own at times, and we can't always help how we feel. Ever try to stop crying? Or stop being frightened? Or stop being nervous before speaking to an audience, or when the siren of a police car suddenly wails near you?

There is a way in which we can bring these negative reactions under control. It is not done by confronting the strong feeling and trying to change it. Instead, we undermine it by giving a positive command to our skeletal muscles: "Release! **Let go** the muscle tension in the arms, the hands, the neck, the abdomen, the back, the legs." As we release the muscle tension of the body and slow down our breathing, an amazing transformation begins to take place in our emotions. Fears calm down, feelings become quieter, the situation begins to be drained of its threat. When our muscles "let go" at our command, the message goes back to the brain: "Everything is all right." This message is relayed to the internal organs. The racing heart slows down, digestion resumes, the headache begins to go away. We feel better.

It is amazing that this muscular relaxation only inhibits **negative** emotions. It never takes away peace, joy, the sense of well being. It is good medicine that brings positive feelings, *The garment of praise* replaces *the spirit of heaviness.*[17] Conscious muscular relaxation goes hand in hand with cheerfulness, tranquility, peace.

Muscle tension and anxiety are Siamese twins. Dis-ease, crossness, anger or being "up tight" are always combined with excessive muscle tension. In any public meeting I can see many "up tight" people. Even their facial muscles are taut. They may not look unhappy but they certainly don't look tranquil, joyful, or at ease! When a tense person trys to act cheerful it seems "fakey," put on. His laughter is too high pitched or too loud, his cheery greeting too warm to seem real. We feel uncomfortable around such a person and want to slip away.

I have explained these things at length because techniques for learning muscular relaxation for childbirth are too often taught as if the techniques were just for birth, but that is not so. Everyone needs to learn these principles and apply them all their lives. When Dr. Edmund Jacobson first published his research on relaxation in book form in 1934,[18] it showed the scientific preventive benefits of relaxation for such health problems as heart attacks, high blood pressure, ulcers, colitis and a host of nervous disorders. Dr. Dick-Read discovered Dr. Jacobson's work shortly after its publication, and applied the principles to his natural childbirth patients. He found the positive results astounding! His principle of birth as a "natural" function had been right, but the best results came only after his patients were taught Dr. Jacobson's system of inducing complete muscular relaxation.

When I first began to learn to relax and breathe properly, in preparation for my first natural birth, my husband learned this deep relaxation also. To his surprise he discovered that this made it far easier for him to fall asleep in all kinds of strange beds when he was away on preaching trips. One time our youngest child, eight years old, said to me, "I'm your best relaxer, aren't I, Mom?" He was, for children are naturally more relaxed and learn the principles quickly.

Right where you are sitting at this moment, stop and think over your body from head to foot, slowly, noticing any tight muscles that you can release. Let your head fall gently forward, shoulders droop, hands and arms rest limply on the arms of the chair or on your lap. Let your stomach sag, your foot stop swinging. Rest your feet on the floor with the soles turned toward each other. Pretend you are a rag doll. Try to become "limp as a wet noodle."

Take slow, deep chest "sleep" breaths as you "slouch into yourself." Notice how restful this seems and stay that way awhile. Do this several times a day, at home or at work, all your life, thinking quietly, "Praise You, Jesus! I love You! I am relaxing and placing all my trust in You, trusting everything will be all right."

This level of relaxation is just the beginning of the depth that needs to be learned for a gentle, comfortable labor. It is too late to learn it when labor begins! The amount of pain in labor is **directly** related to the degree of tension in the skeletal muscles of the body. The pregnant woman should practice relaxing every day, until she can release all muscle tension in only a moment or two.

As relaxation continues, even the pattern of brainwave electrical activity changes. Normal activity produces Beta waves of 13 to 25 cycles per second. As relaxation deepens, the cycles lower to Alpha waves, 8 to 13 cycles per second. This is a state of non-focused thinking, daydreaming.

As the muscles release tension still further, electrical brain activity slows to Theta waves, 4 to 8 cycles per second. This is a reverie, twilight state, usually experienced just before sleep. It is related to creativity, and in this half-dreaming state thoughts and images seem to spring from nowhere, as if the mind were thinking on its own, unrelated to anything going on around it.

Those who practice relaxing diligently will learn over a period of time to recognize each level of relaxation in themselves. When a woman is in labor, it is essential that she be able to relax at **least** to the Alpha (second) level of brainwave activity during the first stage.

Since the steps of learning muscular relaxation are given in detail both in **The Joy of Natural Childbirth** and in **Childbirth Without Fear,** I will not repeat them here, except for the four essential things to remember. First, every portion of the body is to be **completely** supported so that no muscle of the body has to carry its own weight. Second, every joint of the body is to be bent slightly, which relaxes the joints. Even the back is to be curved into a fetal position, similar to a parenthesis: (, this helps the muscles attached to the vertebrae to release their tension.

Third, no part of the body should rest on any other, as this cuts off circulation. And fourth, once settled into a relaxed position, don't move! Resist the temporary feeling of wanting to "get more comfortable" and concentrate on releasing muscle tension more and more instead.

A sensation of floating or pins and needles in the hands and feet will come after a while, as even thought fades to the reverie state. Mind and body are at rest.

Communion with God

There is a tranquility which comes through the relaxation of the muscles of the body but this tranquility will not sustain us through the day. We need more. We need Jesus. We need God to do something **in** us. We need to *wait upon the Lord, so that our strength is renewed.*[19] We need God to ***make*** *us lie down in green pastures, lead us beside the **still** waters, and restore our soul.*[20]

For thus says the Lord God, the Holy One of Israel: in returning to me and resting, you will be protected. Your strength will be found in quietness and confidence. But you would not. You said, "No!..."[21]

We will never find the inner peace we need in Bible study alone, running to endless meetings, rushing about trying to serve God, but in spending quiet time in deep communion with our God. The writer to the Hebrews tells us to *go beyond the first principles of the oracles of God.*[22] He defines these first principles as repentance from sin, salvation through Jesus' death on the cross, the doctrine of baptisms, the laying on of hands, resurrection of the dead, eternal judgment, the charisms, partaking of the Holy Spirit.

The passage says, *let us go **on** to maturity,* and leads the way, right on into the Throne Room of God! Before the exploits of faith later in the book, the next several chapters of Hebrews reveal the open door of the tabernacle of God's presence, with an invitation for us to *come on in!*

Therefore, brothers and sisters, let us have the courage to enter right into the Holy of Holies through the blood of Jesus.... Let us come close with a heart full of the assurance of faith, without shrinking back, for he is faithful who promised.[23]

Our way of praying is to rush into God's presence and give God "a talking to." We give a long recital of all the things we want God to do for us, add "in Jesus' name, Amen." Then we rush out.

Instead, let's go on to maturity and learn a new way of entering God's presence, silent, listening, until God releases us refreshed and full of joy. Choose a time when you are rested and relax in a comfortable chair. Release the muscle tension in your arms, your legs, your back, until completely comfortable. Close your eyes and picture yourself in the throne room of God. The table of holy bread is on your right, the candlestick glowing on your left. The incense of prayer is rising before the Throne of God right before your eyes, and His presence is all around. Keep perfectly silent.

With eyes still closed, picture Jesus kneeling in front of you to wash your feet, taking away all the dust of cares and worries. Look down into His eyes. He is smiling into your eyes. The King of kings, Creator of the universe, has made Himself your servant. See the scars in His hands—scars borne for you. For a long time, picture Jesus present with you and feast your eyes on Him, aware of His strong arms, His gentle touch. For He **is** there. How often we rush out of His presence, leaving Him with His eyes full of tears because we never discerned His loving presence at all!

Another time, imagine the room filled with the golden warmth, love and peace of the Holy Spirit, as if you were a child enfolded in the mother's arms:

Lord, my heart is not lofty. Neither do I exercise myself in great matters, or in things too high for me. Surely I have behaved and quieted myself as a child that is weaned of its mother.[24]

As one whom his mother comforts, says the Lord, so will I comfort you.[25]

And I (Jesus) *will pray to the Father, and he will give you another Comforter, who will stay with you forever, even the Spirit of truth.*[26]

Still another time let us come, wearied with the pressures of life, aware of our own ineptness, weaknesses. As we relax our minds and bodies in His presence, let us picture the Father, strong, powerful, filling the room, the house, the universe, ourselves caught up in His arms in the center of it all:

> *There is none like God who loves us, who rides upon the heavens to help us, and whose excellency is in the skies. The eternal God is your refuge, and underneath are the everlasting arms. He shall thrust out the enemy from before you and shall say, "Destroy them!" Then you will live in safety, with a fountain upon your land of corn and wine. Also the heavens will drop down dew.*[27]

When we remain perfectly quiet in God's presence, words of Scripture will begin to come to us as the Holy Spirit brings to our attention the things Jesus has said in His Word. On leaving the place of communion with God, these words will keep ringing in our ears all day long, until we live and breathe them as our own. Jesus said, *If you abide in me, and my words abide in you, you shall ask whatever you wish, and it shall be done to you.*[28]

Let husband and wife each learn to enter the throne room of God, where He will lead them *from glory to glory.*[29] Before leaving, let each one tell the Lord how much they love Him. The time will come when husband and wife want to enter this Holy of Holies **together** in this new way of praying.

This is the highest form of preparation for childbirth, for when in labor, husband and wife will know how to enter the throne room of the presence of God together. Birth should always take place in this "sanctuary."

And whenever we leave the place of prayer where God has revealed Himself to us, we are more aware than ever of His continuing presence with us:

> *Wherever you go you are pregnant with Christ, and you bring his presence as you would bring the presence of a natural child. For when a woman is with child, people give her special attention. They smile, they offer her a comfortable place to sit down. She is a witness to life. She carries life around with her.*
>
> *Applying this example to the mystery of being pregnant with God (and it applies to both men and women), you have within yourselves a room, a secluded place. You should be more aware of God than anyone else, because you are carrying within you this utterly quiet and silent chamber. Because you are more aware of God, because you*

have been called to listen to him in your inner silence, you can bring him to the street, the party, the meeting, in a very special way.[30]

Therefore leaving the principles of the doctrine of Christ, let us go on to maturing.... For we have a High Priest, who is set on the right hand of the throne of the Majesty in the heavens,... who says to us, "Come on in!"[31]

Vision

A "vision" need not be supernatural, though some visions are. We have been talking about inner vision, seeing Jesus with the mind's eye. And now we will turn from envisioning the real but invisible God to the real but—to us—invisible child within the mother's body, picturing in our minds what only God can see.

You have covered me in my mother's womb. My body was not hidden from you while I was made in secret and being marvelously fashioned in darkness. Your eyes saw my body while it was yet unformed, and in your book all my members were written down before there was any of them. They were gradually fashioned.[32]

At **conception** a human life begins. It does not begin at birth when the infant draws its first breath, nor in the third or fourth month of pregnancy when the mother first feels her baby move ("quickening"). But as soon as the sperm penetrates the shell of the ovum and the nucleus of the sperm merges with the nucleus of the ovum, a living cell is formed which contains all 46 human chromosomes (23 from the sperm, 23 from the ovum). The chromosomes in this single living cell carry all the genetic characteristics of the individual (about 30,000 genes, at least 15,000 from the sperm and at least 15,000 from the ovum). These genes determine the features of a human being, the color of eyes, hair, skin, the tendency to be tall or short, fat or lean, disease-resistant or disease-prone, and the sex of the child.[33]

The genes are so small that their details cannot be seen through any microscope, but they are the remarkable packages of chemical instructions for the design of each and every part of the new baby. The "instructions" are inscribed in the genes' molecular content which is a nucleic acid called DNA. If one imagines the molecule to be made up of symbols, like an alphabet, then one can imagine how these molecule "letters" composed in varying sequences can spell out different instructions in each gene.[34]

The Old Testament is right when it says that all the members of the person being formed have been "written down" before any of them appears. They are written in the genes! The genetic code appeared with the first couple on earth and has been transmitted through all the generations since, so that we really are the brothers and sisters of all other peoples of the world. *God who made the world made of one blood all nations of people who live on all the face of the earth.*[35]

The potential for infinite variety through the combination of the many thousands of genes is so great that every individual is unique, though we are all related.

Although only one sperm penetrates the ovum, the millions of sperm in the ejected semen of the father are thought to help create a protective spherical covering around the ovum. This is called the **corona radiata** (radiant crown). Thus the father's protective "covering" has already begun, even though the child conceived is still but one living cell.

Within 36 hours this single living cell inside the ovum divides into two cells, then four, and continues to increase two by two for several days, like slowly popping corn, until more than 150 tiny, translucent cells have been formed. This is called a "mulberry" cluster.

By the fourth or fifth day this tiny cluster of cells, still protected by the corona radiata, completes its journey through the Fallopean tube to the uterus. There it continues to drift about for another day or two. The "mulberry" ball of cells begins to lengthen, and a central cavity develops, with the cells pressed toward the outer walls. The lining of the mother's womb **(endometrium)** now begins to draw this tiny embryo toward itself. As the endometrium begins to form a "nest" for the embryo, the protective corona, no longer needed, begins to deteriorate and fall away. By the fifth to the seventh day after conception this tiny living organism is implanted in the wall of the mother's womb, drawing nourishment from the mother's blood. The amniotic sac begins to develop around it and the umbilical attachment between mother and infant begins to form.

By the third week after conception the embryo already is a well-proportioned, small-scale baby, the shape of the head apparent and a double heart beginning to form. Within another week the infant will have grown to the size of a dewdrop, and by the seventh week after conception (40 days) it has all the features and internal organs of the future adult, although it is only about an inch long. It has eyes, ears, nose, lip, tongue, arms, hands, fingers, knees, ankles and toes.

All these amazing developments have taken place even before the woman may realize she is pregnant! Because these early days are crucial in preventing malformation of the body or organs of the developing infant, every woman should keep her body healthy, well-nourished and free of all drugs, tranquilizers, sleeping pills and even aspirin, whether she is anticipating pregnancy or not.

At three months, the brain configuration is nearing completion. The infant is about 3½ inches long and would fit in the palm of the hand. By the fourth month the arms and legs have grown long enough for the baby to make his mother aware of his activity, although he has already been actively moving since the seventh week after conception. Scalp hair appears and the sex organs are recognizable. Baby is now about as long as his father's hand and by the end of this month he or she will have reached half the length at birth and is eight to ten inches long.

At five to six months the baby begins to have a chance of survival if born, provided he or she has reached the weight of at least a pound and a half. The most expert medical care is needed to assist survival at this level of prematurity. Every week the baby remains in the womb from now on increases his or her ability to live after birth. Baby keeps growing in length, weight and strength until there is no room to move.

By the end of nine months (40 weeks from conception), it is time to be born. No longer will baby be enfolded in the close, dark, warm waters of his mother's womb, but will be thrust out into a new world of bright lights that hurt the eyes, air that is dry and cold on the skin, an empty world of space which has no boundaries when he moves his arms and legs. But it is all right, for baby's father/priest has prayed over him or her with the mother for nine long months, and now encourages his little one pushing his way out of the womb.

"Come on into the world, child. We will dim the lights for you, hold you close in our warm, loving arms and cradle you against the emptiness. Your mother and I love you. We have prayed for you and looked forward to your coming for a long time. Come on in, child, come on into our world."

NOTES
1. Isa. 40:28-31. **2.** Luke 2:5.
3. Robert A. Bradley, M.D. **Husband-Coached Childbirth.** New York. Harper & Row. 1965, 1974.
4. **Ibid.** P. 113. Reprinted by permission.
5. See the chapter "Awakened Desires" and note #8 of that chapter.
6. Marilyn A. Moran. **Birth and the Dialogue of Love.** New Nativity Press. P.O. Box 6223, Leawood, KS, 66206. Reprinted by permission.
7. Most modern obstetric and pregnancy manuals suggest no limitations on coitus during pregnancy until the last six, or even the last two weeks, if at all.
8. Pfeiffer. **Zinc and Other Micro-nutrients. Op. cit.**
9. Cor. 10:5. **10.** Phil. 4:7. **11.** Ps. 23:1. **12.** Prov. 6:2-23. **13.** Eccl. 5:12. **14.** Ps. 127:2. **15.** Ps. 4:7, 8. **16.** Prov. 15:1, 4, 13, 15; 17:22, 27 RSV. **17.** Isa. 61:3
18. Edmund Jacobson, M.D. **You Must Relax.** New York. McGraw Hill. 1934, 1942, 1948, 1957, 1962 (4th edition).
19. Isa. 40:31. **20.** Ps. 23:2, 3. **21.** Isa. 30:15, 16. **22.** Heb. 5:11-14; 6:1-8. **23.** Heb. 10:19-22. **24.** Ps. 131:1, 2. **25.** Isa. 66:13. **26.** Jn. 14:16, 17. **27.** Deut. 33:26-28. **28.** Jn. 15:7. **29.** 2 Cor. 3:18.
30. Catherine de Hueck Doherty. **Poustinia.** Notre Dame, IN. Ave Maria Press. 1974. Pp. 89, 90. Reprinted by permission.
31. Heb. 6:1; 8:1, 19, 20; Rev. 22:16, 17. **32.** Ps. 139:12-16.
33. Weston D. Gardner, M.D. & Wm. A. Osburn. **Structure of the Human Body.** Philadelphia. W.B. Saunders. 2nd ed, 1973. P. 24: "... the DNA nucleoprotein in the nucleus of **all** cells...bears the genetic characteristics of the individual.... All cells resulting from the first division of the first single cell bear the identification of the new individual's sex in special chromosomal material of the nucleus. It is possible to determine the true sex of any person by analyzing the nuclear chromatin in a very simple microscopic examination of many types of body cells."
34. Geraldine Lux Flanagan. **The First Nine Months of Life.** New York. Simon & Schuster. 1962. P. 25. Reprinted by permission.
35. Acts 17:26.

A Labor of Love

The Lord visited Sarah as he had said, and did to Sarah as he had spoken. For Sarah conceived and gave birth to a son for Abraham in his old age. And Abraham called his son Isaac (laughter).... And Sarah said, "God has made me laugh, so that all who hear of it will laugh with me!"[1]

Then God remembered Rachel, and God listened to her and opened her womb. She conceived and gave birth to a son and said, "God has taken away my reproach." And she called his name Joseph (God adds), saying, "May the Lord add to me another son!"[2]

And Leah conceived and gave birth to a son. And she said, "Now I will praise the Lord!" Therefore she called his name Judah (praise).[3]

I straightened up in the chair and held my breath. That baby was sure stretching! A moment later I relaxed and tried again to pay attention to what my student-preacher husband was saying to our parishioners at the prayer meeting. Before the hour was over I straightened up again, two or three times or more. Baby was really pushing! If baby was so crowded now, what would it be like six weeks from now? I wondered. I was only seven and a half months pregnant.

The hour over, we went to the home of one of the families for dessert, laughed and chatted awhile before climbing into our Model A Ford for the hour long, bumpy ride back home. Baby had kept crowding me while we ate and on the long way back to our little house near the University of California in Los Angeles where my husband was a student. I had enjoyed the dessert, hungry because I hadn't felt much like eating at supper time. In fact, I hadn't felt much like eating all day. When we arrived home we fell into bed, exhausted from the long day. Baby pushed again, hard. Water gushed out all over the bed and I seemed to deflate like a pricked balloon. "Honey!" I cried, alarmed. "The baby's coming!"

Startled awake, my husband dropped on his knees by the side of the bed and began to pray, "Oh Lord, help me! I don't know what to do! Help me!" I began to realize he thought the baby was coming any minute. Wasn't that what I had said? "Honey," I shook his arm to interrupt his prayer. "Hurry and get dressed so we can start for the hospital."

We climbed back into our little rattle-trap and tore off for the hospital, a half-hour's drive away. I scrunched down in the seat, my knees apart, knowing now that it was not the baby stretching I had been feeling all these hours, but labor! The baby was born a couple of hours after we reached the hospital. It was Valentine's Day, 1946.

Almost every young woman in those days was totally ignorant of labor and birth. Not that I hadn't tried to learn. My husband scoured the university library for childbirth books for me, without success except for a little volume thirty years old which told what items to have on hand if the baby was to be born at home. The book said nothing about labor or birth itself, and home birth in the mid-40's was unheard of (though I didn't know that either!).

So, blissfully ignorant, I had gone happily through the greater portion of my first labor, about 15 hours, without any idea that what I was feeling was labor and that birth was imminent.

Through the course of the years since then I have learned many "facts," but more importantly, I have learned that it is not the scientific facts that make birthing so important to a woman. It is the **memory** of the experience that is important. For subconsciously (or consciously) it affects her emotional responses toward her child, her husband, herself, and even toward God. I have yet to talk to a woman who could not recount to me every detail of each birth experience, except for those periods when she was under heavy sedation or anesthetized.[4] Even 80 year old women will begin to describe their birthings if the subject is mentioned. The acuteness of this memory when so many other memories fade demonstrates that a woman's whole personality is affected far more by her childbearing experiences than has been realized.

In this chapter we will "experience" birth, aware of far more than facts, through the mother's thoughts. The following story is a composite of many actual experiences of women in labor. The site of birth and choice of attendants other than the husband are not identified. These alternatives will be discussed in a later chapter.

Although every woman's childbearing is different from that of any other woman, and each birth is different even for the same woman, God's design for natural birthing is generally like this one.

. . . .

Signs of labor

Could it be today, Lord, that our baby might come? These last two weeks have seemed like years, Braxton-Hicks contractions[5] every day, waking me at night. Each time I watch the clock and think that maybe, maybe this time labor is really starting, but then the contractions peter out and disappear! It's hard to sit comfortably, hard to breathe, hard to rest at night, and I keep running to the bathroom every few minutes. Baby's so big there's barely room left in me for food or air or water. And I'm weary, Lord, of people always asking, "Oh, are you still here?"

I've gone over the possible signs of starting labor a hundred times it seems: leaking waters, regular contractions, the mucus plug coming away. Every time I go to the bathroom I check for any mucus discharge, but there's never anything there.

And what would I do, Lord, if my bag of waters leaked, or suddenly broke while I was at the store or in church? I'd be so embarrassed! I almost didn't go to church Sunday for fear that might happen, until You reassured me that *my times are in your hand.*[6]

What would I do without You, Jesus? Please forgive me for griping, for being so impatient, always complaining *how long, O Lord, how long.*[7] I'm grateful that You're the kind shepherd who *gathers the lambs with his arm, carries them in his bosom, and gently leads those who are with young.*[8] I'm tired, Lord. I'm going to lie down a while as if I were a lamb myself instead of the mother, resting my head on Your shoulder while You gather me in Your arms. . . .

Honey, I can't imagine why I felt so discouraged yesterday. I feel great today! I'm going to do some baking, scrub the kitchen floor and maybe clean out some of the cupboards. No, no, I won't work too hard. Don't worry about me. I'll call you at work if I need to.

What a beautiful day! I'm glad I have everything ready for the baby and all my things in order too. I wonder if we're going to have a boy or a girl? Not that it matters. The important thing is that the baby be okay. I wonder how Mary felt, knowing her baby was a boy before He was born. Now I'm *great with child*[9] like she was. I'm proud of that. I've really got quite a profile! I like to look at it in the mirror and imagine how my baby is curled up in me. Sometimes I'd like to walk up and down the street so everyone can see how big I am.

God's ways are really something! The mighty God, Creator of the universe, Lord of lords and King of kings chose to enter the world of human beings in the same way as my baby. His "travel plans" led Him through the "canal zone," the birth canal of a woman like me. And we celebrate childbirth one whole month out of every twelve! "Birth" is the most important experience of the Christian life. Jesus entered our world through a woman like me to lead us back with Him to God in a "new" birth, born of God's Spirit. Birthing really is a "blessed event" for Christians....

I'm tired of trying to time contractions. My uterus has been contracting periodically all through my pregnancy to be in good tone for the birth, but this last week the contractions seem to start and stop any time of the day or night without reason. It's funny though, that I haven't had many contractions today.

My back aches from scrubbing the floor. This pelvic rock on my hands and knees feels good, especially across my sacrum. But it's funny how the back-ache seems to come and go. There it is again. Could this mean, Lord, that my labor is really starting? Please help me know.

Honey? I think I might be starting labor! No, you needn't come yet, but please don't go very far away from the phone. I don't really know yet, but there's this pressure low in my back every once in a while. Here it comes again. No, I gave up trying to time contractions. They haven't seemed as strong today. Okay, I'll try again to time them and then I'll call you back.

I'm glad we bought this rocking chair. It's so comfortable. Maybe if I rock quietly for a while, God will give me the inner assurance that I'm really in labor. This footstool is just the right height to rest my feet on too, my knees falling outward. I'll keep my hands on my abdomen so I can feel any contractions while I relax.

Hey! My uterus is hard as a rock! I didn't even know it was contracting! It's different from the Braxton-Hicks contractions that rise up, upward. And there's that funny pressure low in my back again. What time is it?... There it is again. There's a dull pressure low in front too.

I'd better think through the keys to comfortable labor once more. I'm to totally release all tension in my muscles during every contraction, especially keeping the abdominal muscles loose. My back is to be rounded during contractions, whether I'm lying down, sitting down or standing up, like a parenthesis: (. I'm to breathe deeply into my lower diaphragm, especially during contractions, in deep, slow "sleep" breaths during early labor, and deep "work" breaths during late labor, each breath raising the abdomen off the uterus. Between contractions it's good to be moving, walking or rocking, in an upright position. But I can lie down whenever I'm tired, curling up in fetal position with my back rounded. I can relax more completely when I lie down, relaxing even my face, letting my eyelids droop, my mind drifting off into reverie so that even my brain waves are slowing down....

Honey? Yes, you'd better come now. I'm pretty sure I'm in labor. The last time I was in the bathroom there was a little mucus, and the contractions are about every twenty minutes. I know it may be a long time yet, but I'd feel better if you were with me. I'm so happy! Praise the Lord! I'm going to hurry and finish the baking and the cupboards, now that something's finally happening. Yes, I'll be careful. I won't do too much. But there are all these little things I want to hurry and finish....

Early labor

How I thank You, Lord, for my praying husband. It was such a comfort to have his arm around my shoulders, his hand on my abdomen over the baby while he prayed. Help me remember and treasure his words always: "Father, thank You for this day and its beautiful prospect of the appearance of our child. Thank You for Your promise to bring my wife *safely through childbirth.*[10] I claim that promise, Lord, both for her and for my child. Let it be a smooth, gentle, happy labor.[11] In Jesus' name." Then together we said, *This is the day that the Lord has made. We will rejoice and be glad in it.*[12] Amen!

Now that I'm really in labor, I'm going to trust You, Lord, to make me sensitive to the gentle promptings of my working body. I can do anything I like: eat when I'm hungry, walk or rock or do small tasks, or lie down and sleep. Right now I'm hungry. Let's see. I can have soft or liquid foods, juice, honey, cottage cheese, herb tea, yogurt or things like that. This will help keep my blood sugar normal because my body is working hard and needs energy. I think I'll have a little yogurt and honey....

I can drink all the fluids I want to keep from becoming dehydrated, but I need to remember to empty my bladder often. The contractions have already prompted my bowels to move, twice now. I'm glad for that. If I had let myself get constipated I'd need to give myself an enema, but now it isn't necessary.[13]

Can we go for a walk, Honey? I'm restless. Walking is supposed to stimulate the labor and help move the baby down into good position for the birth. We needn't walk far.

I'm nature's child, am I not? All around us *the earth brings forth grass, the herb yields seed after its kind, and the tree yields fruit, whose seed is in itself, after its kind.*[14] Wait a minute, Honey. Here's a contraction! Hold me so I can lean against you and relax until it passes.... There. Thank you. No, we needn't go back yet. The world has never seemed more beautiful, alive. See those flowers, opening to the sun....

It feels good to lie down. I hope I can go to sleep. I'm glad I've learned to relax on my left side, curled up almost like my baby, my body nestling around his. Roll the pillow a little higher under my right knee. Honey. There, that's better. The more completely I can release all my muscles, the more easily my uterus can pull the cervical muscles up over my baby's head.

Why don't you get a sandwich, Honey? But hurry right back. You can lie down close to me after you eat and doze a while too. You look tired. Don't worry about me. My body will wake me when labor becomes more active.

Help me slow down my breathing, Lord, deep and slow, abdomen rising and falling, deep and slow. Help me fall asleep.[15] *The Lord is my keeper. He who keeps me will not slumber. He who keeps me will neither slumber nor sleep.*[16] I'm releasing my whole weight into Your strong hands, Jesus. You hold the whole world in Your hand, and I am only a feather weight to You. Abdomen, release. Sag onto the bed. Arms, release, elbows, wrists, fingers. There. I can feel the tension in my neck and shoulders leaving, my inner thighs releasing tension, my knees, ankles. I'm letting go, and letting God.... Lower back, release. Perineum, relax.

I'm like a feather floating, resting on the soft air. Eyelids, fall closed.... Sigh....

Active labor

I'm thirsty. No, I'll get it myself. I'm tired of lying in bed. Only three centimeters dilated, after all these hours! I can't believe it. Well, praise the Lord anyway. At least I'm rested. Maybe if I rocked in the rocking chair labor would speed up. How long has it been since I started labor? Yesterday? A year ago? Only this morning? It seems like forever! No, no, I'm comfortable. But I just can't wait to see my baby!

It feels good to be rocking, doing something. I know the constant motion helps increase circulation to my uterus and the baby. Here's another contraction. Pull the stool more under my feet, Honey, so I can release the muscles of my legs and feet better. There. Lean forward, relax my arms on the chair arms, let eyelids droop, breathe slow, deep....

I'm glad my uterus doesn't force my baby's head through the cervix. Maybe baby wouldn't want to go! My neighbor tries to ram her son's head through the neck of his sweater when she pulls it on. No wonder he yells! My womb won't do that to my baby. Gently, gently, it draws the cervix up into itself. Gently, gently, it eases my baby's head through. The more I relax, the more gentle and pleasurable labor is for my baby.

There's another one—lean over—deep breath—relax abdomen—. In my mind's eye I can see how my womb is massaging you, baby dear. Every contraction stimulates your skin, caressing, stroking, comforting your little body and giving you more oxygen, protecting your brain from harm. It is a labor of love, my darling. I have held you in the nest of my body all these long months. How could I let you go too quickly? There is no hurry. With every contraction I am loving you, easing you along your way to the light.

I once heard that there is a Jewish prayer which says God made our bodies full of tubes and openings, and that any wrong opening, or a blockage in any tube causes trouble.[17] How true that is! The circulatory, digestive, reproductive and nervous systems are all hollow tubes. Even our bones are hollow, full of marrow where red blood cells are made. And the muscles of my hollow uterus (full of baby now!) are smooth muscles, like the other internal muscles of my body: my lungs, stomach, blood vessels, intestines. All these smooth internal muscles contract, relax, contract, relax, contract, relax. When they contract, they push their contents on. When they relax, the waste products of their muscles are carried away and their oxygen replenished. Then they contract again. When my uterus contracts it is carrying out its normal function, and there is no more pain than when my stomach contracts—unless there is some blockage, some resistance.

I'm glad I know that pain in labor comes from the skeletal muscles which are **outside** my uterus. If these skeletal muscles tighten up, they press against the contracting uterus and that might hurt. But the pain would be in these **outer** muscles, and I would be causing my own pain. I wonder what would happen if I tightened my abdomen during the next contraction? I'll have to wait for the next one. Here it comes. Tighten, tighten up. Ouch! Let go! Honey, help me relax! Honey! Oh, whew, there. It's over, I sure won't try that again![18] I had no idea tightening my abdomen would make such a difference. No wonder women complain who haven't been taught to relax!

Yes, maybe I'll lie down again. Help me relax. That got me all keyed up and now it's hard to release tension again. Deep breath. Release back muscles. Arms, release tension. Legs,... Slow, deep breath. Abdomen, release.... There, that's better.

Um-m-m, that feels good, Honey. Lord, help me always to remember these loving caresses of my husband during labor, how he strokes the muscles of my arms and legs gently downward to help them relax.[19] Help me remember his gentle caressing of my lower abdomen to help the muscles release. I'm sure he's praying for our baby as he does that. How warm and strong his hand feels on my lower back! And his loving caresses on my ear lobes, throat, breasts, nipples, all stimulate my hormones to "let down" my baby, as a mother "lets down" her milk. *His left hand is under my head, and his right hand is embracing me.*[20] I am leaning on my beloved, under the "apple tree" of the hormones of love. The place of conception—in his arms, is the place of birthing—in his arms.[21] In his loving caresses of my body he seeks nothing for himself. It's all for me, and I'm resting in his love, releasing my baby, letting go....

What a nice, big contraction this is, hard and firm under my fingers. Oh, praise the Lord, this is a good one! Easy now, breathe easy, keep the tummy muscles relaxed. That was a big hug for you, baby dear!

Oh! What's that! Water all over the bed? That really startled me for a minute. It's okay. I'm glad. But let me get up and go change. I'd better go to the bathroom again too. Let me lean on you, Honey, on the way to the bathroom. I'm so relaxed I can hardly stand up. But it feels good to stand up for a change. I'll lie down again in a minute....

I need to be propped up more. I'm supposed to be at least at a 60° angle. Better put an extra pad on the bed under me. I'm still leaking. Don't take the pillows away! I need them under my knees, so I can keep my legs relaxed. I need more pillows under my arms too, so I can stay limp as a wet noodle during contractions even when you're not holding me.

Only six centimeters dilated?[22] Well, that's okay. I'm comfortable, and time doesn't really matter. What a beautiful tree that is outside the window, an old, old tree, there before I was born. Maybe it was there before my mother was born, or even before my grandmother. Maybe it will still be there when my grandchildren are born. *This is the day the Lord has made. We will be glad and rejoice in it.*[23] Time, what does it matter? *One day is with the Lord as a thousand years, and a thousand years as one day.*[24] This is a beautiful time for me, no matter how long my labor may be.

I have a gift to give today—my husband's child.
I've cherished it and nourished it
These many months with my own strength.
Today I give it to the world.
May not indifferent hands, or even kindly hands
Shut me out and take it from me!
My own gift will I bring
In reverent awe and love.

If my strength falters,
My husband's love will give new courage.
He is here to share the moment
Our love-child bursts forth
In fresh, sweet purity.
All the eons of eternity will not
Erase this new life which God has made,
And let us share the making.

"She acts," I heard some say,
"As though none else had ever had a baby!"
How right they are!
No one else has ever borne this child.
It is our own unique gift to the universe,

The living symbol of our faith
In the dignity of life, the destiny of man,
And the reality of an eternal, living God.

Mary also gave a Gift one day.
How little did she know
The greatness of the Gift she brought!
And to her Gift, our Savior,
We offer ours, and pray that through His grace
This child may too bring light, and faith, and hope
To suffering humanity.

Glory to God in the highest, the highest, to God in the highest, and on earth peace, and on earth peace, ... [25] Mary didn't know the angels were watching, all heaven waiting, waiting to burst into song the moment her labor ended and the babe appeared! But she must have thought about the angel Gabriel as she labored, remembering his words. Jesus, I sense Your presence here. Are angels here too? Is my little one's angel already *beholding the face of the Father in heaven*[26] for his every need? The angels' song keeps ringing in my mind, *Glory to God in the highest, the highest*....

Transition[27]

Help me get up again, Honey. Maybe if I got on my hands and knees my back would feel better. Sag, up, sag, up, oh, this pelvic rock feels good across my back! Keep massaging across the sacrum, Honey. I can feel the pressure of the baby through my whole pelvic area. It's comfortable to let my uterus "hang loose" during the contraction. There, it's over. Sag, up, sag, up. All right, I'll get up now. Let me go to the bathroom before I get back in bed....

What tremendous power my uterus has! It's as if my whole body were curled around it, every ounce of energy drawn into this mountainous contraction. It's exciting, Lord! Help me relax and breathe through it, riding the crest with the exhilaration of a surf-boarder. Deep breath, hold, in-and-out-breaths on top, abdomen high and relaxed. There. Whew! Remind me to take cleansing breaths, Honey. I keep forgetting.

My baby is the center of each great wave, my body encircling his, my husband's arms encircling me. The warm pressure of his left hand on my sacrum is like leaning against a big rock, his right hand massaging my lower abdomen gently, a safe boundary to release the muscles against. And all three of us hovered over by Jesus. Here's another wave. Deep breath, hold, in-and-out, keep on top, in-and-out, there. A-whew! That was a good one! Praise the Lord!

God has made everything beautiful in its time.[28] Don't distract me. I want to be totally part of what my body is doing, feel the pressure of my baby's head on my back, feel my body opening down below, ride with awe these waves of power rising in my abdomen. I see You here with me, Jesus. Are You not my Savior? Healer? Comforter? I trust You, Lord, I'm resting my hard-working body on Your strength. Thank You for the wonderful way my body is doing its job, Lord. I praise You! I worship You!

It's getting hard to relax and I half want to push. Prop me higher. There, that's better, Here comes another one, help me grab my knees. Deep breath, hold, **lean** on it. Don't push! Don't push! Who's saying that? The voice is so far away. There. A-whew!... Rest.

I can feel the baby coming down! Now I can push.[29] Oh, this feels so much better!

Birth[30]

We made it, Lord! past the hardest time of waiting, waiting, riding the waves of contractions, letting them carry me where they would without getting frightened and resisting them. Now the quiet, resting times between contractions come, the waves of contractions coming farther apart. Now I can **do** something with each wave. Waiting was the hardest part. *They that wait upon the Lord shall renew their strength. They shall mount up with wings....*[31] Honey, one's starting. Hold me! Cleansing breath, deep breath, hold—keep mouth open—lean over, push down on top of uterus, bear down easy, easy, another breath, mouth open, there....

Oh, I feel so much better! My backache is gone. The stress across the pelvic bone is gone. I can feel my baby now, opening the door of my body. Remind me to keep my Kegel muscle relaxed, opening the "baby door." I'm glad to know it won't hurt, except for a little burning when it first starts to stretch open. Then the pressure of baby's head will provide nature's anesthesia. I have to give the perineum time to dilate, like the cervix, only it won't take as long. Amazing that it's so elastic, an 8 to 1 stretch ration!—opening wide to release my darling.

Hold me closer, Honey, so I can lean back against you. Your legs around my legs are so warm, your arms around my arms so strong, your breast as gentle massage against my back as you breathe, your voice like a soft breeze in my ear. Here it comes —hold me—cleansing breath, deep beath, push down on upper abdomen, mouth open, breathe, push, no strain, easy, breathe, push. A-whew! What's that awful noise? Was that **my** voice? It sounds funny when I leave my mouth open while I push doesn't it? But when my mouth is open, I open up more below too.

My whole body's full of baby, loaded with baby, my vagina stroking him like loving hands, massaging his skin, compressing his chest. I'm like a flower in God's garden, the petals unfolding to reveal its treasure. My baby! It's pressing on the rectum, the head is coming. I feel the burning—it's okay, the baby door has to open, stretch.... There! The burning's gone. Baby must have crowned. Black hair? Can I see? Please, get me a mirror.

Those warm, wet compresses on my perineum feel good, help it relax. Easy does it. I won't push. A-whew, a-whew, softly, softly, blowing out, pausing breaths, easy, breathe the baby out. Honey, I'm releasing this baby into your hands, all my secrets open to you. I'm not ashamed. *Naked, and not ashamed.*[32] *God has made everything beautiful,...* even the flower of my body, opening, opening, releasing its treasure into my lover's hands.

Oh! What a sweet voice! My baby! Let me see! I won't push, a-whew, a-whew, softly, breathe softly. I can feel him turning, the shoulder emerging, the swish of the little body turning. Oh, let me do it! My hands under baby's arms! Soft, warm, wet skin under my fingers as you emerge from my body, you little darling! You're looking right at me! Honey, see! Isn't she beautiful? Why, you're crying too, Honey!

Birth

Laboring to prepare for new life.
A peak. A push. A peek.
An unbelievably beautiful
    miracle unfolding.
Awake. Aware. Alive!
Ecstasy in sharing together
    our new creation.

Tears.
Touching.
Thanksgiving.[33]

After birth[34]

I love you, little one, snuggled against my breast. Daddy did a good job of tying and cutting the cord, severing you from me, taking on his share of responsibility now. God has made us a family! Some day I'll tell you how Daddy was the first to touch you, his touch a benediction of grace from the Lord, and then your body was born into my hands.

Pray, Honey. Pray and give thanks to God. Hand me a tissue first. I'm so happy I can't stop crying....

NOTES
1. Gen. 21:1-6. **2.** Gen. 30:23, 24 RSV. **3.** Gen. 29:35.
4. Surprisingly, women with the most negative memories of birth often are those who had the most medication. Women under sedation are not relaxed, but thrash around in a great deal of pain.
5. The medical term for pre-labor contractions is "Braxton-Hicks." These contractions help uterine muscles keep in good tone for labor, begin thinning out the cervix and provide beneficial stimulation to the baby.
6. Ps. 31:15. **7.** Rev. 5:10. **8.** Isa. 20:11. **9.** Lk. 2:5. **10.** 1 Tim. 2:15.
11. Those who pray for a short, fast labor reflect a negative "get it over with" attitude toward birth. This ignores the fact that the process of labor can be a positive experience for the mother, and ignores the benefits of the labor process to the infant's neurological ability to adapt to survival outside the womb.
12. Ps. 118:24.
13. Early labor contractions often stimulate the bowels to empty and may even cause some diarrhea. If the woman is constipated (as she may be if she has been taking iron), she should give herself an enema in early labor. Hard, compacted fecal matter in the lower bowel obstructs the descent of the baby and can cause much discomfort during late labor and the birth.
14. Gen. 1:12.
15. Those not planning a home birth should wait until they are in the place of birth before falling asleep during labor. Labor moves right along when the mother is fully relaxed and/or asleep. Her body will wake her naturally as she nears transition.

However, if a woman has been given medication, she will need to stay awake in order to stay in control of her contractions. A drugged woman tends to fall asleep **between** contractions, and then awaken tense and out of control at the height of a contraction, unable to relax or get control of her breathing.

16. Ps. 121:5, 3, 4. This thought is mirrored in one of the **Morning Prayers for Shabbath and Shabbath Rosh Chodesh.** Tel Aviv. Sinai Publishing. Pp. 10, 11.

". . . One only God with none second to compare, nor to equal him. He is without beginning and without end, and his alone is the power and dominion. He is my God; my living Redeemer, my sheltering Rock in time of woe. He is my banner, my refuge, a cup of solace when I call upon him. Into his hands do I resign my spirit, asleep or awake; and with my spirit my moral frame also; God is with me and I will not fear."

17. Morning Prayers for Shabbath. Op. cit. P. 11.

"Blessed art thou, Eternal, our God! King of the Universe, who hath formed man in wisdom, and created in him apertures and tubes of various kinds. It is revealed and manifestly known before thy glorious throne, that if but one of them be opened, or stopped, it would be impossible to exist, or to abide in thy presence. Blessed art thou, O Eternal! who healest all flesh and workest wonderfully.

18. I tried tensing my abdomen during a contraction in my third natural birth (sixth labor). I had forgotten how much a contraction can hurt when the abdomen is not relaxed!

19. The presence of the husband provides more than emotional support. His presence is also a stimulus to the hormonal system of her body, for the expulsive contractions of childbirth parallel the expulsive contractions of woman's orgasm in coitus. Not only that, but the reassuring presence and care of the husband help the wife relax so that the cervix and perineum relax, opening the door to let the baby out, just as the female hormones helped relax these organs to let the husband's penis and sperm in.

Uterine inertia can be stimulated by the husband caressing the breasts and nipples. This should be done only if the wife desires it. If the couple has learned good touch communication in love-making, the wife can guide her husband in the touch communication she desires during labor.

Just as the touch of the baby against the breast after birth stimulates the uterus to contract, so the husband's touch during labor stimulates the uterus into more efficient action. In a study conducted in Israel, an attempt was made to induce labor in 300 women by use of a breast pump, operated by the mother. The electrical device was held in place for five minutes on one breast, then on the other, and back and forth for 30 minutes, then a five minute rest before continuing the treatment. The overall success rate was 74.6%. Reported in **Harefuah,** the Journal of the Israel Medical Association, Vol. 87, #2. July 15, 1974. P. 102.

The difficulty with artificial induction of labor either by such devices or by oxytocin derivatives is that this does not relax the cervix. Contractions are stronger, but there is no balancing "let down" stimulation of the cervical tissues which the comforting, relaxing hormonal stimulation of the husband's presence and caresses would also provide.

20. S. of S. 8:3. **21.** S. of S. 8:5.

22. The longest phase of labor is from its onset until the cervix has thinned out and is about 4 centimeters dilated (about the width of two fingers). A relaxed woman should have little or no discomfort during labor until at least 6 centimeters, needing only companionship and reassurance.

From 6 centimeters on labor progresses much more rapidly to full dilation (10 centimeters or about the width of five fingers). A woman may be surprised by the intensity of the contractions during this period, and the husband has a much more active role keeping his wife relaxed and unafraid.

During contractions the woman must be in a rounded, totally relaxed position. For backache, pelvic rocking on her hands and knees helps, the abdomen hanging loose. This position is especially advantageous if the baby is breech or posterior. It may even help to rotate the baby into a better position for the birth.

23. Ps. 118:24. **24.** 2 Pet. 3:8.
25. Lk. 2:14. Luke 15:10-angels rejoice at a "new birth" too!
26. Mt. 18:10.
27. During transition all unnecessary talking should cease except for murmured words of praise and encouragement. The husband should repeat any instructions in his wife's ear from now on through the birth, as she will be less responsive to anyone else. She may seem absorbed in herself, her task, her Lord, perhaps praying softly under her breath. Those assisting her should make sure her body is totally supported at all times so there is no muscle tension anywhere in her body.
28. Ecc. 3:11.
29. Elizabeth Noble advocates a slow steady exhalation, the lips pursed as in trumpet blowing, the throat open in sustained soft moaning or groaning as the air moves through. The **upper** abdominal muscles are to be contracted, the mother slumped over, leaning on the air in the lungs above the diaphragm. The face is to be kept relaxed, eyes and mouth open, exhaling slowly and continuously while bearing down. She can inhale as necessary and continue. The open mouth and throat help keep the birth outlet open and relaxed also. See Elizabeth Noble. **Essential Exercises for the Childbearing Year.** Boston. Houghton Mifflin. 1976.
30. As baby moves down the vagina the smallest circumference of his head appears first (where the "cow's lick" grows). As his head is born it turns to the side, so that he faces his mother's inner thigh. Now the wide shoulders can come through the narrow passage sideways, one at a time. Our Lord thinks of everything!

As the body is born the baby continues rotating until he is facing his mother. She can reach down under his arms and lift him to herself, looking right into baby's eyes.
31. Is. 40:31. **32.** Gen. 2:25.
33. Mary Rodning. Printed by permission.
34. If no episiotomy has been done, the tight perineum compresses the baby's chest so that as the body emerges, mucus pops out of his nose and throat with the sudden release of pressure, like a cork out of a bottle.

When an episiotomy has been performed, the infant more often needs the excess mucus in his nose and throat suctioned out by the attendant.

The mother often experiences chills after the birth because of the loss of body fluid. She must be kept warmly covered even before the afterbirth comes (each leg covered separately). Baby at the breast stimulates the uterus to contract and expel the afterbirth, and she can also gently massage her own abdomen to keep the uterus firm under her touch.

The mother often feels exhilarated and hungry after the birth. This exhilaration is an important part of the birth process, quickly stimulating the whole body back to good functioning.

The Way of Wisdom

Where shall wisdom be found? Where is the place of understanding? Man does not know its price, nor can it be found in the land of the living. Gold and silver cannot equal it, nor sapphires, corals nor pearls. Its price is far above rubies.

From where then does wisdom come? and where is the place of understanding? God understands the way of wisdom, and to man he says, "Behold, the fear of the Lord, that is wisdom."[1]

In that night God appeared to Solomon and said to him, "Ask me what you want me to give to you."
And Solomon said to God, "... Give me now wisdom and knowledge, that I may discern between good and bad."[2]

If any of you lacks wisdom, let him ask God, who gives generously to all men without reproaching, and it will be given him. But let him ask in faith, with no doubting, for he who doubts is like a wave of the sea that is driven and tossed by the wind.[3]

Childbirth is one of the most powerful spiritual experiences of life, one in which those present at the birth often become aware of the presence of the Creator. It is a holy time, and the rightful place of birth, a sanctuary. A former radical, who turned to faith in Jesus Christ, says:

The most powerful, single breakthrough, in my Communist-held position, was the birth of my children.

For me, each one was sort of a cosmic, spiritual event. A miracle... first, Macea, and then my daughter. I didn't come out of the Marxist philosophy all at once. But this crack appeared like a breach in the wall—and the crack which never closed was the affirmation of life that gripped me at my children's birth and kept saying to me: here is a soul, here is a link in the chain of life.[4]

Childbirth is not only a spiritual experience, but it can also be a beautiful, rewarding physical experience when the woman has learned to give birth in harmony with God's natural law. It can in truth be said that normal, physiological childbirth is not painful.[5]

God has created our world with orderly, consistent and beneficial natural laws. When these natural laws are flouted, serious consequences follow. We do not discard the laws of good nutrition because some people are malnourished and others refuse to eat properly. We do not scoff at the necessity of rest, exercise and good hygiene because some people get sick. Neither can we invalidate the principles of painless childbirth in harmony with natural law because many women suffer due to ignorance, or because difficulties occur to a small percentage in every species.

In childbirth, when God's orderly, consistent, beneficial natural law is violated at any point during the process of labor or birth, serious consequences may follow, one of which is pain.

The importance of pain

If childbirth is not meant to be painful, then we have to ask the question, "What causes the pain?" For some women have suffered great pain. But first we must ask the question, "What is pain, and what physiological purpose does it serve?"

Pain is something which "hurts." The physiological purpose of "hurting" is to warn that something is **out of harmony with nature.** Pain is an important, efficient, life-preserving signal that something is wrong. If we touch a hot stove with our finger, the pain signal warns us to take it off. The body reacts even before we consciously think about it. Limbs can be seriously burned or injured in diseases such as leprosy where the pain signal is absent.

Pain in labor is one of the most efficient diagnostic tools available to alert attendants to a problem, warning them that something is out of tune with the natural processes. Yet in our society pain in childbirth is considered to be a "normal" part of the process! Its usefulness as a diagnostic tool is ignored.

There are several major causes of pain in childbirth. The first is **physiological**. In a small percentage of births there will be disproportion (baby too large for the mother's bony pelvis) or malpresentation (wrong part of the baby's body coming first). Other physiological problems that might occur are toxemia, some disease such as diabetes, poor health, fatigue, laceration of tissues, dehydration or any other unnatural physical conditions. Pain may be one of the earliest indications that medical attention is needed.

A brilliant young friend of mine entered childbirth confidently, looking forward to a comfortable birth. Labor progressed well at first, but as it advanced, pain began and gradually increased in intensity. Nothing she could do controlled the pain, nor could her husband help her. It was impossible to relax, for the pain was too great. Hours and hours went by on into the next day, hospital attendants and the doctor coming in and out while she was literally torn apart with agony, screaming for help, but none came. The medications administered were ineffective.

Finally a cesarean was performed and then the doctor apologized, saying that the baby's head was too large for him to have been born normally! The mother had been traumatized by suffering long hours of unbearable pain, even though her body had been efficiently proclaiming all along that there was a problem. Pain was ignored as a diagnostic tool by her birth attendants, because it has come to be expected during birth in our society.

There are three **functional** causes of pain in labor, the first two directly brought on by the woman's negative emotional state: incomplete muscular relaxation and improper breathing. The third functional cause is the improper physiological position of the mother for labor and/or birth.

The uterus itself has few pain receptors, but is smooth muscle like the rest of the body's internal organs, the stomach, heart, lungs, etc. Contractions are not actually felt in the uterus, but in the pressure of the uterus **against the surrounding muscle tissues** of the abdomen, back and pelvic area. These surrounding muscle tissues are liberally supplied with pain receptors. If the contraction causes pain, it is because these muscles are tightening across the uterus and **resisting** its rise in the abdomen. Thus the uterine muscles must work even harder to overcome the outer resistance, and pain increases. This outer muscle tension interferes with the normal circulation of oxygen and the carrying away of waste products, not only in the tense muscles but also in the uterus. Abdominal pain due to tension is a signal that the uterus and baby are not receiving enough oxygen.

The remedy is to concentrate on **releasing** all muscle tension in the abdomen, lower back and pelvic area. The more the mother consciously "lets go" the muscle tension in these areas, the better she will feel, and the more smoothly and rapidly will the birth proceed.

Improper breathing contributes to muscle tension. The rapid, shallow breathing of a nervous, frightened woman not only causes a lack of oxygen to the uterus and baby, but causes toxicity and pain in all the skeletal muscles. Ask such a woman where she hurts and she will likely reply, "All over." This is not exaggeration. Her head aches, her neck hurts, her legs may be cramping, even the muscles of her hands may be aching from gripping the sides of the bed.

The third functional cause for unnecessary pain in labor is the improper position of the woman. A woman in labor must never be kept flat on her back with her legs out straight. This position inhibits the blood flow to the uterus and baby by as much as 20 per cent. And it is impossible to relax the abdominal and back muscles adequately in this position. It also causes the uterus to work harder, against the laws of gravity.

In all stages of labor when the mother is at rest her back should be rounded like a parenthesis: (. Whether she is lying on her side or in a semi-sitting position, every joint should be flexed —neck, elbows, wrists, hips, knees, etc.—because this shortens and relaxes the skeletal muscles, especially across the abdomen.

In early labor, when not sleeping or resting, the mother should be sitting in a rocking chair or walking around. This mild activity stimulates the uterus to work more efficiently and adds the benefits of gravity. If her waters have broken, this upright position helps engage the baby's head through the weight of gravity and helps avoid a prolapsed cord (cord coming through the cervix first and being compressed by baby's head). During contractions she can quickly lean over in the "parenthesis" curve, to completely relax the abdominal muscles.

If she is in bed, she should be propped to at least 60 degrees for this same maximum gravity in late first and second stage, in a simulated squatting position. Every part of her body should be

fully supported. This nearly upright, rounded body position provides the best mechanical advantage for the birth.

Another unnecessary cause of pain in labor is **iatrogenic,** pain caused by procedures done to the mother by medical attendants. Enemas, blood tests, rectal or vaginal exams, the use of oxytocin, injections, or thoughtless words and actions on the part of attendants all contribute to discomfort.

Not only are these procedures uncomfortable, but they may disturb, frighten or make the laboring woman unhappy. This in turn activates her sympathetic nervous system, which disrupts the functional harmony of the birth process. The circular muscles of the cervix are linked to the sympathetic nervous system and thus are directly affected by the woman's emotional state. Even slight anxiety triggers adrenalin,[6] causes the heart to beat faster and blood pressure to rise. Relaxation is disrupted, breathing is faster and more shallow. Most serious of all, it causes the cervix to **tighten** and become resitant to dilatation! When the uterus has to work against a resistant cervix severe pain soon sets in, causing further cervical tightening. **Thus anything which disrupts the mother's peace, even to a slight degree, has a direct, negative physical effect on the progress of her labor.**

How many times other remedies, including cesareans, are applied because of a "resistant cervix," with no consideration given to its cause! The emphasis should be on keeping the mother relaxed and undisturbed so that the cervix will also relax and open and the birth proceed smoothly and comfortably to a healthy conclusion.

A false foundation

The belief that childbirth pain is normal is a false foundation upon which to build safe birth experiences. The medical answer to the expected pain is to try to relieve it with analgesics or anesthetics, although most physicians try to give only minimal amounts, hoping this will bring relief. They are aware that larger amounts may be harmful to mother or baby. If the "safe" amount of medication does not relieve pain, the mother just has to endure it.

But this medication sabotages the body's pain signals, just as we sabotage other pain signals by "popping pills." For a headache, we take aspirin; for an upset stomach, antacid; for constipation, a laxative; for sleeplessness, a sleeping pill; for childbirth pain, medication. We do not bother to discern the

causes of the headache or sleeplessness and change our way of living. Instead, we go on blotting out the signals with medication and eventually reap the consequences of impaired health. In the same way, medication for childbirth pain without diagnosing the **cause** (muscle tension, anxiety, wrong position, a serious physiological problem), sabotages nature's signal. When the cause of pain has been properly diagnosed, then the appropriate measures can be applied to relieve it.

There is mounting evidence that no obstetric medication is without negative effects on the newborn, whether given orally, by local injection, or by general anesthesia. This negative effect is directly dose-related and potency-related, with greater or lesser long-lasting effects.[7] During the first year of life the strongest effects are in gross motor abilities, learning to sit, stand, move around. The marginal brain damage also removes the normal "brakes" on the infant's behavior, so that he is less able to **stop** crying when comforted or to stop responding to distracting stimuli.

Marginal brain damage due to medication in labor may not be evident until the child is in school. Here it may be manifested in a short attention span, hyperactivity (no "brake" on behavior), and the inability to learn well. It is the development of the higher skills of language and other cognitive abilities that are the most affected.

Drugs during labor and delivery rapidly cross the placenta and easily reach the unborn child's brain, because the "barrier" that screens the human brain from many substances in the blood is not fully developed in the newborn. And once the drugs enter the baby's blood stream they are cleared away only slowly, for the newborn's liver and kidneys are not fully functioning at birth. The toxins remain in the newborn for hours and even days, continuing to cause damage.

A current popular approach to childbirth admits the dangers of medication, and proposes enlightened, scientific means to make childbirth painless. The difficulty is that this approach is based on the same false foundation of believing childbirth painful. It proposes to teach the woman how to **rise above** the pain so that she will not feel it, **distracting her** from the pain.

The principle of distraction assumes that childbirth is painful, thus denying the goodness of the Creator, so that one must mentally "escape" the pain of the contractions. In order to "escape," the woman is taught to focus her eyes on some object, or some spot in the room, and **concentrate** on carefully patterned breathing in the upper chest, keeping her mind off the abdomen and what is happening below. With the woman's attention distracted from the contracting uterus, her labor becomes "painless."

The prefix "dis-" is a negative one, associated with words like dis-ease, dis-appointment, dis-like. It brings a negative word into an experience which should be a positive one of praise and peace. Distraction techniques are not natural, physiological childbirth, although they do decrease the need for medication.

When the mother is distracted so that she does not "feel" the pain in the abdomen, her labor is still being inhibited and the baby failing to receive adequate oxygen. For just as medication fails to relax the abdominal and cervical muscles, so "distraction" leaves them unrelaxed. It is impossible to release abdominal muscle tension enough to reach a natural, lower plateau of brain-wave activity, with the eyes focused and the mind working at "concentrated" breathing. Concentration implies greater brain activity, which increases residual tension throughout the body.[8]

The muscles of the woman's eyelids should be relaxed so that they are drooping, closed or almost closed (not squeezed shut), her eyes unfocused, her mouth relaxed and open, her abdomen relaxed, her perineum relaxed. This does not "distract" from pain, but prevents pain from occuring in the first place. If she needs a little guidance in her breathing during contractions, an attendant can guide her breathing by breathing with her. She can easily hear and follow the guided breathing with her eyes remaining relaxed and closed.

A more serious objection to these distraction techniques is that focusing one's eyes on an object while concentrating on a rhythmical activity (such as breathing) is one of the ways in which hypnotism may be induced. An obstetrician who sometimes uses hypnotism in therapy for disturbed gynecological patients pointed this out to me. (I am not condoning his use of hypnotism! It appears to be forbidden in Scripture.[9]) It is true that a temporary distraction will prevent one from feeling pain in another part of the body. A momentary distraction is not hypnotism. But the technique as often taught can lead toward a hypnotic state when continued for any length of time. This is something conscientious Christians will want to avoid.

It cannot be stressed strongly enough how important it is to diagnose correctly the **cause** of a woman's pain in labor, rather than resorting either to medication or to distraction techniques. Ignoring pain in labor by blotting it out with medication or distracting the woman's attention from it is like silencing a ringing phone without answering it to see **why** it is ringing.

Is the pain beginning to occur because the mother is being disturbed too often? Is she alarmed by something? Is she breathing normally, her abdomen, back and pelvic muscles well relaxed? Is she in a comfortable, correct physiological position? During contractions the woman should be in a rounded, relaxed position, the abdomen loose. If she is walking, she can rest her arms and head on the back of a chair, or mantle, or lean against her husband, closing her eyes and letting the abdomen hang limply forward. If sitting, she can rest her head and arms on a table about chest height to keep her knees and inner thighs relaxed, her muscles relaxed all the way up through the perineum and abdomen, her eyelids relaxed and her mouth open.

If her breathing, relaxation, body position are all correct, the room quiet and her attendant affirming yet unobtrusive, and there is still pain, her attendants should be alert to a possible physiological problem which needs attention.

Women who have conscientiously learned natural relaxation and breathing patterns can look forward to a safe, comfortable, unmedicated birth with no need to "escape" through distraction. The mother in labor can place her trust in Jesus, the divine Deliverer, resting as if in His arms, "letting go" and "letting God." She is trusting in a sure Foundation.

The obstetrics of fear

When a woman is admitted to the hospital in labor, the maternity staff goes into action according to custom. An enema is administered, the pelvic area shaved, blood tests taken, and pills and/or injections may be given for a variety of reasons. In addition, a fetal monitor may be attached to her and an intravenous needle inserted into her hand or arm. She may not be allowed food or liquids until after the baby is born, may be confined to her bed, and of course periodic vaginal or rectal checks will be made to determine the progress of her labor.

The difficulty is that all this can be upsetting even to a prepared woman, and it disrupts the smooth course of her labor from the very outset. Obstetrics in the United States has become defensive medicine, each routine procedure carried out "for fear that..." An enema is given (even when it is not necessary) **for fear of** contamination during the birth. Pubic hair is shaved **for**

fear that the hair might harbor germs. Labor is induced **for fear of** postmaturity, or **for fear that** the baby will not arrive at a convenient time (for mother or doctor), even though the Food and Drug Administration warns of the dangers of induced labor.[10]

Fetal monitors are used **for fear of** fetal distress that might not be recognized. The intravenous is inserted **for fear that** the mother might become dehydrated, in order to supply her with glucose or dextrose and water, or **for fear that** she might need a transfusion. Medications are given **for fear that** the mother might have pain without them. A cut is made in the perineum (the "episiotomy") **for fear that** the vaginal opening might tear. Forceps may be used **for fear that** the baby might come too slowly—or too fast. The placenta is forced out quickly **for fear that** hemorrhage might occur. The newborn is placed in a "warmer" heated by infrared radiation, rather than in the mother's arms, **for fear that** he might lose too much body heat.

Cesarean sections are now being performed in some hospitals as often as one out of every four or five labors,[11] **for fear that** the birth might not continue normally, or the baby might be injured by a vaginal delivery. It is insisted that birth must take place in the hospital **for fear that** complications might occur.

No sensible person would deny that the very best medical care should be available for every birthing woman. However, this **routine** intervention causes many more problems than it solves. For example, an epidural given for the mother's comfort can cause weak muscle tone in the newborn.[12] The fetal heart beat drops dangerously low just after a paracervical is given.[13] Placing a woman on her back for the attachment of monitors and intravenous needles decreases the flow of oxygen to the uterus and baby by as much as 20 per cent.[14] The cesarean newborn is more likely to suffer from premature birth, asphyxia, and respiratory distress syndrome,[15] and the mother must recover from this major surgery. The nation's pediatricians are now being warned by the American Academy of Pediatrics of the dangers to the newborn of radiation from the radiant warmers which may not appear until later, including eye diseases.[16] And of course, many of these interventions upset the mother and make her tense, giving rise to pain, slowing down the labor, reducing oxygen to the baby and risking brain damage.

Unhappy consequences may follow even when these medical techniques result in a healthy baby. Who can say how many couples have experienced marital problems because the wife has pain during coitus after having had an episiotomy? This complaint is made by 39 per cent of women who have undergone this surgical procedure.[17] As time passes, the pain may ease, only to recur again after menopause when the tissues are more fragile and there is less natural lubricant. The hard scar tissue does not stretch properly and again causes pain in coitus.

Though many doctors feel there are various medical reasons for the necessity of the routine episiotomy, there are non-medical reasons as well. One doctor's wife (who is also an obstetrical nurse) once was overheard saying that they disliked "all that waiting around" when no episiotomy was performed. Her husband preferred to get the birth over with and get home.

And what of the psychological after-effects of all these procedures? One time at a seminar a young woman with a healthy, beautiful six months old daughter approached me. Although she was successfully breastfeeding, she was still traumatized by the birth experience. She had been well trained, was relaxed throughout, breathing correctly and was comfortable, her labor proceeding slowly but at a steady pace. From the time she entered the hospital she was periodically threatened that if she didn't "hurry up," a cesarean would be performed because the baby was in a breech position.

Each time she pleaded that she was comfortable, enjoying her labor, and did not want the operation. All the signs of both mother and baby were stable. After twelve hours of labor she approached transition, still relaxed, comfortable and in full control. But over her protests she was wheeled away and the baby taken by cesarean, **for fear that** delaying any longer might lead to problems.

Now, six months later, she still could not shake off depression over the birth. We talked together about the need for the healing of this memory. First we prayed that God would help her forgive those who had wronged her, and then asked His grace in helping her forgive herself for not objecting more vigorously. We prayed that *no root of bitterness*[18] might be harbored in her mind toward those who had grieved her so deeply.

Then we looked at the grief itself, accepting the fact that she had been going through the normal stages of grief, even though her baby was all right. She had experienced that shock of being robbed of the birth experience that was rightfully hers, the disbelief that a good labor could be so arbitrarily terminated, the helpless anger of not being able to change what was being done to her without her consent. Depression followed and the recognition of loss. I assured her that it was all right to grieve, for something precious to her had been lost. Nonetheless, Jesus could lead her on to acceptance of what could not be changed, and to peace of heart. Later I received a long letter from her in which she said in part:

> *I have intended to write to you since last spring when you were such a help to me with my childbirth experience.... I unburdened myself to you and it was one important step in a long process of healing over the disappointment and trauma of a surgical childbirth.... Women in our area get far too much manipulation and technological intervention and no one is warning them that it isn't necessary (pitocin, breaking of waters, monitoring, etc.).... Every pregnant woman ought to consider the "what if's" and discuss them with her doctor or birth attendant and know her rights, that she doesn't have to have her birth experience manipulated if she chooses not to.*
>
> *...Thank you for being there to help when I really needed it. "Loving my baby real good" is helping me to heal also. What an absolute joy, thrill, fulfillment to have and nurse our baby. The miracle of creation is a constant reminder to me of God's love and presence. Praise the Lord for the wonder of life, for friends and their help.*[19]

This friend did not know that most physicians now insist on a cesarean for all breech babies, and that there are many medical students who are never taught how to vaginally deliver a baby that is in a breech position. Cesareans are sometimes also performed when babies are in the normal position if labor passes an arbitrarily set number of hours.

> *Whereas once the radical procedure of a Caesarean, which puts extra stress on the mother and baby, was reserved for specific medical conditions, now this operation is done frequently to spare the baby the "stress of labor." These (medical students) were told nothing about the massaging effects of normal, unstimulated contractions, or about the increased oxygenation of the placenta produced by normal, rhythmic contractions. Confirming the information that had been circulating for months, the students were told that 20 per cent of the deliveries in this*

hospital are now done by Caesarean section. One third of these are scheduled ahead of time, and the rest are unplanned. General anesthesia is used for approximately half of the Caesareans, and spinal anesthesia is used for approximately half. For a few the epidural is used, because the epidural had already been given and the Caesarean was unplanned.

One out of five pregnant women who walk through the doors of this hospital will undergo major surgery. At one of the smaller hospitals a nurse who worked there told me that because of the convictions of one man, the rate was approaching one out of four deliveries.[20]

In defense of doctors it must be said that many of these interventions in normal childbirth are due to consumer pressure. There are women who want to have "nothing to do" with the birth and ignorantly expect the doctor to "take care of everything." Consumer expectation often is that medication will take away any discomfort, and that labor can safely be induced any time it is convenient for mother and doctor. Women have requested forceps and even cesareans to "get me out of this," or "hurry up and get it over with."

Combined with this false concept by consumers is their false appraisal of the power of the doctor. If anything "goes wrong," it is assumed to be the doctor's fault, and the physician may be sued for malpractice. This has driven the doctors' insurance costs incredibly high, and has led them to intervene more often with cesareans, etc. **for fear that** they might be sued for malpractice if anything is wrong with the baby. Thus consumers as well as the medical profession share responsibility for promoting the obstetrics of fear.

Christian couples need to take a careful look at all the current obstetric procedures carried out in hospitals in their area, learn the pros and cons of each procedure, and seek the wisdom of the Lord Jesus in learning when to say "no thank you." They should not question the good motives of the health care provider, but should question the necessity of certain **routine** procedures. Is that "routine" necessary in every case?

If the birth is to take place in the hospital, the physician should be asked to prepare a **written** list of procedures ahead of time for the hospital, with a copy in his office and a copy in the couple's possession with his signature on it. This list could, for example, state no enema, no shaving, no Pitocin, no medications, no relaxant, no monitor, no intravenous, no epidural, no paracervical, no stirrups, no episiotomy, etc., without the doctor's **express** permission **at the time** he felt it was necessary. This will help protect the woman from unwanted procedures until the doctor arrives at the hospital. An attendant who insists on any of these procedures (including the doctor) should be able to fully explain and justify the reason to the couple. Even then, the woman's **consent** is required or the hospital can be found at fault.[21] If the couple have found a doctor with whom they have good rapport, they will be able to trust his judgment if he feels, at the time, that one of these procedures is necessary.

The privilege of standing by

The Christian husband and wife need further wisdom from the Lord in deciding where He wants the birth to take place, and what persons should be given the privilege of attending it. The woman who carries and gives birth to a child is not sick, nor suffering an injury, but is carrying out one of the most healthy, normal functions of the human body.

The role of the obstetrician is defined by his title, which in the Latin, **ob stare,** means "to stand by." Similarly, the term "midwife" means to be "with" the wife. Those who are given the privilege of being present at the birth are by definition there to encourage the mother in giving birth to her own child, standing by to give assistance if it should be needed.

Not only must a cooperative physician be found but also a hospital with policies compatible with the philosophy of unmedicated natural births. It is important to know both the policies concerning the mother and those concerning the husband and the newborn. For example, will the husband be allowed to stay with his wife throughout the labor and birth? Will baby be allowed to stay with his parents for the important bonding period in the first hour after the birth? Is rooming in available, with baby staying in mother's room? If not, will her baby be brought to her for breastfeeding whenever he is hungry? Will the nursery agree to give the baby no glucose and water before the mother's milk comes in? Some nurseries have even been known to give the infant (without the mother's knowledge or consent) a "whiskey nipple," 50cc's of whiskey in a nipple (about a teaspoonful) to keep the baby quiet. The "whiskey nipple"[22] came into use as a sedative for babies who were to undergo some unusual medical care, but it could be a temptation for nurses to also use it for restless babies who cried "too much." (Some hospitals prohibit the use of "whiskey nipples" because of possible liver damage to the babies.)

A joint position statement by five professional groups has been prepared, called **The Development of Family-Centered Maternity/Newborn Care in Hospitals.**[23] This position statement also has the endorsement of the American Hospital Association. It is valuable not only as a guide to parents looking for the right hospital, but also as a guide in helping hospitals re-evaluate their own policies.

Some hospitals have established "birthing rooms" in which the woman labors and delivers in the same bed, in the same room. She may be under the care of either a physician or a certified nurse-midwife.[24] The nurse-midwife is qualified to attend the delivery but has the back up services of a physician if this is needed. Nurse-midwives are gaining wide acceptance in medical facilities throughout the United States, and women who go to them are enthusiastic about the care they receive.

Birthing rooms are a vast improvement over the usual odyssey from home to labor room, to delivery room, to recovery room, to maternity ward. But even where hospital birthing rooms are available the woman may still be subject to the intervention of nurses, interns (especially in a teaching hospital) and others, who may not share the couples' views. In any hospital setting, the couple has the least control over who the actual attendants will be for most of the labor, for the physician often is called only when the birth is imminent.

Birthing centers are springing up across the country, removed from the hospital setting with its subtle atmosphere of sickness and injury, yet with more facilities for birthing than at home. Those who give birth at these centers usually go home within a day after birth. Birthing centers operate under physicians and certified nurse-midwives. These nurse-midwives have obstetric nursing experience and also graduate training in midwifery. They oversee the woman's care through the pregnancy and birth. If unforseen complications develop, the mother is transferred to a hospital and a physician's care.

Birthing centers often allow family members and friends to attend the births (depending on the couple's wishes). Their warm, home-like atmosphere brings enthusiastic responses like the following:[25]

My birth experience has proven to me that the single most important factor in a positive natural birth is to have people there who care about you. I did, and it made it the most rewarding, wonderful time of my life. Because I ended up at the hospital, I was unaware of some of their "policies" but I felt prepared to make independent decisions because of previous information given to me at the Birthplace. (mother)

I chose the walnut room, feeling closer to the generations of African women who birthed their babies in a natural setting. I felt reassured at the Birthplace and appreciated the constant support and comfort. (mother)

I was part of the scene. Many people seem to think fathers should be left out of the birth/mothering aspects. But not at Birthplace. (father)

The whole experience was astounding for me and my enthusiasm is unbounded. I learned a great deal that morning and am grateful to you for myself and for my children and grandchildren. (grandmother)

A job well done! (grandfather)

Thousands of responsible young couples are not choosing any of these options, but are having their babies at home. It is more difficult to find qualified attendants for a home birth. Physicians who attend births at home may suffer ostracism from other physicians and even risk losing hospital privileges. Certified nurse-midwives are often forbidden to attend home deliveries or are refused medical back-up if they do.

Of necessity this has led to the return of lay persons as birth attendants. Those who are actively involved in home births are called "lay midwives." In some states they can be licensed to attend the births, working under the supervision of a physician, in touch with him by phone. Many of them are well-trained[26] and competent, and their numbers are growing rapidly throughout the country.

Spiritual realities

It seems that there is still a tremendous spiritual conflict going on between Satan and the woman which centers around the birth of a child. For each battle overcome, a new problem appears! Now there is a peril new to Western culture. As natural childbirth and home births have become more accepted, spiritism has begun to make inroads into childbirth philosophies, *superstitions from the east, divination like the Philistines.*[27] The appearance of this danger has been so subtle it has scarcely been recognized by Christians, for too often they fail to realize that not everything "spiritual" is of God.[28]

Many "psychic" experiences are shadow images of the true gifts of the Holy Spirit of Jesus, our crucified and risen Savior, whose blood saves us. These counterfeit "religious" experiences include hypnotism, extra-sensory perception, clairvoyance, transcendental meditation, seances, levitation, ghost-writing, mind control, and other "out of the body" experiences.

The Bible teaches that we are like ignorant babes in a universe of spiritual realities and warns: "high voltage—keep out!" Satan parades not as a devil but as an angel of light, his false prophets *showing signs and wonders, to seduce, if possible, even the elect.*[29] Spiritualism and spiritism are not Christian, but are terms used by some who deny either the deity or humanity of Jesus Christ, or both, and deny the necessity of His blood to cleanse us from sin. The cross of Jesus Christ is the "lightning-rod" of safety for us, grounded in the Bible, the Word of God. Only Jesus Christ can lead us into deep, powerful, **safe** dimensions of spiritual power.

It is unwise to have a person present at the birth who *gives heed to deceitful spirits and doctrines of demons,*[30] or who *practices divination or sorcery, interprets omens, engages in witchcraft, or casts spells, or who is a medium or a spiritist who consults the dead.*[31] The Bible warns, *What fellowship has light with darkness? What communion has Christ with demons?*

Therefore come out from among them, and be separate from them, says the Lord, and touch nothing unclean, and I will receive you. I will be a Father to you, and you shall be my sons and daughters, says the Lord Almighty.

*Because we have these promises, beloved, let us cleanse ourselves from every defilement of body **and spirit**, and be completely holy in the fear of God.*[32]

In his book **The Power to Heal,** Francis MacNutt says that "in most nations and cultures—including the United States—there are witches or spiritualists who claim to curse and also to heal. . . .

> *I see no reason to deny that there is a power in spiritualism that works.... freedom from sickness can come through the same demonic force that originally imposed it.... My own experience leads me to a firm conviction in the reality of the demonic realm and of its power to curse and to heal. These powers are ultimately destructive and enslaving; it is important to recognize them, rather than to deny them, and to learn to apply the power of the Holy Spirit in healing, so that sick people will not be driven to seek help from an alien and dangerous source.*[33]

There are certain words that give early clue to someone's possible involvement in such things: karma, reincarnation, astrology, tea-reading, palm-reading, energy field around the body, energy blocks, mantra, mandala, hatha, yoga, polar energetics, life force, life creation, nirvana, rebirth, etc. (This "rebirth" is **not** what Christians mean by the new birth!)[34] The phrase "holistic" or "wholistic medicine" is popular with these practitioners, referring to the healing of the whole person, body, soul and spirit. Since this term is also being used by some Christians in medical practice, it is important to find out if what is meant is spiritually compatible with one's own faith.

We need to ask the Lord to give us discernment about such things, and to heed any inner warning He might give, such as an uneasiness in our spirit. It is necessary to look behind the "beautiful thought," the gentleness of many of those involved in various aspects of spiritism, the "peace" they radiate, for it is not the peace of the Holy Spirit. They are usually vegetarian, proponents of non-violence, and nice people. But they are trapped in spiritual deception.

Another precaution we need to make is to cleanse our environments of anything which might be an invitation to unclean spirits. **Nothing** should be in our homes, our churches, or our places of giving birth which is symbolic of the demonic realm. This includes pictures and toys of things like snakes, owls, frogs, dragons, etc. Snakes and dragons are symbols of Satan in the Bible. Frogs are associated with unclean spirits.[35] Owls are among the unclean birds and animals associated with the haunts of demons.[36]

Owls are considered an evil omen in many primitive cultures. In Shakespeare's story of Julius Caesar, an owl is hooting in the middle of the day as an omen of Caesar's impending death. The primitive Navajo Indians linked sickness to the presence of owls. It is said of an Indonesian tribe that:

> *"The basis of their religion is the messages they receive from birds at night."*...
> *"What kind of birds," I asked.*
> *"The owl," he replied. "The owls not only tell them when a visitor is coming, but whether or not he has been there before, and whether or not his intentions are good or bad."*[37]

The spread of Eastern mysticism and spiritism in Western culture has been paralleled by an increase in "decorations" such as owls which we have accepted innocently. Thank God, He overlooks our ignorance of these things and forgives us! But when we become aware of the negative symbolisms they carry, we need to cleanse our surroundings of them. It is good to go through each room of our home and ask, "Lord, is there any thing before our eyes that does not please you?"

When I first learned of such things I didn't want to believe it. But after praying about it, I felt led of the Lord Jesus to go all through my house and throw out anything I felt uncertain about, until a great peace came into my heart that nothing was there of such a nature. We need not be rigid with others about this. For example, I sat next to the teacher's wife in a Sunday school class. Owl earrings dangled from her ears. I said nothing to her, but quietly said a prayer for her to be protected and forgiven.

When one of our daughters and her husband bought a new home, they discovered that every cupboard knob in the house was decorated with a sign of the zodiac. They went to the builder and said, "We're Christians, and we don't want these signs in our home!" Not only did the builder replace all 40 knobs, but thanked them for pointing this out to him. "I'm a Christian too," he said, "and I hadn't noticed this." Not only was their home cleansed of these symbols of astrology (which is forbidden in Scripture[38]), but they found new fellowship with the builder.

Television of course is one of the most flagrant intruders into the home with the increasing number of ads for occultish and terror programs sandwiched into segments of the most innocent program. As much as possible, let's "decorate" the walls of the inner temple of our minds only with that which is pure and holy, remembering that everything we or our children see is imprinted on the subconscious mind.[39] Let's keep our homes clean of any item related to the occult, as the Psalmist declares, *I will not set any base thing before my eyes.*[40]

> *The graven image of their gods you shall burn with fire; you shall not desire the gold and silver that is on them, nor take it for yourself, . . . neither shall you bring an abomination into your house, lest you become an accursed thing like it . . . .*[41]

Blessed indeed is the infant whose godly parents have made every preparation for his or her arrival under the guidance and wisdom of the Holy Spirit.

> *I will sing a new song unto thee, O God: upon a psalter and an instrument of ten strings will I sing praises to thee.*
> *Deliver me from the hand of strange children, whose mouth speaks vain things, whose right hand is a right hand of deception, so that our sons may be as plants grown up in their youth; that our daughters may be as corner stones, polished like the stones of a palace. . . .*
> *Happy is that people whose God is the Lord.*[42]

NOTES
1. Job 28:12-28. **2.** 2 Chron. 1:7; 1 Kgs. 3:5ff. **3.** Jas. 1:5-8.
4. Eldridge Cleaver. **Soul on Fire.** Waco, Texas. Word Books. 1978. P. 135. Reprinted by permission.
5. Flora Hommel, founder of the Childbirth Without Pain Education Association of Detroit explains: "Under normal circumstances, the normal, healthy, well nourished woman whose baby is in a left occiput anterior or right occiput posterior position should have a painless birth."
6. See the explanation of the effect of the sympathetic nervous system on the cervix of the woman in labor in **Childbirth Without Fear,** 4th ed., **op cit.** Part IV, "The Physiology of Childbirth."
7. Yvonne Brackbill, Ph.D. did research on 50,000 births in a longitudinal study lasting several years, called "Lasting Behavioral Effects of Obstetric Medication on Children." Her article was submitted to the Senate Subcommittee on Health and Scientific Research on April 17, 1978. Some new studies are under way by others.

8. Dr. Edmund Jacobson has demonstrated through the equipment in his laboratory that the electrical impulses from muscles of a person who is under hypnosis or whose mind is not at rest show incomplete muscle relaxation.

9. Deut. 18:9-13; Lev. 19:26. The words "charm," "enchant," or "a spell" refer to a hypnotic state in which one is under the control of another.

Hypnosis is being increasingly used for therapy, even by some Christian doctors. They have their patients relax and begin to picture some lovely scene such as the seashore or a warm fireside. In this "daydreaming" state with one's muscles relaxed a person is more open to suggestion and less aware of their fears.

This "daydreaming" or "absent-minded" state is common to us all in everyday experience, whenever we are preoccupied with something. It is a **normal** state of mind. Counselors would do better to call it by its real name, "daydreaming," rather than to label it hypnotism.

Although this normal state of mind may parallel the beginning stages of hypnotism it is unfortunate to make the public think that hypnotism is an acceptable practice. The phone books of every city are full of charlatans who are "professional" hypnotists.

10. Reported in "The Federal Monitor," Vol. 1, No. 4, Oct. 28, 1978. Published by Maternal and Child Health Legislative Alert, Inc., Drawer Q, McLean, VA, 22102.

11. ICEA News. Vol. 18, No. 4, 1979. Published by the International Childbirth Education Association, 1410 Fleetfoot Drive, Waukesha, WI 53186. Most of this issue is devoted to the discussion of cesareans.

12. Constance Bean. **Labor and Delivery: An Observer's Diary.** Garden City, NY. Doubleday. 1977. P. 5.

13. Ibid. P. 41. **14. Ibid.** P. 42. **15.** ICEA News. **Op. cit.**

16. Reported in "The Detroit Free Press." January 27, 1978.

17. Niles Newton. "Psychological Aspects of Female Surgery." Excerpts reported in "Dateline: U.S. Midwest." June 1979. Newsletter of the U.S. Midwestern Region, ICEA, P.O. Box 20852, Milwaukee, WI 53220.

18. Heb. 12:15.

19. Personal letter, January 1979. Printed by permission.

20. Bean, **op cit.** P. 194. Reprinted by permission.

The American Board of Obstetrics and Gynecology (ABOG) reported in **Ob. Gyn. News,** Vol. 14, No. 10, in comparing the cesarean rates in 1977 and 1978 showed that cesarean rates for physicians with mixed ob/gyn practices rose 3% (from 16% to 19%); for physicians primarily in obstetrics it rose 6% (from 18% to 24%); for physicians primarily in gynecology it rose 22% (32% to 54%).

21. "The Pregnant Patient's Bill of Rights." For a complimentary copy send a stamped, self-addressed envelope to the ICEA Committee on Patients' Rights. Box 1900, New York, NY 10001.

22. Babies born to alcoholic parents may already be alcoholic, predispos-

ed to the need for alcohol. This is true even if the mother is only a "social drinker." The alcohol quickly reaches the baby's bloodstream through the placenta before birth.
23. Prepared by the Interprofessional Task Force on Health Care of Women and Children. Participating organizations were the American Academy of Pediatrics, American College of Nurse-Midwives, American College of Obstetricians and Gynecologists, American Nurses' Association, and Nurses Association of The American College of Obstetricians and Gynecologists. Copies may be obtained from any of the participating organizations or from the Interprofessional Task Force Secretariat, ACOG, One East Wacker Drive, Suite 2700, Chicago, IL 60601.
24. Barbara Brennan, CNM and Joan Rattner Heilman. **The Complete Book of Midwifery.** New York. E. P. Dutton. 1977. This book includes a directory of Nurse-Midwifery services in the United States.
25. Comments from families of infants born at Birthplace, 635 NE 1st Street, Gainsville, FL 31601. Reprinted from Birthplace Newsletter by permission.
26. There are some places where lay midwives can receive training in midwifery and conduct deliveries under the supervision of competent physicians. Many of these are not publicized because of legal complications. A "Directory of Alternative Birth Services and Consumer Guide" by Penny Simkin, RPT is available from NAPSAC, P.O. Box 267, Marble Hill, MO 63764.
27. Is. 2:6 NIV.
28. Ina May Gaskin. **Spiritual Midwifery.** Summertown, TN. Book Publishing. Stephen Gaskin is the head of a "religious" community known as "The Farm." Farm midwifes have delivered over 1000 babies in the last eight years at the Farm, and there are now 14 other Farms around the country. The "religious" aspect does not measure up to the warning in 1 Jn 4:1-3.
29. 2 Cor. 11:13-15; Mk. 13:22. **30.** 1 Tim. 4:1. **31.** Deut. 18:10-13 NIV.
32. 2 Cor. 6:14-7:1.
33. Francis MacNutt. **The Power to Heal.** Notre Dame. Ave Maria Press. 1977. Pp. 74, 75.
34. For example: "The breath is the bridge between you and the universe; the Body is just the universe which has come to you" (from Bhagwan Shree Rajneesh). These "trainers" claim to assist the expectant mother in working through the areas of her life that need "clarification" through the process of breath, so that she can totally experience her "divine self."

A young woman who had practiced karate before she became a Christian says that at times she had actually felt "otherwordly," and believes her spirit left her body during those times. Christians need to beware of all such mind-altering "spiritual" experiences which leave them vulnerable to the influence of evil spirits.

A young man who had practiced transcendental meditation before becoming a Christian said that the "mantras" he was given to recite were the names of demons. One of my daughters once heard a woman telling (after she became a Christian) what her mantra had been. Since my daughter had spent two years in the Philippines and knew some of the Filipino dialects, she felt a chill when she heard the woman's mantra. It was a Filipino word for death! The woman had had no idea what the word she had been reciting meant.

35. Rev. 16:13

36. There are five different Hebrew words translated as "owls." In Isa. 34:14 it is *lilith,* "bird of the night." "Lilith" is represented in Jewish mythology as "a female evil spirit, roaming in desolate places, attacking children." In Isa. 34:13 the word translated owl is "daughter of howling" (hooting). *It shall be a habitation for dragons, and a court of owls, ... and the satyr ... the screech owl ... and the great owl.... There shall the vulture be gathered* (to feed on the dead). Rev. 18:2 says, *Fallen, fallen is Babylon the great! It has become a dwelling place of demons, a haunt of every foul spirit, a haunt of every foul and hateful bird; ...*

37. Reported in New Tribes Mission magazine. October, 1980. Sanford, FL 32771. P. 9.

38. Deut. 4; 19; 17:2, 3; Isa. 19:13; 47:12-15; Jer. 2, 3a.

39. Halloween customs are grossly inconsistent with Christian principles. Dr. James A. Borror, senior pastor of First Baptist Church of Lakewood, California correctly points out that "the whole process of making pretend that we are witches or monsters or ghosts and producing fear by projecting that which is grotesque or evil is at odds with the biblical statement that perfect love casts out fear or the prohibition to have anything to do with the occult or witchcraft or the demonic." Dr. Borror suggests that children's ministries sponsor biblical character parties or Reformation parties, or other fall festivities that are compatible with true faith.

40. Ps. 101:2, 3 NAB. **41.** Deut. 7:25. **42.** Ps. 144:9-15.

No Place Like Home

And the king of Egypt spoke to the Hebrew midwives and said, when you perform the office of midwife to the Hebrew women and see them ready to give birth, if it is a son, kill him. But if it is a daughter then let her live.

But the midwives feared God and did not do as the king of Egypt commanded them, but saved the boy babies. And the king of Egypt called for the midwives and said to them, "Why have you done this?"

And the midwives said to Pharaoh, "Because the Hebrew women are not like the Egyptian women, but are strong and healthy, and give birth even before we get to their homes."[1]

There was a knock on the front door. I tore my eyes away from our newborn son Daniel, two hours old, walked to the door and opened it. Our pastor stood there. He looked shocked to see me and stammered, "But, but, I thought you had your baby this morning!"

"Yes, I did. Won't you come in?"

Flustered, he shook his head. "No, I'd better not," he said and hurried away. I was disappointed. I would have liked for him to come in, see our beautiful son and pray God's blessings over him. I was dressed in my robe and had already put the house in order, including the bedroom where our son was born. But our pastor was not able to overcome his astonishment that I was at home rather than in the hospital, for this was 1956 and home births were unheard of.

Now this son is grown and gone from home, but I still treasure a comment he made in a college research paper. "Perhaps the most wonderful moment of my life," he wrote, "was one I don't remember, but one which my mother cherishes. Her account of it always leaves me warm and peaceful inside."

The decision

When an expectant mother asks me, "Do you think I should have my baby at home?" my answer is no. I will not take the responsibility of making that decision. If she is so unsure in her own heart that she has to ask someone else, a home birth is probably not for her.

If an expectant couple says to me, "We want to have our baby at home. What do you think about that?" I would counter with another question. "Why do you want to?" If the reason is because a home birth is supposedly cheaper than the hospital I would have to say that that is not a valid reason.

If the wife has reservations about staying home and the husband is pressing for it, they need to pray more about it. If her reservations remain, she probably belongs in the hospital.

On the other hand, if the wife feels strongly that she should have her baby at home and the husband is hesitant, then a home birth should be given serious consideration. Perhaps if the husband can be reassured by gaining additional information and becoming better prepared, he will change his mind. But if by the time of birth he is still resistant, then it is better for his wife not to defy his husbandly authority and move out from under his spiritual protection by refusing to go to the hospital.

A couple who have prayed together and are united in their decision for a home birth must weigh the consequences of their decision. What back-up plans will they have for a possible medical emergency? Are they willing to learn what to do during the birth and to make all the preparations necessary? No one else will do this for them. And they must face the question which some one will be certain to ask them: "What if the baby or the mother dies?"[2]

In modern American hospitals today, about 13 babies die out of every thousand births. Friends are sympathetic, birth attendants consoling, comforting the couple in their loss. Not so if the baby dies in a home birth. Even if the baby is stillborn or dies because of gross deformity, the prevailing attitude among friends and family will not be one of sympathy but of judgment: baby died **because** of being born at home. Can they face that?

There are three basic criteria that give me peace about a couple's decision to have a home birth:

1. "We have prayed about this and really believe this is what Jesus wants us to do."

2. "We have qualified persons to assist us at the birth and medical back-up plans for any emergency."

3. "We are willing to make all the preparations necessary, to learn everything we can in advance, and to accept the consequences of our decision."

A fourth criteria would add to my confidence concerning their decision: "We have Christian friends who have agreed to be in prayer during the labor and birth."

The preparations

There are four areas in which preparations should be made. The first is childbirth education and birth training for both husband and wife. Second is the choice of birth attendants. This includes persons to look after the household, care for other children, prepare any necessary meals, etc. Third is gathering the necessary supplies, and fourth, the parents' spiritual preparation for the birth.

A couple who chooses to stay home for the birth of their baby needs to read widely[3], gather information concerning the various stages of a normal birth, master the relaxation and breathing patterns through practice, and go through a "birth rehearsal" a few times. The "birth rehearsal" will bring up questions such as, What is the most comfortable place for first stage? Where should the rocking chair be placed—in the bedroom or in some other room? Where are the best places for the wife to rest her arms and head when she needs to lean over to relax during a contraction while walking around? Is the bed firm enough to give birth on? Can the head of the bed be arranged as a back rest, or should a back rest be made? Or would it be more comfortable giving birth in a reclining chair? Or in a bean bag chair by the fireplace? As the couple thinks through the sequence of labor in the circumstances of their own home, other such questions may come to mind. These decisions need to be settled ahead of time.

Those who are to be present in the home for the birth must be selected carefully. Prenatal care for the mother is essential, for only those women who are considered "low risk" should consider home birth. But even those women who show no indication of a possible problem need a qualified medical attendant present in the home, not to take over the couples' responsibilities, but to be available to answer their questions, diagnose possible problems, and make suggestions when necessary. The medical back-up plan would include a physician (if the medical attendant is not a physician) and a hospital in which the patient will be cared for if the need arises. A station wagon with a full tank of fuel should be at the house, and friends available to help carry the woman to the car if this should become necessary. Or if ambulance services are nearby, they can be alerted at the time labor begins that their services might be needed.

Other persons present in the home can look after the house, prepare meals, care for other children, answer the phone or handle any other details. They must be persons with whom both husband and wife feel comfortable and secure, who will respect the privacy of the couple and not intrude unless called for. A list of phone numbers of all attendants should be placed by the phone for immediate reference when labor begins and should include emergency numbers that might be needed during the labor.

Unless the mattress is quite firm, a sheet of plywood should be on hand to slip under the mattress for support during the birth. The mattress can be protected by a rubber sheet or a clean, old shower curtain under the sheets. Clean sheets should be on hand to put on the bed when labor begins and also to replace wet or soiled sheets, if necessary, during the labor. Disposable bed pads will be needed under the mother. These can be absorbent old towels or old sheet squares, with rubber pads or layers of newspapers underneath. Or disposable toddler diapers can be used.

Sterile washcloths, soft cotton cloth pieces of towels should be at hand to keep the mother clean and comfortable. Any of these cloth items can be sterilized by putting them in a brown paper bag and placing them in a 200^0 oven over a pan of water for an hour. (But don't try to sterilize rubber or plastic items in this way as I did, and have them melt all over the oven!)

Sterile gauze squares will be useful during the birth to support the perineum. Olive oil should be on hand. Ample newspapers can be used to make a path to the bathroom so the mother need not worry about dripping on the floor. A large bowl or pan will be needed for the afterbirth, as well as sanitary napkins and belt for the mother to wear afterward.

Items for the baby include sterilized white cotton shoestrings to tie the cord, sterile scissors (sterilized by dipping in alcohol) to cut the cord, a rubber ear syringe (no plastic parts) to suction baby's throat and nose if necessary, and disposable diapers or diaper liners. The baby's first bowel movements are dark and sticky, so that it is better not to use cloth diapers without the liners the first few days, as they will be hard to get clean.

In addition, clean clothes for the mother both during and after the birth and blankets for the baby need to be on hand. The baby's clothes and blankets should all be softened by prewashing. All the washed and sterilized items can be placed in plastic bags and set aside for the day of birth.

An antiseptic soap should be on hand so that the couple and attendants can wash their hands and arms (up to the elbows). They should also make certain that their fingernails are short and clean.

Every Christian husband should become knowledgeable enough to lead his own wife through labor and childbirth, whether at home, in a birth center or in the hospital. The "husbandman" of the flock is the one who attends the births. The husband who loves his wife enough to accept this God-given responsibility will find tremendous rewards, in his marriage, in his own self-esteem, and in his relationship with the infant which was born by his wife into his own hands. No matter who else is present at the birth, this should be his awesome joy. The importance of the husband's presence and participation in the birth of his child has been documented in psychological research:

> *...the sharing husband is seen as busy, active, important, strong, competent, involved, performing important physical and emotional functions. He is described by his wife or by himself as interested, excited, pleasantly surprised by his own attitudes, and thrilled at the experience of sharing childbirth.*
>
> *These findings relate to the man himself and to his own psychological growth. But there is another and larger context in which my survey results are meaningful. The material assembled has major implications for certain basic attitudes in our culture and for long held views in the field of psychology. Most strikingly the results suggest that some differences between men and women are not as great as had been traditionally thought. Contrary to popular and academic notions about "masculinity" and "femininity," the husbands studied expressed strong interest in the whole area of childbirth, wanted to and did*

participate and had positive feelings about having done so.... It may be, then, that in some ways men and women are psychologically more alike than had been felt. Men may have a greater need to play a role in birth than had been realized....

A second point, also of great importance, is that this greater male involvement in childbirth by no means represents the "demasculinization" of men. The husband involved in childbirth is not "sissified," as common thinking might expect. On the contrary, the natural childbirth husband emerges as strong, competent, important and someone on whom in most cases his wife can lean and depend. In contrast, it is the uninvolved father, the non-natural childbirth one, who shows up as weak, impotent, childlike, someone to be worried about rather than depended upon at this time.[4]

An excellent book called **Childbirth at Home** stresses the importance of the husband's involvement in delivering his own baby:

*No known American institution yet follows the example set by Nesbitt Memorial Hospital in Kingston, Pennsylvania. There, patients of obstetrics chief William Hazlett take classes where they learn natural childbirth techniques. During the delivery, Dr. Hazlett stands by—**while the husbands deliver their own babies.***

During the past seven years, over one thousand fathers have delivered their own babies at Nesbitt Memorial. But some of the do-it-yourself deliveries have also taken place in Dr. Hazlett's office across the street....

"There's nothing on earth like it," beamed a young construction worker who delivered his baby daughter under Dr. Hazlett's supervision.[5]

The husband's role in his wife's labor and delivery is not to be that of observer, or even the important one of emotional support only, but is of far greater importance to the smooth progress of his wife's labor than is often realized. As has been mentioned earlier, the contractions of the uterus and expulsive actions of the vagina in childbirth parallel those of female orgasm.[6] The "love hormone," oxytocin,[7] stimulates orgasm in both men and women, and is essential to the normal functioning of labor and breastfeeding, causing not only uterine contractions but also helping the mother "let down" her baby and "let down" her milk. This normal let-down reflex is blocked if the woman is tense or worried. The reassuring, loving presence of her husband assists not only in stimulating the release of oxytocin in the mother's system but also the necessary emotional relaxation in his protective presence. Perhaps it is no surprise that labor most often begins at night, when the mother is sleeping close to her lover.

Because the loving, touch relationship between husband and wife is so crucial to the normal progress of labor, it is essential that their privacy be protected for their uninhibited interaction during labor. She can release the tension in her skeletal muscles at his gentle touch, letting go all anxiety and tightness, leaning on his strength. Kissing helps relax the birth outlet. His caresses not only keep the uterus contracting normally[8] but help relax the cervix as she yields peacefully to his touch. He can be taught how to massage the perineum with olive oil to help her relax the birth outlet—"opening the door" to let the baby out—returning to him his gift of love nine months earlier.

It cannot be overstated that an **essential** need for the laboring couple is **privacy!** The interaction between the husband and wife during labor is a most private affair into which no one should intrude without permission. This privacy is most easily attained at home, but it should be respected wherever the birth is taking place. In a hospital, the door should be closed, with **no** one entering without first knocking on the door and receiving permission to enter. If a couple is assured of this privacy, their interaction during the labor will not be inhibited by the fear of intrusion, a fear that prolongs the labor and increases problems. Anything that embarrasses or inhibits the mother's free expression of her sexuality adversely affects the progress of her labor, for childbirth is a sexual experience.

But while privacy is important, let no young couple assume that birth is something they can manage "on their own."[9] Qualified attendants are essential to answer questions, to give guidance, to ascertain from time to time that all is normal. Although expectant parents can be taught how to hear the fetal heartbeat and how to determine the progress of labor, they both need the experienced wisdom of qualified birth attendants at hand for reassurance and safety. With a first baby, the mother may be overwhelmed by the intensity of late labor and transition contractions, and may need a more experienced labor companion than her husband to help guide her breathing and relaxation through this short but trying period. This person would not replace the husband, but assist him in guiding the wife comfortably on into second stage labor.

The Christian couple preparing for birth will want to take time each day to pray about these things. They will seek God's wisdom about the place of birth, about the choice of attendants, about the preparations He wants them to make. They will pray for the safety of mother and child, and for His guidance through every moment of that very special coming day.

> *If you listen to these instructions, and keep and do them, then the Lord your God will keep His promise to you, and the mercy which He promised with an oath to your forefathers.*
> *And he will love you and bless you, and multiply you. He will also bless the fruit of your womb, and the fruit of your land.... You will be blessed above all people. There shall not be male or female barren among you, and the Lord will take away from you all sickness, and will put none of the evil disease of Egypt, of which you know, upon you.* [10]

A family affair

One of the decisions a Christian couple must make in advance is about whether they want their other children to be present for the birth of their baby. Some couples may prefer privacy through the entire experience. Others may want the moment of birth to be a "party," with close friends, parents, or their children participating in the "celebration." Children who are to be present must be well prepared in advance. They should know, for example, that the groaning sounds Mother might make are only because she is working hard. A friend wrote to tell of her home birth and the responses of her two little boys who were present for the birth:

> *... I am a registered nurse, and my husband is an auto dealer. We have 3 children, Aaron, 7 yrs., Benjamin, 5 yrs. and Andrea, 6 mon. ... The Lord has given me a real ministry in teaching childbirth classes in my home and a real freedom to share with couples my true motivation for teaching the last 5 years—that I believe birth to be more than a physical/emotional experience. We found it to be a*

spiritual experience as well, and especially meaningful to us because of our relationship to Jesus Christ.

... I had a growing desire to have a baby at home, because of wanting to experience birth to the fullest and to have the people who loved me present who could offer me spiritual support during birth. Psalm 37:4 ("Delight thyself in the Lord, and he shall give thee the desires of thine heart") became a reality to me as the months went by. At one point I did feel the Lord asked me if I was willing to give up the desire of my heart for Him. I had come to the place of being willing to do that, as strong as the desire (for the home birth) *was. When I was able to honestly do that—the miracle occurred.*

... I woke up at 3 a.m. to go to the bathroom and had quite a bit of thick mucus discharge. I went back to bed but was unable to sleep. At 3:30 I was up to the bathroom again and membranes ruptured on the toilet. At 4 a.m. fetal heart tones were regular through contractions. I listened to them with a stethoscope. I couldn't sleep so I got up and moved to the living room to read the Psalms between contractions and have a quiet time with the Lord....

10:32 a.m. Dr. called and on his way. I felt I needed my husband now to stay with me. It was getting harder to relax. 10:45 Dr. arrived, rushing to set things up ... 11 a.m. Began to push. My husband got up on the bed behind me and I leaned against him. The boys were brought in for the birth after a "refresher" course by Barb with a midwives' textbook. (Barb is a nurse friend who was staying with us to help at the time of birth.)

11:06. Ben's comment, "I hope the baby comes out head first." Dr. "Why is that?" Ben, "So the baby will be able to see mom."

11:10. Crowning. Aaron announced the color of hair was black. 11:12. Tear, and Dr. "You're not going to make it," and did a small episiotomy (1½ in.). Aaron left as head was born and returned for birth when my husband called him. I felt I wanted the boys to be a part of the birth experience if they wanted to, but not force them. I asked Aaron later why he left and he said, "Because I was scared." I asked why he was scared and he said, "Because there was a lot of blood (from the episiotomy) *and when you lose all your blood you die." He felt free to express himself and is apparently comfortable with what he felt he had to do.*

The phone rang twice and the alarm clock went off from this point until birth, approximately nine minutes. While baby was being born it occurred to me to ask Barb if she had remembered to take a cake out of the oven. There was some struggle delivering the typical head (big) our children have, and the shoulders. Once the shoulders slipped out, her whole body swished out covered with vernix and some blood. Dr. dried her well, cut cord and laid her skin-to-skin on my tummy with warm blankets on top. I had my hands under the blankets on her and will never forget the feel of that little bottom in my left hand and my right hand on her head which was on my breast.

11:25. Placenta delivered—episiotomy repaired.... I was totally at peace with myself. Instead of laughing or crying at the moment of birth, I just felt very quiet and restful after a hard day's work. Thank you, Jesus![11]

Childbirth in the Sanctuary

I have seen the labor which God has given to the children of men to be exercised in. He has made everything beautiful in its time. Also he has put eternity into their heart.[12]

A "sanctuary" is a sacred place for safety. And what better place for a child to be born than in the sanctuary of the presence of the living Lord Jesus? Wherever a child is born he or she should be surrounded by the loving prayers of God's people, and the atmosphere of the room of birth as peaceful as a chapel.

The importance of intercession was brought forcefully to my attention during the first labor of our oldest daughter. I was not able to be with her, but at three in the morning her husband called to say they were on their way to the hospital. Two hours later the phone rang again. He had called to say she had asked him to call me for prayer, as she was having a great deal of pain. I asked how far dilated she was and could hardly believe my ears when he said only 3 centimeters!

I hung up the phone with an uneasy feeling. Pain at only 3 centimeters was clearly a warning that something was wrong. As I prayed quietly in bed, the phrase *Fathers of spirits* kept coming to my mind again and again. The prayer burden grew so heavy I could no longer stay in bed but went into the study for more intercession. The burden became incredible! I prayed *with my understanding*. I prayed *in the Spirit*,[13] I *groaned with words which cannot be uttered*,[14] but the burden did not lift. Finally I said, "Lord, what is going on!" I picked up my Bible to see what He would say. It occurred to me to look up the phrase *Father of spirits* which had been put into my mind. I found it in Hebrews 12, but did not like what I read!

> *For whom the Lord loves he chastens.... Shall we not be in subjection to the **Father of spirits**, and live?... Now no suffering at the time is joyous, but grievous. Nevertheless, afterward it yields the peaceable fruit of righteousness....*[15]

These words confirmed the burden of prayer I was feeling. My daughter was indeed having a hard time. For over an hour and a half the prayer burden weighed me down, as I prayed in every way I knew. By the time the rest of the family was awake and wanting breakfast at about seven the burden was beginning to lift a little. I continued praying quietly in the Spirit as I worked. At 7:15 I hurried back into the study to pick up the prayer burden again in greater intensity, but no prayer would come, only peace. I could not get back under the burden of prayer no matter how I tried.

At 7:30 the phone rang. It was my son-in-law, saying our little granddaughter had been born at 7:15. No wonder the prayer burden was gone! The answer had already come. Later I learned that my daughter's baby had been in the posterior position (face up instead of face down), causing severe back pain.

My daughter had gotten on her hands and knees and had spent most of the time in this position. During contractions while on her knees she would hold her breath slightly and "lean on it" without pushing. The doctor had come in at 6:15, and after examining her, quietly told her husband that it would be at least another four hours or more before the baby was born. Then he went off to surgery. Fortunately, she had not overheard this discouraging remark!

Forty-five minutes after his comment she was rushed to the delivery room and the baby born in the normal position shortly after. Her hands and knees position and "leaning on it," had effectively caused the baby to rotate into normal position as it moved down the birth canal and the birth was uneventful. She had no medication and no intervention, except for the presence of an all-wise God who prompted her to do the right things, and who had answered prayer by quickly bringing the birth to a safe conclusion.

One Christian couple felt strongly led of the Lord to stay home for the birth of their third child. Labor began on a Wednesday morning, but contractions were weak and ineffective for nearly two days. By Friday morning the whole church family was alerted to prayer through their telephone prayer chain and entered into intercession for the safety of mother and child. Soon after this concerted prayer effort began the mother went into active labor and the child was born shortly after.

This mother, who is a nurse, later told me she would never have been allowed to be in labor so long in the hospital without her labor being stimulated by injections. "And if it had been stimulated," she said, "I know my baby would have died." She explained that signs were present at birth indicating that the placenta pulled away as the baby entered the birth canal. If her labor had been induced, it would most likely have caused too early separation of the placenta, and the baby could not have been delivered in time to save its life.

This couple had a fourth child at home and are now expecting their fifth child, once again seeking God's guidance:

I am expecting our 5th child, due around May 13th. Home deliveries are almost unheard of in these parts. The thought makes most women "cringe," I have found. We are only 25 miles from my parents now,... My talk about our desire to have home birth here has caused much antagonism in my parents (mom a nurse 30 odd years) and anxiety in my sister, also a nurse. Thru much prayer and seeking the Lord, C_____ and I are strongly led to have this baby in the hospital. I am under the care of my old family doctor. Prayerfully and hopefully he will allow me to have the baby as naturally as possible. We believe that God had us move here in Oct. to be close to C_____'s parents and mine so family relationships could be mended and restored. A home delivery would work against this purpose. Nevertheless, I am saddened because of pending hospital birth. I am working at letting God be God in this area of my life, as well as other areas. At times it is quite a struggle between self and God....[16]

Recently a Christian couple gave birth at home who chose to have two friends come who would pray *in the Spirit* during the period of active labor. It was a beautiful labor and the rejoicing parents named their baby boy Judah. Later the grandfather, who was not a Christian, came to visit them. "Judah," he exclaimed. "What kind of name is that?"

They explained that it was a Bible name which meant "praise," and they had chosen it because they were praising the Lord for their baby. "Oh," he said. "That's nice!"

A letter dated December 8, 1979 arrived just as I have been working on this chapter. This mother's first birth had been most traumatic, and I had had the privilege of praying with her and her husband for the healing of this bad memory, and of guiding them to the truths of unmedicated natural birth. She wrote:

Well, I wanted to share with you our tremendous news: another baby girl!—the Lord has blessed us with. We had her at home and it was the most wonderful, enriching experience L_____, and I have ever shared. L_____ got to "catch" her, then cut the cord. Our midwives were tremendous: we were thrilled in every way with this birth. For me—as a mother again—this birth fulfilled my motherhood and womanhood in every possible way.

There were times of anxiety but God gave us peace that we were right to stay home.... I had mild contractions Tues. night and Wed. night becoming stronger Thurs. AM. My hard labor was only 2 hrs.—so when things finally got going it was a relatively short time until she was born. I was able to walk up until 2 hrs. before. L_____ was a terrific labor coach helping me with my deep chest breathing and panting.

*I felt so tremendous and elated after the birth—I took a shower and then sat around until 8 PM admiring our new daughter. I had no episiotomy, but a slight ½" outer surface tear along my old episiotomy scar.... I want to thank you so much for your generosity in sending me your book. It and Dick-Read's book have been invaluable. One thing I appreciate **so** much is your diligence in the Heb. and Greek survey regarding "pain" in the Bible. It all makes so much more sense.... "Behold, children are a gift of the Lord; the fruit of the womb is his reward."*[17]

A Christian couple discovered that the wife was carrying

twins during her second pregnancy. A month before the birth ultra-sound pictures were taken to verify it. "One will be born normally, and one will be breech," the parents were told and it was explained to them that a twin born breech is sometimes at high risk.

A month later labor began while the mother was at a baby shower. After she left for the hospital the shower turned into a prayer meeting in her honor. When the doctor arrived at the hospital the mother informed him that she was going to have two normal deliveries. "You see," she explained later, "I had talked to the Lord about it, and one night just before going to sleep, I felt Michael somersault. I do not think the doctor really understood or believed me until 1:31 a.m. and 1:48 a.m. when both precious little ones were born normally,... both in perfect health. Praise the Lord!"[18]

> *Even the sparrow finds a home,*
>   *and the swallow a nest for herself,*
>   *where she may lay her young,*
>   *at thy altars, O Lord God of hosts.*[19]

NOTES
1. Ex. 1:15-19.
2. Maternal deaths occur most frequently when the mother is toxemic, in which case she would not be having a home birth; and from hemorrhage. If a hospital is near by, it is improbable that the mother could not be taken there in time for effective treatment.

Infant death may occur from the complications of **placenta previa,** in which the placenta is too close to the cervix and comes away first. There is usually advance warning of this as the cervix begins to dilate. **Placenta abruptio,** in which the placenta comes away before the baby's head is born, cutting off his oxygen, is a danger. The third danger is a **prolapsed cord,** in which the cord precedes the baby. Baby's head compresses the cord and cuts off his oxygen. All three of these major complications take the lives of infants being born in hospitals too, but in the hospital there is more rapid access to emergency procedures which may help to save the baby's life.

Most couples who choose to stay home do so because they believe it is **safer** as well as more pleasant. There is less possibility of germs, less disruption of the labor through interference and inhibitions, etc. Statistics demonstrate that **planned** home births have far fewer infant deaths than the hospital, but this comparison is not entirely fair because high risk mothers most often give birth in the hospital. For discussions of hospital versus home birth see **Safe Alternatives in Childbirth** by David and Lee Stewart, available from NAPSAC. P.O. Box 276, Marble Hill, MO 63764. This book received the 1976 "Books of the Year" Award from the American Journal of Nursing.

3. For further information see **Home Oriented Maternity Experience,** H.O.M.E. 511 New York Ave., Takoma Park, Washington, D.C. 20012 and **Emergency Childbirth** by Gregory White, M.D., available from La Leche League, 9616 Minneapolis Ave., Franklin Park, IL 60131.

4. Dr. Deborah Tanzer. **Why Natural Childbirth?** Garden City, NY. Doubleday & Co. 1972. Pp. 205, 207. Reprinted by permission.

5. Marion Sousa. **Childbirth at Home.** Englewood Cliffs, NJ. Prentice-Hall. 1976. Pp. 74-75. Reprinted by permission.

6. See chapter "Awakened Desires" footnote # 8.

7. See chapter "Awakened Desires" footnote # 9.

8. See **Obstetrics and Gynecology,** Vol. 41, # 3, March, 1973, pp. 347-350.

9. In 1964 I attended my first ICEA convention (and was elected president for the term 1964-1966). One couple attending the convention had come even though the wife was a week overdue with her first baby. On the second day of the convention the baby was born in their hotel room.

Dr. Carolyn Rawlins, that selfless, supporting natural childbirth obstetrician who was one of the founders of ICEA was called to check the mother during labor. Then the husband locked her out of the room until after the birth! She stood just outside the door giving instructions until he had delivered the baby. Only then did he unlock the door and let her in. She was not offended by his action, but on the contrary, understood it.

When the couple arrived at the banquet that evening with their new baby people were shocked. The couple said they had already been out for a walk that afternoon, after the baby was born! But out of respect for the feelings of the others at the convention, they did not appear at the meetings again.

10. Deut. 7:12-15.

11. Personal letter, June 9, 1979. Printed by permission.

12. Eccl. 3:11 AV & RSV. **13.** 1 Cor. 14:14, 15.

14. Rom. 8:27. **15.** Heb. 12:6-11.

16. Personal letter, Mar. 7, 1980. Printed by permission.

17. Personal letter, Dec. 6, 1979. Printed by permission.

18. Reported in "Call to Prayer." World Gospel Mission. Marion, IN. April, 1980. P. 3.

19. Psa. 84:3 RSV.

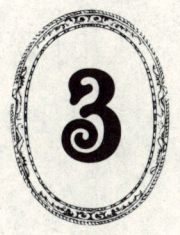

The Circle of Love

Baby Makes Three

> *And it came to pass in those days that a decree went out from Caesar Augustus that all the world should be taxed. And all went to be taxed, everyone to his home town.*
>
> *Joseph also went up to the city of David which is called Bethlehem, because he was of the house and lineage of David. He went to be taxed with Mary, his espoused wife, who was great with child.*
>
> *And so it was that while they were there the time came for her to give birth. And she gave birth to her firstborn son, wrapped him in strips of cloths and laid him in a manger, because there was no room for them in the inn....*
>
> *And the shepherds hurried to Bethlehem, and found Mary and Joseph and the baby lying in a manger.*[1]

The most significant journey a human being ever makes is the few inches from the mother's womb into the light of day. The Spanish speak of birth as **dar a luz,** "to give to the light."

What awaits the child given to the light? Recent research shows that the first few moments after birth, the first few days, the first few weeks, are far more important than ever before realized. Medical science has focused so much concern on the physical aspects of the newborn that the extremely important psychological and intellectual and spiritual factors have too often been ignored.

The laying on of hands

Before a baby is fully born, before he hears a voice, before he takes his first breath, he receives the most basic human response to his presence. This is the touch of someone's hand as he emerges from darkness into light. It may be the father's touch as the head is born, and then the mother's as she reaches down to take the baby into her own hands as his body is born. Or perhaps the first touch is that of the birth attendant and then the parents. Thus the initial response to the appearance of the child is the "laying on of hands," touching.

Continued touching by loving hands is an essential need of the newborn. The skin, which is the largest and most sensitive of the sense organs, has been extensively stroked during the journey from the womb through the vagina into light. This stimulation quickens the baby's nervous system to adapt to life outside the womb.

Animals instinctively lick their young all over their bodies as soon as they are born. This licking stimulates the functioning of the digestive and elimination systems. A puppy taken from its mother before this licking occurs often fails to survive.

What is the first thing a new mother instinctively does when the baby is placed in her arms? Her hands begin to move. She touches the baby's head, his cheek, his arms. It has been observed that a mother usually explores the baby first with her fingertips and then proceeds on to stroking with her whole hand. The sooner she has the infant after birth, the more quickly this progression takes place, so that before long she is stroking the whole body of the infant cradled in her arms. This stroking instinct is so strong and so natural that she is probably not even aware of her moving hands.

The symbolism of the laying on of hands can be seen even more clearly in the father's unpremeditated response to the newborn in the mother's arms, if he has been present at the birth. He lays his whole hand upon the baby, on its head or on its body. No fingertip touching for him! The first spontaneous response of the new father is to "lay hands on" his newborn. How naturally does the Christian father become the priest before God for his own child, from the first instinctive touch!

Psalm 22:9, 10 says of the Lord, *You are the One who took me out of the womb. You made me hope when I was on my mother's breasts. I was cast upon you from the womb; you have been my God from the time of my birth.*

The Hebrew literally says, *upon You was I thrown from the womb.* This refers to the ancient custom of placing a newborn baby in the father's arms or on his lap, so that he could acknowledge that it was indeed his own baby. This is a beautiful custom which every newborn and every father ought to be able to experience. During the first half hour after birth the parents should be alone with their newborn (assuming all is well) for this important time of the "laying on of hands," touching, stroking, blessing.

The laying on of hands in Scripture has tremendous spiritual significance. It is a sign of **belonging.** It identifies a claim of God upon the one so touched, with all the rights and privileges which He bestows upon His own. *When they brought infants to Jesus, he touched them.... Then brought them to him so that he would put his hands on them, and pray.... And he laid his hands on them.*[2]

The Christian father will make his instinctive touch a conscious act of blessing upon his child, a visible sign to the seen and the unseen world that this child is bonded not only to the parents but to the Heavenly Father as well. All heaven will witness that this is so, for Jesus said,

> *Be careful that you do not despise even one of these little ones. For I say to you that in heaven their angels are always beholding the face of my Father which is in heaven.*[3]

Eye to eye

Most infants born to relaxed, unmedicated mothers do not cry, but are peaceful, breathing quietly. When the baby emerges he or she should be covered with a warm blanket and left lying below the level of the cord on the bed until the cord stops pulsing. Blood from the cord can supply as much as one third of the baby's total blood volume.

After the cord stops pulsing the baby can be lifted to the mother's breast, if the cord is long enough, the cord still untied. Whether the child suckles or not is unimportant. The sensitive touch of the baby's mouth on her nipple stimulates the uterus to contract and expel the afterbirth. The cord should not be pulled, nor should the abdomen be pummelled, as these maneuvers may cause incomplete separation of the placenta, unnecessary bleeding, and "after pains" the next day or two as the uterus tries to expel clots and bits of tissue left behind.

There is no hurry in tying the cord. Sterile, soft cotton ties (sterilized shoe strings will do) should be tied in a square knot in two places around the cord, a few inches from the navel. The cord can then be cut between the two knots, with sterile scissors. The daddy cutting the cord is a symbolic gesture of the baby's separation from total dependence on the mother. Both parents are now involved.

The newborn baby often looks right into the eyes of his mother and father. The infant can not only see them, but can mimic facial expressions such as a smile, frown, or yawn. During this first hour after an unmedicated birth his sensitivity is heightened to every external stimulus. He hears, sees, smells, feels, and responds, storing away these impressions during this crucial "bonding" period.[4] It is now scientifically verified that during the first week a baby not only sees, but has visual preferences,[5] consistently choosing the orderly features of a human face to "scrambled" features and soft, round lines to harsh, sharp corners. The newborn also prefers some colors to others. Nothing should be done to the baby which will interfere with his natural ability to focus his eyes clearly not only in the hour after birth, but also during the crucial first few days of his life.

There is a new, "humane" approach to the newborn which has the infant immersed in water for the first 20 or 30 minutes after birth, gently massaged by the physician (sometimes by the father). Certainly this is preferable to the usual treatment in which the baby is washed, weighed, stretched out for measuring, his foot poked for blood, his eyes blurred by silver nitrate; and after all these indignities, bundled into a blanket and hurried to the isolation of the nursery.

But soaking the baby in water removes the protective coating **(vernix caseosa)** on the baby's skin which should be allowed to be absorbed into the skin gradually. It is a natural protection against infections of the skin. A more serious objection to immersing the newborn in warm water is that it takes the baby away from the mother during this crucial bonding period. In the first moments of life baby should feel the mother's loving hands, the taste of her nipple, the scent of her warm body, the intonations of her voice, the look in her eyes as he focuses his eyes on hers.

The attempt to ease the baby's birth "trauma" reflects a negative attitude toward the birth, paralleling the negative attitude that birth is a "trauma" for the mother. A baby is not to return to the environment of the womb from which he has just emerged, but to experience the loving feel of skin upon skin, the healing, soothing touch of another human being. He needs to enter into touching relationships and not to withdraw from them at the very outset of his life.

Night and day

The initial bonding of infant to parents has been shown to be almost as important for the parents as for the baby. Studies show that infants kept in the hospital for a lengthy time after birth are among the children most often brought in as battered children later on. Of course this does not imply that all parents of infants who were separated from them at birth (premature, ill babies etc.) become abusive, but it does demonstrate that bonding deprivation affects the parents as well as the child.

For example, how many fathers feel aloof from their infants until they are several weeks or even months old? The father may be afraid to touch his baby, afraid he might hurt him or her (though he might never admit fear!). The mother becomes confident through her continual touching and handling of the baby, but the father continues to be deprived of this experience. Rather than admit his timidity, he may claim that he "doesn't want to be bothered."

The father's bonding to the infant may be deepened by having the baby in the parental bed.[6] The baby's bassinet or crib may be in the parents room, but keeping the baby in their own bed whenever they wish keeps the parents from jumping up and down during the night to check on the baby, cover him, pick him up or bring him to the mother to nurse.

A breastfed baby does not sleep through the night, fortunately, for if he did his mother's breasts would be engorged and uncomfortable by morning and she would be more vulnerable to breast problems. With baby in the bed, it is a simple matter to let him or her nurse several times during the night without disturbing anyone. The mother need not even turn over to nurse the baby on alternate breasts, unless she chooses to. She can nurse first on the breast which is next to the bed, then turn slightly toward the baby and nurse on the other breast. The mother's body should be in the curved position used for labor with her knees drawn up. Baby is to be pulled in toward her, with his feet on her tummy, to align him correctly with the breast while nursing.

A passage in 1 Kings expresses a common misconception that babies who sleep with others might be smothered in the night.[7] But what has often been thought to be smothering of an infant (whether in his own bed or wherever he is) is now known to be the Sudden Infant Death syndrome, in which a baby simply stops breathing because the breathing reflex fails to function. Parents of a child who died in this way need to know that they are **not** at fault, whether the child was alone or not. Fortunately, this syndrome is uncommon, and researchers are continually studying ways in which to identify which infants might be subject to this problem.

Even a tiny baby will object strongly to being rolled on or being buried under the covers. The breathing instinct is one of the most powerful of the survival instincts, so that the baby will squirm or cry (as when his nose is wiped) until the problem is resolved. The mother especially is more likely to be awakened by the baby squirming for air in their bed than if he is struggling alone in his own crib, entangled in the blankets.

For nine months the baby has been in constant contact with another person, rocked in the womb as the mother moved around, caressed by the moving waters of the amniotic sac and the frequent contractions of the uterus, soothed by the sound of the mother's heartbeat and other internal noises. This close association needs to be continued after the birth, with baby close to mother and daddy both night and day, smelling their distinctive odors, hearing the sounds of their breathing, feeling their warmth.

The phenomenon of a child being placed in his own bed, in his own room, from the time of birth on is found only in affluent societies—societies with the highest rates of alienation and suicide.[8] Through most of history in every culture children have slept with their parents. The infant Jesus snuggled between Joseph and Mary in the warmth of the manger. He was fortunate that he had "no crib for a bed." Poverty may be the cause of families sleeping together, but there are compensating emotional benefits of which the isolated, untouched child is deprived. Tine Thevenin, author of **The Family Bed,** suggests that one reason so many teenagers are jumping into bed together may not be simply a desire for sex, but an unconscious search for the closeness and security of the parental bed which was denied them as infants and small children.[9]

Jesus tells the story of the man who would not get up at midnight to answer his friend's knock at the door. *Don't bother me,* the man said. *The door is already locked, and my children are **with** me in bed, so that I cannot get up....*[10] Some modern translators have "culturized" this statement to read, *My children and I have gone to bed,*[11] but this is not what the text says. Because the children were sleeping with their daddy, he could not get up without the risk of disturbing them.

Jesus is aware of our need for "closeness" when He says, *I will never leave you nor forsake you!*[12] The Psalmist says, *My help comes from the Lord.... He who keeps you will not slumber.*[13] *He gives sleep to his loved ones.*[14] *I will lie down peacefully, and sleep, for you, Lord, keep me in safety.*[15]

One of the most devastating human feelings is that of being forsaken. The infant has no concept of the ever-present God. His security is found in the closeness of his parents day and night. A lawyer friend said to me that he and his wife keep their baby girl in bed with them at night so that she will never know fear as an infant. Whenever she wakes up, she can look into one of their faces, or if it is dark, can reach out and touch them.

What's in a name?

A name is an important symbol of a deeper reality—the person. A name is more than a convenient label to tell people apart. People in western cultures often choose names simply because they "sound nice," but many other cultures are more creative in their choice of names. Some have used names as simple as One, Two, Three, Four, giving the children names in the order in which they were born into the family. Indian children have often been named for items in the physical world such as Gray Squirrel, Red Fox, Crying Wind, etc. The child is thought to have some of the qualities of the item for which it is named.

In the Philippines new names are often coined uniquely. Our daughter Margaret spent two years in the Philippines in the Peace Corps. One of her Filipina friends named her little boy Marwel, a combination of Margaret's first and last names. When her second child was born, she named him Felmar, after her sisters Faith and Marion. A Filipino evangelist named his new daughter Charisse, because she was born while he was conducting a charismatic crusade. Another Filipina friend is named Saigua, because her father had been both in Saigon and Guam in the months before her birth. These are all delightfully creative ways of assigning distinctive names to a child.

Names are important, for they are the symbols of our unique identities before God and man. An inspiring name becomes a self-fulfilling prophecy, something to live up to. Several cultures wait a month or more before naming a baby in order to find out what the personality of the child is like before choosing a name to fit. However, parents need to decide upon names for their children which not only have positive meaning to the parents, but will not offend the child later. It is helpful to check the meanings of common names in an unabridged dictionary list, in order not to choose one with negative overtones. Who, for example, would want to be named Jezebel?[16]

When God created man and woman, *he blessed them and called **their** name **adam**.*[17] This identified men and women as people of the earth *(adamah)*. The name Noah means "comfort." *For this boy will comfort us concerning the toil of our hands....*[18] Abraham means "father of many nations."[19] Sarah means "princess of God,"[20] Isaac means "laughter,"[21] Samuel means "asked of God,"[22] Jesus (Hebrew: Joshua) means "savior" (Jah saves).[23]

Names are so important that God will give each of us a "new name" one day,[24] different from that of any one else and known only to Him and to us. This will be His intimate, endearing, special name for us, such as the special name we give to someone we love dearly. For example, no one outside our family would know which of our children we call "Beezer," but the family knows.

Christian parents may want to agree on a name before birth, so that the newborn already has some identity when he or she appears. One couple decided on two names if their third child was a boy. If he was slender and fair he would have one of the names, but if husky and dark haired, he would be named Seth. The moment the baby appeared the father exclaimed, "It's Seth!"

The comforting breasts[25]

The new baby needs to be put to the breast as soon as possible after birth. The touch of baby's mouth stimulates the uterus to contract and expel the afterbirth. For the child, the touch of the mother's nipple on the most sensitive part of his body—his mouth—insures that he will quickly learn to recognize the source of supply for his needs. Even a two or three day old baby who has been bonded from birth may refuse an alternate source such as a finger or a rubber nipple. The baby already knows his own mother by smell, touch, and taste.

The baby should be nursed frequently (every 1½ to 2 hours) during the days following the birth. This gives baby the benefits of the colostrum (the secretion in the breasts which precedes the appearance of milk) and helps the milk to be produced more quickly with less engorgement of the breasts. Colostrum and breast milk are absorbed much more quickly by the baby than formula, so that he needs to be fed more often than the bottle-fed baby. He can suck as long as he likes each time. He needs the sucking, even if he is not getting much at first. If baby won't take the breast, or won't suck, it may be because he is being given glucose water or formula in the nursery.

After childbirth there is additional fluid in the breast tissue which is caused by the total hormonal changes in the body. If the milk is not "let down" as it begins to form in the breast, stimulated by the baby's frequent sucking, the breasts can become engorged and extremely uncomfortable. After a week or two the breasts will have become smaller and less firm. Some mothers fear that they have "lost their milk" when this occurs, but this is not true. Only the initial swelling of the tissues has receded, and there is still milk in the breasts. The more baby sucks, the more milk there will be, as milk production is stimulated by the sucking.

Sometimes the baby's sucking makes the nipples sore after a day or two. Several techniques can help avoid this problem. First, it is important the position of the baby's mouth on the nipple be correct. The baby's mouth must be well up on the breast, around the darker section of the nipple called the **areola,** not just on the end of the nipple. Also, it is essential that baby's tongue be **under** the nipple, and not curled back in his mouth above the nipple. (This only occurs occasionally. Most babies instinctively grasp the nipple correctly.) Never pull the baby off the breast, but insert a clean finger between his gums in the corner of his mouth to break the suction, and then remove the nipple. Air dry the nipples after nursing, and if they seem tender, apply a recommended nipple cream. Often these protective creams are not needed, for natural lubrication is provided by the tiny Montgomery glands around the nipple area (the little bumps around the nipple which are more obvious when the woman is cold). These glands produce a secretion which softens the skin of the nipples and kills undesirable bacteria. Nothing stronger than water should be used on the nipples (soap is drying and removes the natural secretions). Plastic bra liners and plastic-backed nursing pads should be avoided, as plastic does not allow the skin to "breathe" adequately. It also prevents evaporation so that cracked and sore nipples may result. Prenatal nipple preparation can be helpful in preventing soreness. Massaging nipples with a dry towel and rolling them gently between the fingers are good "toughening" exercises.

In Houston hospitals 90 percent of the newborns going home with their mothers are being breastfed, according to Dr. Buford

Nichols, a pediatrician who is head of nutrition and gastroenterology at the Baylor College of Medicine in Houston. These women are urged to continue breastfeeding for six months or more. There are benefits for the breastfeeding woman as well as the baby. Dr. Nichols points out that "there is a lot we do not know about lactation, but we do know that the breast cancer rate in mothers who breastfeed their children successfully is only one-seventh what it is in women who do not."[26]

Babies can and should be breastfed even in special situations such as prematurity, twins or triplets, malformations, developmental problems, adopted babies, and so forth. Dorothy Brewster has published an excellent book on how to cope with these problems successfully.[27]

In many earlier cultures babies were carried continually in touch contact with another human being day and night. As the baby grew older, he or she was carried by the father, older brothers and sisters, and grandparents. But most often it was the mother who kept the baby next to her body, letting him nurse not only when hungry but whenever comfort was needed.

> *Rejoice with Jerusalem and exult in her,*
> *all you who love her;...*
> *Then you may suck and be fed from the*
> *breasts that give comfort,*
> *delighting in her plentiful milk.*[28]
>
> *As nurslings you shall be carried in her arms,*
> *and fondled in her lap.*[29]

The breastfeeding mother can learn a variety of comfortable positions in which to breastfeed the growing baby: lying down, sitting up, or walking around with the baby tied to her in a sling or cloth baby carrier. The above passage in the King James' Version reads, *you shall be borne upon her sides, and dandled on her knees.* This is the picture of an older nursling astride his mother's hip, for one does not carry a newborn on the side or bounce him on one's lap! The older baby is still close to the mother, never far from the *breasts of comfort,* even if he only wants to lean his head against their soft warmth or suck for comfort.

The baby can be fed discreetly in public with none being the wiser, unless they happen to lift the edge of the blanket to peek at the "sleeping" baby.

Every church should have resource persons who will help guide the younger breastfeeding mothers. Paul aptly says, *Let the older women...teach the younger women....*[30] in practical ways, helping young wives to fulfill their responsibilities to husbands and children. Breastfeeding may be "natural" but a young woman will have many questions from time to time. Although there now is a wealth of helpful literature for the breastfeeding mother,[31] there is also a need for "mothering the mother."[32] How helpful it is to have a trusted, experienced woman to whom the new mother can turn for practical as well as spiritual advice!

A living fountain

A perfect substitute will never be found for breast milk, for it is a living substance, flowing from the mother's living tissues into the living baby, providing antibodies and friendly bacteria. Attempts to analyze it in the laboratory are imperfect, for stored breast milk is not the same as that which goes directly from the mother's body into the body of the baby. Subtle changes occur when it is allowed to stand that make complete analysis impossible, and research techniques also may be imperfect.[33]

Because breast milk is living tissue similar to the baby's own tissues, if he chokes on it and aspirates it into his lungs it is readily absorbed. Any other substance, even water but especially formula, is toxic when aspirated into the lungs, causing fluids and swelling to develop which may lead to serious respiratory ailments or pneumonia. It is common knowledge that breastfed babies, especially prematures, have unexpected immunological and biochemical advantages over bottle fed babies.[34] They have fewer allergies, fewer digestive upsets, fewer skin disorders (such as eczema) and fewer respiratory infections (such as colds, bronchitis and pneumonia).

Now it is being discovered that chemicals in human breast milk stimulate the normal development of organs such as the intestinal tract. For example, it helps prevent circulatory problems in later life by changing the way in which the body handles cholesterol. Harvard researchers have shown, in a longitudinal study begun fifty years ago, that babies who were breastfed exclusively for more than two months have less cholesterol in their blood as adults than babies who were bottle fed.[35]

The breastfed baby also appears to have an intellectual advantage. Dr. Gerald Gaull, pediatric researcher at the New York State Institute of Basic Research in Mental Retardation, explains that the human brain is relatively immature at birth, having acquired only 25% of its mature brain weight by that time. "After birth, the baby is still in his phase of most rapid growth, and there is a great demand for specific essential nutrients. Nutritional requirements are, therefore, critical."[36]

One of the more important of these substances in human breast milk is taurine, a nonprotein nitrogen compound 30% to 40% more abundant in breast milk than in cow's milk. There is considerable evidence that the taurine in breast milk "may be a neurotransmitter or neuromodulator substance in brain and retina."[37] The human fetal and infant brain requires a high concentration of this substance, higher than that of the mature brain. Yet the newborn has limited ability to utilize taurine from sources other than the mother's milk, although it is essential for the development of his brain.

One of the tragedies of our modern world is that women in third world countries are turning in large numbers from breastfeeding to formula feeding of their infants with disastrous results. Not only are their infants deprived of the advantages of breast milk, but infant illnesses and deaths are soaring. Formula is so expensive that often it takes so much of the family income to feed the baby that the rest of the family cannot afford adequate food. Unlearned mothers will add water to the formula to "stretch" it. Not only is this starving the infant, but the water is often from unsanitary supplies. Bottles may be improperly washed, the milk not refrigerated and easily spoiled. Malnutrition, gastrointestinal illnesses, low resistance to disease and mental retardation are increasingly common.

Dr. William Hodges, a missionary pediatrician in a hospital in Haiti says that when he first began his practice there in 1958, he tried to teach the families of babies whose mothers died in childbirth to make formula at home. But the babies did not thrive and were soon sick with diarrhea and dehydration. Soon he also discovered that children from the city of Cap Haitien were being hospitalized far more often with problems than children from the country. He discovered that the city mothers were being encouraged to stop breastfeeding between six and nine months.

The results were obvious. One could almost go out in the clinic waiting room and guess where the patients were from by the general condition of the babies! The Cap Haitien baby of one year was often underweight (10-12

> *pounds), was a little puffy from hypo-proteinemia, and
> had a peculiar coloring of the lips due to vitamin deficien-
> cy. The peasant baby, on the other hand, frequently weigh-
> ed 20 pounds at one year and was doing quite well....
> Thus, it was that by 1960 this hospital began to scream in
> a loud voice about giving breast milk to all babies until
> they were two years old.*[38]

I was astonished, when traveling through the Philippines in the 1970's, at how few Filipina women breastfed their babies. When I asked why, I was told that no one wanted to be like the poorest of the poor, who couldn't afford to buy formula. Formula feeding was a "status" symbol! Unfortunately cultural lag has again made our example a disadvantage to the world's people. They are copying a custom we are now turning from, for breastfeeding is coming back into favor in the United States, as the great advantages for both mother and baby are becoming known.

Breastfeeding involves not only the milk itself, this living substance, but the relationship between the mother and her baby. The skin-to-skin contact—baby's mouth to mother's skin—stimulates subliminal responses in them both, stored away in the subconscious mind, impossible for either of them to experience in bottle feeding.[39] An emotional intimacy develops between mother and baby that far exceeds the simple act of providing the baby with physical nourishment.

The living fountain from the breast is one of the most intimate of the symbols of the believer's relationship to God. Once more God appears in Scripture as mother, this time not as giving birth to spiritual children, but as nourishing them from the fountain of the female breast. The profound intimacy experienced between a breastfeeding mother and her baby is pictured in Scripture as also occurring between the believer and God:

> *As newborn babies, desire the pure milk of the word, so
> that through it you may grow, now that you have tasted
> that the Lord is good.*[40]

This is a reference to the Psalm which says, *O **taste** and see that the Lord is good.*[41] What does it mean to "taste" the Lord? It is a picture of the infant tasting the skin of his mother's breast as well as the milk, even as the new believer "tastes" the Lord in drawing milk from the living fountain of Christ the mother.

Too many Christians are "bottle-fed." Everything comes to them second hand, drawn from Christ perhaps, but passed on by someone else rather than coming to them fresh from the original source. The new believer needs to draw life and comfort from Christ, the living fountain.

Women as well as men are made in the image of the eternal Spirit of Christ, women's life-sustaining breasts symbols of God's own life-sustaining nature. We need not be offended at this symbolism any more than at the symbolism of eating Christ's body and drinking His blood:

> *Jesus said to them, I tell you the truth. Unless you eat the flesh of the Son of man, and drink His blood, you have no life in you. Whoever eats my flesh, and drinks my blood has eternal life, and I will raise him up at the last day....*
>
> *Does this offend you? For there are some of you who do not believe.... From that time on many of his disciples went back, and would not follow him any more.*[42]

These profound symbols relate our most elemental human experiences to spiritual realities. We need to receive spiritual sustenance directly from the true source, the living God.

NOTES
1. Lk. 2:1-20. **2.** Lk. 18:15; Mt. 19:13-15. **3.** Mt. 18:10.
4. Marshall Klaus and John Kennel. **Maternal-Infant Bonding: The Impact of Early Separation or Loss on Family Development.** St. Louis. C.V. Mosby. 1976.
5. Film, "The Amazing Newborn." Cleveland, OH. Ross Laboratories. 1976.
6. Tine Thevenin. **The Family Bed.** P.O. Box 16004, Minneapolis, MN 55416. 1976.
7. 1 Kgs. 3:16-18. *This woman's child died in the night, because she lay on him.* The woman in this passage is relating to King Solomon what she **thought** happened. But it was most likely a case of Sudden Infant Death syndrome.

8. Suicide rates have been shown to be statistically related to the standard of living. The higher the standard, the more suicides there are. Sweden has the highest standard of living (per capita income) in the world and the highest suicide rate, as of this writing.
9. Thevenin, **op. cit. 10.** Lk. 11:7. **11.** For example, NEB. **12.** Heb. 13:5. **13.** Ps. 121:4. **14.** Ps. 127:2. **15.** Ps. 4:8. **16.** 1 Kgs. 18:4, 19; 19:1-3; 2 Kgs. 9:30-37. **17.** Gen. 5:2. **18.** Gen. 5:27. **19.** Gen 17:5.
20. The Hebrew word *sar* means "prince." The name Sarai (Gen. 11:29) adds the feminine ending, meaning "princess." God changed her name to Sarah (sar-Jah), "princess of God" (Gen. 17:15).
21. Gen. 18:10-15, 21:1-7. **22.** 1 Sam. 1:20. **23.** Mt. 1:21. **24.** Rev. 2:17. **25.** Isa. 66:11.
26. Reported in the **Minneapolis Star and Tribune,** 1979.
27. Dorothy Patricia Brewster. **You Can Breastfeed Your Baby—even in Special Situations.** Rodale Press, P.O. Box 2003, Palos Verdes Peninsula, CA 90274. 1979.
28. Isa. 66:10, 11 NEB. **29.** Is. 66:12, 13 NAB. **30.** Tit. 2:3-5.
31. The La Leche book, **The Womanly Art of Breastfeeding** is a classic resource. La Leche League also provides many reprints of pertinent articles, local groups for breastfeeding mothers and telephone counseling. 9616 Minneapolis Ave., Franklin Park, IL 60131.

A number of helpful pamphlets on breastfeeding are also available from Health Education Associates, 520 School House Lane, Willow Grove, PA 19090.
32. Dana Raphael. **The Tender Gift: Breastfeeding. Mothering the Mother—the way to successful breastfeeding.** New York. Schocken Books. 1973.
33. For example, for a long time researchers claimed there was no vitamin D in breastmilk. They were looking for it in the lipid fraction, because it's a fat-soluble vitamin. Medical World News magazine (McGraw-Hill, Feb. 9, 1979, vol. 20, #3, p. 71) reports that they happened to test for it in the aqueous fraction and found it there.
34. W. G. Whittlestone, D. Sc. "The Biological Specificity of Milk. Cow's Milk For Cows, Human Milk For Humans." La Leche League Information Sheet No. 14, November, 1976.
35. Reported in "Science confirms suspicion: Mother's milk is best for baby," **Minneapolis Star & Tribune,** Dec. 9, 1979.
36. Reported in **ICEA Communications West,** 8322 Maybell Lane SW, Tacoma, WA 98498.
37. "Science confirms suspicion:...," **op. cit.**
38. Reported in **Insight: A Special Report:** "International Milk Companies and Breast Feeding." International Ministries, American Baptist Churches in the USA. Valley Forge, PA 19481. November 1979.
39. Those who have bottlefed in the past need not feel guilty, but can thank the Lord that young mothers today have access to both information and personal encouragement that help them to choose breastfeeding far more often.
40. 1 Pet. 2:2, 3. **41.** Ps. 34:8. **42.** Jn. 6:47-66.

New Identities

Blessed are all who fear the Lord,
  who walk in his ways.
You will eat of the fruit of your labor;
  blessing and prosperity will be yours.
Your wife will be like a fruitful vine
  within your house;
your children like olive plants
  around your table.
Thus is the man blessed
  who fears the Lord.
May the Lord bless you from Zion
  all the days of your life;
may you see the prosperity of Jerusalem,
  and may you live to see your children's children.
Peace be upon Israel.[1]

The arrival of the first baby changes a "couple" into a "family," the most dramatic adjustment of a lifetime. While still only a couple, husband and wife learn to give and take, yielding to the desires of the other or being yielded to. This mutual joy of **being** loved is still in the realm of self-gratification.

But when baby comes, for the parents it is **all** give, give, give, twenty four hours a day. For some new parents, this is the first time in their lives that they have experienced the need for the total renunciation of their own desires for the sake of another. The husband has become a father for the rest of his life, whether he wants to be or not. The wife becomes a life-long mother. Even if the child dies or grows up and moves away, even if the parents separate, the father is still the father and the mother is still the mother, responsible before God for their child. One might say that God gives children to parents to help the parents "grow up," turning their thoughts outward, away from self, in a new dimension of personal growth.

Father of compassion

God does not leave the new father without a model for his behavior, but is Himself the perfect model. *Praise be to the God and Father of our Lord Jesus Christ, the Father of compassion and the God of all comfort, who comforts us in all our troubles.*[2]

The picture that most of us have of God as father is as provider, protector, disciplinarian, "boss." Those are all secondary aspects of God as father, but the first and primary one is that *God is love.*[3] This love is expressed by His constant presence and involvement with us, just as the human father is to be close to and involved with his children from the time of birth, carrying them in his arms, holding the infant skin-to-skin, sleeping with him or her, building a relationship from the moment of birth. God as father is pictured as this loving, caring person:

> *He shall gather the lambs with his arm and carry them in his bosom.*[4]
> *You have been my burden since your birth, whom I have carried from your infancy. I will carry you from the womb to the grave.*[5]
> *When Israel was a boy, then I loved him; I called my son out of Egypt.... It was I who taught him to walk, I who had taken them in my arms, drawing them with love-bonding. I had lifted them like a little child to my cheek, I had bent down to feed them.*[6]

One of the loveliest thoughts in Scripture is that of God singing over His children. One can picture a father rocking or walking with his baby in his strong arms, singing to him or her:

> *The Lord your God is strong. He will save, he will rejoice over you with joy. He will rest in his love, he will joy over you with singing.*[7]

One of our sons likes to sing to his nieces and nephews. He takes the tiny, fussy squirmer from the weary mother and begins to sing. They **listen.** If the baby is fussing in his bed, jumper or play pen, he doesn't pick the baby up but sits down near him and starts singing softly. That loving, bass voice does wonders! The baby quiets down, turns, and gazes into his eyes, soothed and comforted by his singing. *He will joy over you with singing.*

The closeness of father-child bonding benefits the father as well as the child. My son-in-law is unaware of the profound changes that have been taking place in him through touch contact with his small children. They can fall asleep together anywhere, in the rocking chair, on the floor, snuggled together. In this same way many fathers are being healed of their own touch-deprivation suffered from infancy.

Bath time provides the father with an opportunity for good interaction with his baby. He can not only give the baby his bath, but when the infant is old enough, take him or her into the tub with him, skin to skin in the warm water, splashing and playing.

It all sounds beautiful, but it isn't easy! God's children often bucked and kicked and tried to throw off the bonds of love![8] It's easy to love the peacefully sleeping baby, but the halo begins to slip as days go by. The baby keeps daddy awake at night. He isn't used to any disruption of his sleep and drags out of bed exhausted in the morning. The song fades, and human nature asserts itself. One time a young couple who lived in a little house near ours were blessed with their first baby. Three weeks later I was startled awake in the middle of the night by the new father yelling at his crying baby, "SHUT UP!" I could hear him yelling even though our houses were two hundred feet apart. Of course the baby went right on crying, harder than ever.

The problems that arise are promptings to the father's primary role as spiritual head of his household, the intercessor. Moses, that great leader of the people of Israel, complained that the Lord had overburdened him in a parent role. He turned to the resource of prayer in his distress.

> *And Moses said to the Lord, "Why have you afflicted me, your servant? Why have I not found favor in your sight, but instead you laid the burden of all this people on me?*
>
> *"Have I conceived all these people? Have I given birth to them that you should tell me, 'Carry them in your bosom as a father of a breastfeeding infant carries his sucking child?'*
>
> *"I'm not able to carry all these people alone, because it's too much for me! If you're going to treat me like this, please kill me! I can't take it any more!"*[9]

Children are a mixed blessing. It is a wise father who takes his complaints to the Lord and does not inflict his wife and children with his irritations, as most human fathers do. The Bible says, ***be angry, but don't sin.***[10] The feelings of frustration and anger are normal. It's what we do about them that counts. Moses took his anger to the Lord, except once. On that one occasion he lost his temper at the **people:** *Listen to me, you rebels!....*[11] And with those angry words, he lost the right to enter the promised land! *It went badly with Moses because of them, for they provoked his spirit so that he spoke unwisely with his lips.*[12]

A man cannot be a loving father at all times unless he is a loving person, filled with the love of God toward everyone. *Everyone who loves is born of God and knows God. He who does not love does not know God, for God is love.*[13] Dostoevsky writes of this in **The Brothers Karamazov.** The saintly, dying priest Zosima is speaking:

> *Every day and every hour, every minute, walk round yourself and watch yourself, and see that your image be seemly. You pass by a little child. You pass by, spiteful, with ugly words, with wrathful heart; you may not have noticed the child, but he has seen you, and your image, unseemly and impious, may remain in his defenceless heart. You don't know it, but you may have sown an evil seed in him and it may grow, and all because you were not careful before the child, because you did not foster in yourself a circumspect, actively benevolent love. Brothers, love is a teacher; but one must know how to acquire it, for it is hard to acquire. It is dearly bought, it is won slowly by long labour. For we must love not only occasionally, for a moment, but for all time. Every one can love occasionally, even the most wicked can....*

Working fathers?

In many simpler, less industrialized societies families were together all day, carrying out a trade at home or farming together. This kind of family life is seldom possible today, so that most fathers are away from home for long hours at a time. The conscientious father will want to find creative ways in which to compensate his children for the deprivation caused by his absence at work.

Some have suggested that one of the troubles with America as a nation is that whole generations have been raised by women, first in the home, then in preschool and on into the elementary grades. This pattern of deprivation (robbing both fathers and children) is paralleled in the sex and age segregation of our churches, where men teachers are seldom in evidence before children reach junior high age. (The men are too busy with the important "work" of the church?) Thus the generation gap begins with the cradle.

Father-infant bonding which begins at birth should be continued through the early weeks and months. The more the daddy handles his baby, changes diapers, walks the floor with, talks to, sings to his baby, the more his own self-esteem grows, and the more confident he becomes in his ability as a father. His closeness to the child will give him insights into the child's needs and behavior, making his expectations more realistic. His work will not be the center of his life, nor will he need to find other things to do after work so he won't have to be "bothered with" the baby.

Joseph, the husband of Mary, is a beautiful example of a godly father who placed the needs of the child above his own, and it was not even his own child! When Joseph learned that Mary was pregnant, his first thought was not one of anger, but of kindness. *Because he was a righteous man, he did not want her to be publicly disgraced.*[14] While he was meditating on what to do about this seeming tragedy, his heart was so open to the Lord that an angel came to him in a dream and told him what to do. Joseph obeyed the Lord, and took Mary as his wife.

Again, when the angel of the Lord warned him that the child's life was in danger, he took the child and his mother to a place of safety. He was willing to give up his professional contacts for the sake of the child. He was a carpenter in Nazareth, where he no doubt had built up a clientele. All this was sacrificed when he left Bethlehem for Egypt rather than returning to Nazareth after Jesus was born. How many men would leave their jobs and move to another community—or to another country as Joseph did—for the sake of their baby? Yes, there are fathers like that. Joseph was one of them, giving up his business for his adopted son. For what is the purpose of a good income anyway?

> *The ground of a certain rich man brought forth an abundance. And he thought to himself, "Now what shall I do? I will pull down my barns and build bigger ones, so that I have room for all my produce and equipment. Then I will say to my soul, 'Soul, you have enough stored up for many*

years. Take it easy now. Eat, drink, and be merry!'"
But God said to him, "You fool. This very night your soul is required of you. Then whose will those things be that you have provided? So it is with everyone who lays up treasure for himself and is not rich toward God."[15]

While a man may say he has to work to earn a decent living for his family, his motives are often mixed. His profession gives him a sense of self-worth. The money he makes adds to his (false) feelings of importance. His wise investments make him feel "secure" for the future. This is not the way of blessing!

Children should not save up for their parents, but parents for children. I will gladly spend myself and be spent for your sake. If I love you too much, will I be loved the less for that?[16]

A father's investment in his child is not to be just money, but the investment also of himself, spending time and energy, showing interest and affection. God has promised to meet every need of a father who walks in the way of such faith and obedience as Joseph's, even in times of financial panic or collapse. *Blessed is the man who trusts in the Lord, and rests his confidence upon him. He shall be like a tree planted by the waterside.... In a year of drought it feels no care, and does not cease to bear fruit.*[17]

Nor does a Christian father's investment of himself and his money end with his own children. *Pure religion which is undefiled before God and the Father is this: to visit the fatherless and the widows in their affliction, and to keep himself unspotted from the world.*[18] The passage does not say to "give money to" the fatherless children and the widows, although that is part of what is meant. It says to *visit* them, to give of one's **self** and not just give a handout. God as father again provides the example, for He is called *a father of the fatherless, and a defender of widows. He gives a home to the forsaken.*[19]

Joseph had such a heart for God that he was able to receive guidance for the welfare of a "fatherless" child, Jesus. Twice more the Lord guided him by a dream, first to return to his own nation and then warning him not to go to Judea but to return to Nazareth. Both times he obeyed, raising his foster son in the workshop beside him, guiding him in the ways of faith to the best of his ability until the Lord took him home.

The priest/father, the protector, provider, intercessor, the loving, caring, touching father will one day stand before God to answer to the responsibility which God has given him. How wonderful if he can truthfully say, *Here I am, and the children you have given to me.*[20]

The "insulator"

The new father needs to allow his own natural "mothering" instincts to flourish toward his wife as well as his baby. His companion may seem like a different person for a while! Her first concern always seems to be the baby. Meals may or may not appear on time, the washing piles up and he has to rummage in the dryer to find his own clean socks. It is a wise husband who will share the new responsibilities not only by caring for the baby, but quietly making his own lunch (or breakfast or supper), helping take care of his own clothes, picking up the house and even throwing a load of diapers in the wash himself.

This self-denial on the husband's part will bring him rich dividends. His wife, who seemed so independent and self-sufficient before, now needs someone to lean upon, someone to share the decisions and work. A wise husband will enjoy the new esteem that comes to him from a wife who finds him dependable in this way.

It won't be easy, for his wife seems to be taking less notice of him. The baby always seems to be at her breast, even at night. It may seem as if he didn't exist to her, as if he had no sexual needs, for the baby is always in the way. He may feel jealous of his wife giving the baby so much attention, jealous of the baby enjoying his wife's breasts.

These negative feelings are perfectly normal, for things are not the same as they were before. Grantly Dick-Read points out that in crisis situations, such as shipwreck, a man's first thought is for the safety of his wife. But her first thought is for the safety of the children! Only later will she think of him. When a husband realizes that his wife's attentiveness to the child is a God-given instinct for the survival of the race, it will be easier to be patient.

Everyone seems to be drawing from the mother. The baby feeds on her body, older children clamor for attention, the husband may be impatiently waiting for his meals or wanting sex. Such a wife feels drained from all these demands on her. The wise husband rises to her need and ministers to his wife, encouraging her, and sharing the work load.

This sets a pattern for the years that follow, in which husband and wife work as a parenting team. I am reminded of my own husband and the many ways in which he helped when our children were small, such as grocery shopping together—hauling babies and grocery bags up the hill to the house with me, helping in the kitchen. One time several of our small children were sick with the intestinal flu, all at the same time! We spread sheets around over the floor, around the beds and on the path to the bathroom—for those old enough to walk seldom got there in time. Not once did I have to leave a sick child. For while I held them, comforted them, or rushed to the bathroom with one of them, he was gathering up the stinking sheets and bed clothes, spreading clean ones, and washing out the filth in the laundry. He did it voluntarily, and said not one word of complaint.

In simpler times everyone worked at home to provide for the needs of the household, but in our industrial society this is seldom possible. Many mothers work away from home out of economic necessity. This makes it all the more imperative for husband and wife to be a parenting team. When we had five children under eleven years of age, my husband wanted me to go back to college for a B.A. degree, which had been interrupted by our marriage. At first I hesitated, but began to feel it was what the Lord wanted me to do. For two and a half years he juggled his schedule as a seminary professor to come home and care for the three little ones under school age, so that I could take my classes at the college. Only twice during those years was it necessary for me to take the children to a sitter for a class hour, because of a conflict in our schedules. Because of the continuity of care in the home, either mother or daddy always there, the children didn't even notice the coming and going. I was able to finish my degree and go on to graduate school. My husband invested himself, his time and his helping hands in our family, not only by his professional skills but as a husband and father.

Jill of all trades

The care of a new baby is an awesome responsibility for a first time mother, especially if she has never been around babies. A new mother wants to do everything **right.** Inevitably this makes her overprotective of the first child, but that's all right. It's baby's first experience at being mothered, and he or she will adjust to the kind of mothering being given. The physical care of the first baby is tiring—washing, changing, burping, feeding, clothing, covering with blankets. The exhaustion comes not so much from the work involved as from the emotional energy expended trying to be the "perfect mother."

Not only that, but the regular routine also must go on, the housecleaning, the meals, the family wash, the shopping. Daddy may be a willing helper, but even he can't do it all. Relatives may move in to help, but much wisdom is needed in this, for they may displace the father's role and add tension to the marriage. Diaper service for the first few weeks is a wise investment, or disposable diapers can be used until the new mother feels she has things under control.

It is important to let some things go! Schedules no longer matter. Clothes will get just as clean on Thursday as on Monday. Beds can be made at night rather than in the morning. The mother must learn to ignore the uneasy feeling of being continually behind, put baby's needs first and take care of other tasks as she can. The household will gradually return to normal sooner than she thinks, although that "normalcy" will be different from her previous ideal conception of it.

The biggest identity crisis in a woman's life comes in this transition from person to mother, although she may not be aware of this right away. Her personhood becomes lost in the tangle of responsibilities to others—wife, mother, housewife, nursemaid, cook, dish washer, bed changer, secretary, chauffeur and on and on through the years—with no direct financial return and often little or no words of appreciation or confirmation. She becomes of necessity a Jill of all trades.

One of our daughters taught at a university before her marriage. After the birth of her first child she met a woman friend she had known at the university. When asked what she was doing, my daughter replied that she was married and at home with a new baby. "Yes," her friend replied, "but what do you **do**?" Mothering didn't count as "doing" anything important.

Center of the universe?

One of the risks of this role change is that a woman becomes so absorbed in her baby that the baby becomes the "center of the universe." Every mother should remember that children grow up and go away, but her spouse is the one who will share all the years of her life with her. This is not the time to shut him out, but to draw him in!

When bottle feeding was more common, some fathers greatly enjoyed giving their baby the bottle. The father of a breastfeeding baby does not have this privilege and can feel left out unless he is allowed to develop a close relationship with his baby in all other ways. He can talk or hum to him or take naps with baby snuggled close to him. And of course there are always those prosaic activities for him of walking the floor, burping the baby, talking to him and looking into his eyes while changing diapers, and so on.

Many mothers are unconsciously selfish and prevent the father from sharing these responsibilities. The mother feels he "can't do anything right" and shuts him out. Or she fears that the baby will bother him and refuses to give him enough responsibility. Often a husband intuitively senses his wife's fear of his handling the baby and isolates himself from contact during the early weeks and months.

The first year of a child's life he needs to be near his mother most of the time, for the security of continuity of care. If it is financially necessary for the mother to work it is even more important for the father to be actively involved with his baby, to help compensate for this maternal deprivation.

It has been said that the first five years of our lives are the most important in determining our emotional ability to cope with the stresses of life. These are also the most formative years. If both parents must work, they need to pray for wisdom in finding child care from people who share their Christian faith and their philosophy of family life. The more the environment in which the child will be cared for is like his own home, the better.

Even school age children need the security of finding mother or daddy at home by the time they come from school, full of things to tell about their day. A high schooler needs to be able to walk in the door and call, "Mom! I'm home!" and hear a familiar voice reply.

It is possible for a working mother to breastfeed her baby, and this helps overcome some of the handicap of separation. Baby can be nursed before she leaves for work and nursed frequently after she returns home and through the night. This frequent nursing after working hours keeps her milk supply adequate. She can express her milk during the day while she is at work and store it for the baby's use.

In the future it may be that both mothers and fathers will once again work at home, thanks to the computer age:

> .... *A whole group of social and economic forces are converging to transfer the locus of work.... Since large numbers of workers are involved in moving tangible symbols and information rather than physical goods, it is no*

longer necessary for them to go to the central location to do their jobs.

Even today, production engineers report, 35 percent to 50 percent of the work force in some advanced manufacturing centers could actually perform their work at home if we chose to organize production in that fashion. Many others could work a few days in the office and a few days at home.... "Telecommuting" may well replace commuting.... In many homes, the family may well become a work-together production unit, as it typically was before the Industrial Revolution.[21]

Breastfeeding and sex

The new father still has sexual needs which must not be overlooked. A wise wife will not neglect these needs, although her own desires may be temporarily sublimated through breastfeeding, or she may be too weary to want love making, or fearful of pain if an episiotomy was performed. Even in the early days and weeks after childbirth, touching and closeness between husband and wife should continue, and love-making without coitus until the allotted time has passed for the mother's safety (two to six weeks). Fulfilling a husband's needs during this time is a way of reminding him that "I still care about you too."

Recent studies indicate that breastfeeding mothers tend to be more willing to resume sexual relations than do bottle feeding mothers.[22] A woman who substitutes her baby for her husband to fulfill her emotional needs is sending a signal that there are **other** problems in the marriage relationship. Breastfeeding is not the cause of the problem, but may bring an existing problem to the surface.

Sexual relations during breastfeeding may require a little ingenuity. For example, a baby will often cry when the mother is becoming sexually aroused, even though the baby is in another room! The baby seems to sense that the mother's attention is focused on someone else. This subconscious link between mother and breastfeeding baby is a profound one.

And what can one do about the baby in the parental bed? Obviously the baby need not be there **all** the time. During the day he will learn to sleep in his own bed and from time to time during the night. Before coitus, it is best to breastfeed the baby and put him to sleep in another room. If a pillowcase on which the mother has slept is put in the baby's bed, the smell of the mother's pillowcase will help to keep him content.

Breast stimulation increases sexual desire, but the breastfeeding mother may find her nipples leaking during sex play. This is another good reason for breastfeeding first, which also makes the breasts softer and more comfortable. They are not "off limits" to the husband, and he may caress them in the same ways as before.

Hormonal changes may make the vagina a little dryer than usual, but this can be overcome with a clear vaginal cream for lubrication. If an episiotomy was performed and coitus causes discomfort, the scar tissue should be gently lubricated and massaged before insertion of the penis, to relax the tissues and prevent pain. If pain persists, the doctor should be consulted.

Since the breasts produce milk continuously as long as lactation occurs, it is essential that a couple not wait until weaning for re-establishing normal coitus relations. Ingenuity and a sense of humor can sustain the continuity of this relationship and overcome minor problems, not only during the early weeks after the first baby, but also in the months and years to come when additional children are in and out of the parental bed.

Her own vineyard

The bride in the Song of Songs complains, *they made me keeper of the vineyard, but my own vineyard I have not kept.*[23] The demands of being wife and mother can become so overwhelming that one's own personal needs—physical, emotional, mental, and spiritual—are overlooked. This gradually leads to disastrous consequences. Either the woman becomes a non-thinking, boring drudge as time passes, or she begins to neglect her family responsibilities and is drawn toward self-assertion and self-satisfaction. In either extreme, her *own vineyard* is neglected.

It is essential that she care for her physical needs: sufficient rest, the right food and exercise. The most difficult of these is the need for rest, especially when there are several small children who never all nap at the same time and who wake up at various times of the night. Sometimes the husband can take care of the children in the late afternoon or early evening so his wife can nap. Or a friend may look after the children for awhile during the day while the mother sleeps. No woman should allow her need for rest to get beyond the point of no return or she will be "tired all the time" and heading for a breakdown of her health.

Her emotional needs must be met. If she was active in the work force before the baby was born the transition to being home all the time may make her feel "stir crazy!", as one young wife complained. It is not that her baby is loved any less than the baby of a young woman who "loves" housework. A new mother needs to find ways to maintain her own identity. She needs little pockets of time each week to go somewhere, to think, to take part in a favorite activity. Unless it is necessary for her to work, the tiny, breastfeeding baby goes with mama, but not the toddlers. Some young mothers have a Saturday morning "walk out," leaving the children home with daddy while they meet somewhere for breakfast and/or to do the weekly shopping.

At one time we had five children under ten, with three babies under two-and-a-half, all in diapers. Each day when my husband walked in the door in the late afternoon he met me on the way out! For a half hour or so I would walk away from it all, up the hill overlooking the city. After a while the fresh air, the exercise, the quietness, restored my composure and I was eager to return to pick up my responsibilities again. In the meantime, the children enjoyed playing with daddy after his absence all day. A quiet supper and evening followed. This worked far better than for daddy to romp with the children after supper, making them over-excited and unable to sleep.

But above all, the mother needs to keep God in first place in her heart. The baby must not become her idol, displacing not only her husband but her Savior. The vineyard of her innermost being must be kept well-cultivated and watered by prayer, praise, and meditation on the word of God.

The breastfeeding mother will find that her communion with God is not disrupted but can be enhanced by her communion with her baby. Baby needs no other food than breastmilk for the first six months of life, and even after other foods are introduced, breastfeeding remains the most delightful time of all for both mother and baby. During this time communion is developing between the two. The baby receives not only perfect nutrition, but enjoys the feel of his mother's flesh, the expression on her face, the sound of her breathing and even her heartbeat. The marvelous thing about all this is not only what it does for the baby, but what it does for the mother! She can meditate on how she is made *in the image of God*[24] who said, *Can a woman forget her sucking child, that she should not have compassion on the son of her womb? Even if they forget, yet I will not forget you. I have written your name upon the palms of My hands.*[25]

Do you know what it is like to have someone look lovingly into your eyes? The breastfeeding baby has continual eye contact with the mother. (A bottle fed baby does not, unless the mother is aware of the need for eye contact and turns the baby to face her.) Looking at the mother becomes habitual for the breastfed baby. He will stop nursing to smile at her, pat the breast, affirming her. She is the most necessary, special person on earth to at least one other person, her nursing infant.

Those of us who are experienced in observing mothers with their babies can often tell a breastfed from a bottle-fed baby, without being told, by the way the baby looks at his mother, or by the special look that passes between them. This developing communion not only hastens the baby's sociability, but enhances the mother's own poise and self-confidence.

This time with the baby also provides the mother with ample time to *pray in the Spirit* and softly *sing in the Spirit*.[26] Baby will love it! When he or she begins to coo and make sounds (at about three months), mother and baby can talk back and forth in the language of heaven while the angels gather around to listen.[27] Jesus quotes the Psalmist by saying that baby's first language is perfect praise, sounds full of meaning but without intellectual content, sounds coming from the heart rather than from logical thoughts formed into speech. *Jesus said to them, Listen, have you never read: "Out of the mouth of babes and sucklings you have perfected praise."*[28] Mother understands the baby's language of love. Even so, our prayers *in the Spirit* may bypass our understanding, but God, *Who searches the hearts knows what is the mind of the Spirit.*[29] He interprets the heart cry, or the song of our heart that we cannot even form into words.

When the mother (and father) learn to worship the Lord while loving the little one at the same time, a good pattern is set for the months and years to come. From the time they were toddlers, my children often came into the room where I was praying, wanting my attention. Even as teenagers they would sometimes come near and wait for me to notice them. The temptation sometimes was to say, "Don't bother me now. Can't you see I'm praying?"

But the thought always came to me that if I sent them away, maybe Jesus would leave with them!

> *They brought infants to Jesus, so that he would touch them. When his disciples saw it, they rebuked them. But when Jesus saw it he was much displeased, and said to them, "Let the little children come to me: for of such is the kingdom of God. I tell you the truth, whoever will not*

receive the kingdom of God like a little child will not enter into it." And he took them up in his arms, put his hands on them, and blessed them.[30]

NOTES
1. Ps. 128 NIV and NAB. **2.** 2 Cor. 1:3 NIV. **3.** 1 Jn. 4:16. **4** Isa. 40:11.
5. Isa. 46:3. **6.** Hos. 11:1-4. See NEB. **7.** Zeph. 3:16. **8.** Deut. 32:15.
9. Num. 11:11, 12. **10.** Eph. 4:26. **11.** Num. 20:10. **12.** Ps. 106:32, 33.
13. 1 Jn. 4:7, 8. **14.** Mt. 1:18-20. **15.** Lk. 12:16-21. **16.** 2 Cor. 12:14, 15 NAB. **17.** Jer. 17:7, 8 NEB. **18.** Jas. 1:27. **19.** Ps. 68:5. **20.** Heb. 2:13.
21. Alvin Toffler. **The Third Wave.** New York. Wm. Morrow. 1980. Reported in "The Minneapolis Star," April 9, 1980.
22. "Fathers Ask Questions About Breastfeeding." Pamphlet available from Health Education Associates, 520 School House Lane, Willow Grove, PA 19090. 1978.
23. S. of S. 1:6. **24.** Gen. 1:27, 28.
25. Isa. 49:15, 16. See NAB.
26. In 1 Cor. 14:14, 15 Paul contrasts praying in the Spirit to praying in words which we can understand. He adds that when we *bless in the Spirit, we are giving thanks well,* even though others cannot understand us and are not "edified." With the baby no such barrier exists for he does not understand speech anyway. He understands expression, tone of voice, the language of love that needs no "explanation." Thus it is when we bless God in the Spirit. God hears and interprets our "song without words," knowing our hearts.

A lovely discipline in praying in the Spirit is to memorize Scripture in another language which we do not understand. I love to listen to Psalms read in Hebrew or songs of worship sung in Italian, although I do not know the meaning of the words being sung. My spirit is refreshed and blessed.
27. Mt. 18:10. **28.** Ps. 8:2; Mt. 31:16. **29.** Rom. 8:26, 27. **30.** Lk. 18:15-17; Mk. 10:13-16.

The Way of a Child

Even at play a child reveals whether his actions will be pure and right.[1]

Instruct a child in the way he should go, and when he is old he will not turn from it.[2]

Love the Lord your God with all your heart and with all your soul and with all your strength. Fix these words of mine in your hearts and minds; tie them as symbols on your hands and bind them on your foreheads. Teach them to your children, talking about them when you sit at home and when you walk along the road, when you lie down and when you get up. Write them on the door frames of your houses and on your gates, so that your days and the days of your children may be many in the land that the Lord promised to give to your forefathers, as the days of heaven upon the earth.[3]

Our children do not belong to us. They belong to God, but are entrusted to us for a time with the responsibility of bringing them up to love and follow God. The difficulties we sometimes undergo in carrying out this responsibility—our hopes, fears, dreams, questions, anxieties, disappointments and sometimes grief over our children—make us realize our own need of God.

There are no perfect parents. When we recognize from the beginning that as parents we are both a blessing and a liability to our children, then we will be more fully aware of our total dependence upon God for wisdom, discernment, mercy and forgiveness. We are sinners, and although we do the best we can, it is never good enough. Thus our greatest responsibility as Christian parents is to walk in the ways of God day by day in the care of our children, trusting the Holy Spirit for guidance, pleading His mercy to bless them even through our mistakes.

Consecration

Our first requirement as Christian parents is that we consecrate ourselves to God. *They first gave themselves to the Lord, and then to us by the will of God.*[4] The heart of the Christian home is Jesus. Our own personal godliness and obedient walk with the Lord is central to our ability to be good parents. We will not seem "saints" to our growing household, for they will see all too clearly our feet of clay, but that must not discourage us. We can commit ourselves to Him as parents and commit our children to His care, believing that *He is able to **keep** that which we've committed to him.*[5]

I've often reflected on the encouraging thought that the Lord is behind me, helping to rectify my mistakes, as well as in front of me pointing the way. The Psalmist says, *Lord, you go **behind** me and before me, and lay your hand upon me.*[6] And Isaiah says,... *righteousness will go before you, and the glory of the Lord will be behind you.*[7]

We all need forgiveness for the harm we sometimes do in our attempts to do right. We need Jesus going "behind" us to place His healing balm upon our children for the times we have misunderstood and hurt them. And we must forgive our own parents for their "mistakes," for our resentment against our parents will be reflected in the way we raise our children. Either we will repeat their mistakes, or over-react and make mistakes in the opposite direction. If we want our children one day to *forgive our sins,* then we must forgive our parents for the times when they unwittingly *sinned against us.*[8]

But although we are imperfect, yet we have been given authority by God to bring our children up in the ways of God. Our awareness of our imperfections is not to make us hesitant and fearful in rearing our children, but to keep us humble. Brother Lawrence has said that "he who has not learned to obey is not fit to rule." Our God-given authority over our children comes out of our own obedience to His authority over us—out of our willing submission to His loving discipline.

The centurion whose child Jesus healed from a distance understood the meaning of authority. He said to Jesus, *I am a man **under** authority, and I say to my servant, "Go," and he* *goes.*[9] This man recognized Jesus' authority over sickness because he himself not only gave orders, but knew what it was to be under orders.

The principle of submission to authority is one of the greatest spiritual principles of all Scripture. The Bible says that Jesus humbled Himself and *became obedient.*[10] To whom was He obedient? To God? Yes. But in obedience to God He humbled Himself to be born in the flesh and to be submissive to his parents, to his teachers, and even to the religious authorities in his "home church." Surely, during all those growing up years, Jesus, the perfect child, could see the flaws in His parents and elders and at times inwardly questioned their wisdom.[11] Yet He humbled Himself to be obedient to their authority, learning the Scriptures from their lips.

Our children are to be brought up "by the Bible." This does not mean laying down rules and regulations, but living with the Scriptures so naturally and freely that the child is hearing the Word of God even before he can talk. Bible songs and stories are to be interwoven into every day of the child's life and not left for Sundays only. The inner lives of small children can be nurtured by the sounds, rhythms and atmosphere of holy things even in the earliest years. As they grow, their parents can teach them Bible stories and songs and help them memorize Scripture. These words of Scripture stored in the child's mind will come back to him or her with new force when in later years their minds can comprehend these truths more fully.

Devotional classics can also be read to children, appropriate to their level of understanding. I spent hundreds of hours reading such stories to our children, until they were old enough to read them for themselves. When our youngest son was in first grade, I began reading C.S. Lewis' Narnia tales[12] to him, those marvellous allegories of spiritual truth. His reading vocabulary was not equal to the task, but his comprehension was tremendous when read to. At bedtime each night I read to him—all the way through all seven of these books, and then began with the first one again! Then we went on to other inspiring literature.

One evening when he was in sixth grade I called him to come indoors, as it was time to read before bedtime. He hurried into the house, closed the door behind him so his friends could not overhear, and then whispered, **"Sh-sh-sh!** Mother! Big boys' mothers' don't read to them!" He was embarrassed to have his friends know how much he loved to be read to. How poor they were in comparison to his knowledge of the Scriptures and of ennobling literature!

But the book which our children read most clearly and accurately is our lives. They "know us like a book!" *You are the letter of Christ, written not with ink, but with the Spirit of the living God.... Not that we are capable by ourselves, but our ability is from God, who makes us able teachers of his word; not of the letter, but of the spirit: for the letter kills, but the spirit gives life.*[13]

> *There was a child went forth every day,*
> *And the first object he look'd upon, that object he became,*
> *And that object became part of him for the day or a certain part of the day,*
> *Or for many years or stretching cycles of years....*
> *His own parents, he that had father'd him and she that had conceiv'd him in her womb and birth'd him,*
> *They gave this child more of themselves than that,*
> *They gave him afterward every day, they became part of him.*
> *The mother at home quietly placing the dishes on the supper table,*
> *The mother with mild words, clean cap and gown, a wholesome odor falling off her person and clothes as she walks by,*
> *The father, strong, self-sufficient, manly, mean, anger'd, unjust,*
> *The blow, the quick loud word, the tight bargain, the crafty lure,*
> *The family usages, the language, the company, the furniture, the yearning and swelling heart,*
> *Affection that will not be gainsay'd, the sense of what is real, the thought if after all it should prove unreal,*
> *The doubts of day-time and the doubts of night-time, the curious whether and how,*
> *Whether that which appears is so, or is it all flashes and specks?...*[14]

Affirmation

God as the parent gives loving attention, leads, teaches, keeps His children close to Him, carries them in His arms, does not say "Go do such and such" without adding, *I will never leave you nor forsake you.*[15] The infant and child need the affirmation of touch, of loving voices talking to him, the security of being held, of frequent eye contact, of being fed when hungry and soothed when uncomfortable or afraid.

Yet even a tiny baby can learn a certain amount of responsible behavior so that a mother need not leap to her feet at his every whimper. It is normal behavior for an infant to fuss and squirm a little when going to sleep or when waking up (don't we sometimes toss around before settling down to sleep?). If the parents jump at baby's every whimper, they will wonder why baby seems so demanding as the months pass, making the days and nights miserable for everyone.

Parents should listen when the baby fusses, before deciding what is needed, and learn to distinguish a sleepy fuss, a hungry cry, a sharp cry of pain or a lonesome cry. Then they can respond accordingly. A baby crying of hunger should be put at once to the breast. If it is a sharp cry, look for an open pin, or pick him up, burp him and help him overcome colic pains. A lonesome baby should never be allowed to cry but should be held and cuddled. If it is just a sleepy fuss, set a timer for ten minutes and wait until it goes off to go to the baby. Often he will have fallen asleep before the time is up. If not, quiet him, and put him down again.

Whenever feasible, pick the baby up when he is **not** crying, talk to him, feed him, make eye contact, cuddle him and then put him down. Baby soon learns that his **non-**crying behavior is rewarded. It is easy to ignore the "good" baby. But if he is picked up only when he cries, his negative, crying behavior is reinforced and everyone soon wearies of it.

A toddler who is secure, loved, had all his needs met and his negative behavior unreinforced still becomes "difficult." As soon as he or she is able to move around, he can climb precariously, fall down stairs, "get into" things, and so on. This is a time for setting safe boundaries.

A home should be a happy place, with as few negatives as possible. Rather than say "no-no" to the young child, make a suggestion instead. "Let's do it this way." Put breakables out of reach, unless you don't mind his exploring them and the possibility of destruction. A child's intelligence grows by his exploring, looking at, handling and examining objects. He learns the feel of textures, shapes, temperatures. The environment should be one in which he may safely explore nearly everything within his reach. Exceptions are stoves, electric cords and other items of danger, which are **always** "no!"

Safety is the key factor in setting the boundaries of a toddler's increasing freedom of movement. The Lord's *rod and staff* of which the Psalmist speaks is not used to beat the sheep, but to safeguard and comfort. *Thy rod and thy staff* **comfort** *me*.[15] The shepherd uses the crook of the staff to lift the wandering lamb out of danger. He lays the long side of the staff against the erring sheep or lambs to push them back toward the safe path. The rod is used against predators to keep them away from the sheep.

The wise parent makes as few rules as possible, but enforces the rules that are made. Too many rules create so many prohibitions that a child could not possibly remember them all. Another mistake is to "make allowances" for the child when he breaks one of the few necessary rules, so that he quickly learns that if he cries hard enough, long enough, he'll get his own way—if not now, then a half hour from now. Soon everything the parent requests is ignored. The child won't sleep, won't stop crying, won't eat, won't be quiet in church, won't put away toys or clothes, won't get ready for school on time, won't make his bed, won't wash dishes, won't come in at a reasonable hour.

Look at all the negatives! And how do we respond? More negatives. Actually, parents begin the negative cycle: don't-don't-don't—, followed by the child's response: won't-won't-won't.

Much of what we consider "problem" behavior is the failure of the child to accept certain responsibilities by the time **we** expect him to. This occurs from early childhood through the teen years. Parents need to ask themselves: "Are my expectations unrealistic for a child this age or for this particular child?" "Have I been confusing the child by too many rules, and being inconsistent in carrying them out?" "Have I been continually affirming and reinforcing my child's self-esteem by commending his responsible behavior?"

A certain amount of rebellion is normal, typical of certain age levels, a sign of growing independence. The child is learning to make decisions for himself. The wise parent will provide choice options rather than supply opportunity for a negative reaction. For example, if the parent asks, "Shall we go to bed now?" the child says, "No!" He has made a choice!

But choice making is part of growing up. It would be better to say, "It's time to go to bed now. Would you like to wear the red pajamas tonight, or the blue ones?" This gives the child an opportunity to make an acceptable choice. The same choice technique can be used at the table. "Would you like a banana or an apple?" For if one says, "Would you like a banana?" the child can too easily say "No." If we ask the question, then we should accept his choice!

In the grocery store, one can fill the child's hands with items rather than keep repeating "don't touch." "Would you hold this for mommy?" In this way busy hands are kept out of mischief and he can be affirmed, "You are such a big help!"

Much of a child's behavior is copied from us. Does the child say, "Just a minute." "I'm busy now." "Don't bother me"? How many times a day have we said these same words to our child! Since he learns by imitation, we can respond to his requests with the same respect we want him to show us. If we are continually telling him to "wait a minute," it is unfair to demand an instant response when he echoes it. It is better to say, "In a few minutes we are going to...," thus giving the child a little time warning. Then his "wait a minutes" are not justified.

Do we stop and listen when he wants us, giving him our full attention? Inattentiveness is a form of rejection, a way of saying, "You're not important enough to listen to." A parent might set a goal of spending 10 minutes several times a day, giving **full** attention, looking into the child's eyes. Doing this a half dozen times a day provides the child with an hour's worth of quality attention every day. And if the parents listen to the child, the child will more readily listen to the parent. Parents who listen attentively to their three-year-olds will find their children sharing more with them as teenagers.

Motivation

God the parent lets us learn from our own mistakes, enduring the painful consequences of our disobedience. But even here, His sheltering hand protects us from devastation. He did not stop Peter from denying the Lord, but left the door open for forgiveness and reconciliation. Peter's terrible grief over what he had done was punishment enough.

Our goal as parents is to provide motivation for the child to **want** to be good, not out of fear of punishment, but out of a real desire to please the parents and later on to please God. The child's obedience is not to be like that of the trained dog, unthinking, undiscerning obedience to authority, or he might one day end up obeying a Hitler.

The child's assertion of his will is part of his struggle to grow up, to be a person, independent of his parents. This is healthy and good, but channeling the child's will constructively is not an easy task. We want our children to develop the desire to do right, to learn to *choose* between the good and the evil.[16]

When we discern that a child's misbehavior is due to his childishness, then we can ignore his cries of protests, his verbal arguments, for there are things he **must** do, whether he chooses to or not! This does not necessarily mean spanking, but it does mean that the child must carry out the requested behavior. He has no choice in the matter. My small sons would scream when put into the bathtub, and protest just as vigorously when it was time to get out! Ignoring the cries, we firmly lifted the rigid little bodies in or out of the tub anyway, calmly, quietly. Occasionally a little swat was necessary, but they soon learned that it was futile to "buck the system." Certain things we **do** when mama or daddy says, whether we want to or not.

There are other, often more effective ways than spanking to discipline a child for childish misbehavior. For example, the best cure for antisocial behavior in a small child is to remove him from the social environment. It is futile to tell a small child to stop crying. He or she will only cry louder or go into a tantrum. But what good does it do to yell up a storm if nobody pays any attention? The child can be firmly put into his room and told he may come out when he is through crying. (The bed should never be used for punishment. It should have only good connotations, a place of rest and comfort. And it is cruel to put a child in a dark closet or frightening place.)

"If you want to keep crying, you must stay in your room until you finish, because it hurts our ears." Affirmation should follow quickly when the crying stops. "I'm so glad you feel better! Why don't we...." Hug the child and spend some time in a fun activity, reinforcing the fact that he **stopped** crying. One of our little granddaughters sometimes says, "I think I'm getting mad, so I'd better go in my room for awhile."

Children can learn that certain actions bring undesirable consequences. One son had difficulty remembering things. When our children reached a certain age they were given their lunch money at the beginning of each month. Their responsibility was to remember to take some of it to school each Monday when lunch tickets were sold for the week. One Wednesday I received a phone call from our son, then in fifth grade, begging me to drive to school with his lunch money. (He had already borrowed from his teacher for Monday and Tuesday and was too embarrassed to ask again.) Although it pained me to do so, I refused.

A few minutes later the phone rang again. This time it was the principal. He had found our son sobbing his heart out by the telephone in the hall, but he couldn't get him to explain his problem. When I told him my son was crying because he had no lunch money and I refused to bring it, he commended me, and loaned him the money he needed for that day. The following morning I did **not** remind my son to take his lunch money, but he didn't forget! There were many times later when he forgot again, but he never asked me to bring it. He took the consequences himself. Often he forgot to return his library books, but I never reminded him to take them (when he was old enough to remember). Of course he had to pay the fine himself, out of his allowance. He was learning responsibility by having to take the consequences of his own behavior.

The Bible says, *Foolishness is bound up in the heart of a child, but the rod of discipline will drive it far from him.*[17] The Hebrew word translated "rod" is **shebet,** which literally means "sceptre." *He who spares his sceptre **(shebet)** hates his son: but he who loves him chastens him at times.*[18] The rod or sceptre is a symbol of authority. It is the parents' responsibility to teach the child respect for their authority.

Wise parents will ponder the thought that *whom the Lord loves he chastens, and disciplines every son he receives.... For if you are without discipline, then you are not sons.*[19] The difference between God chastening us and our discipline of our children is that we often punish *for our own pleasure,*[20] while God disciplines us only because He loves us. We must admit that much of our discipline of our children, especially spankings, is done in anger, in irritation with the child, in frustration, rather than out of love and a pure desire to do what is best for him.

Spankings should be reserved for actions which threaten the child's safety (such as running in the street), or for **deliberate** rebellion and disrespect. One should never spank a child for accidents, or for new discoveries. We need to discern between a child's willful defiance, and his childishness, and to discern the **cause** behind unacceptable behavior before deciding upon the appropriate reponse.

For example, is a child's refusal to go to bed caused by too early a bedtime, so that he is restless lying awake, unable to sleep because he is not tired? Is daytime misbehavior due to boredom, with too little variety in interesting activity, or too few opportunities to play with other children?

Is he jealous? If so, he needs more personal attention alone with one or the other parent, rather than to be pushed further away or punished for acting rejected. Is he cross because he is not feeling well? fatigued? hungry? overstimulated? overburdened with rules he does not comprehend?

One important cause of misbehavior is frustration, the inability of the small child to make himself understood. Or he may be showing anxiety through misbehavior. Spanking may silence the child, but it does not heal his frustration or anxiety and only causes him to feel misunderstood. The child's will is to be molded, not broken. A strong will is an asset when brought under self-control. It helps provide the courage to endure martyrdom as Stephen did, or to obey God rather than men, as Peter and John did.

Dr. James Dobson warns of the danger of breaking a child's spirit and explains the important differences between willful defiance and childish irresponsibility:

> *The will is not delicate and wobbly. Even for a child in whom the spirit has been sandbagged, there is often a will of steel, making him a threat to himself and others as well. Such a person can sit on a bridge threatening to jump, while the entire army, navy, and local fire department try to save his life. My point is that the will is malleable. It can and should be molded and polished—not to make a robot of a child for our selfish purposes, but to give him the ability to control his **own** impulses and exercise self-discipline later in life....*
>
> *On the other hand (and let me give this paragraph the strongest possible emphasis), the **spirit** of a child is a million times more vulnerable than his will. It is a delicate flower that can be crushed and broken all too easily (and even unintentionally). The spirit, as I have defined it, relates to the self-esteem or the personal worth that a child feels. It is **the** most fragile characteristic in human nature, being particularly vulnerable to rejection and ridicule and failure.*[21]

Yet there are times when a simple spanking clears the air, and is a catharsis which settles the emotional climate. Parents who hesitate to spank often substitute anger, yelling at the child, losing their temper, saying unkind things about the child. "You're such a bad boy!" Can't you ever mind!" This becomes a self-fulfilling prophecy, entering the child's mind and determining his subsequent behavior: "I'm a bad boy. I never do anything right."

When a child has deliberately, willfully misbehaved and knows he is wrong, he knows that he deserves the correction, whatever form it may take. After a Quaker mother spanked her child she looked at him and said, "I'm going to spank thee again, for what thee is thinking!" She recognized his rebelliousness, even after correction.

There are times when nothing seems to work. One child can be corrected with a word or tap on the hand. Another child becomes more rebellious the more he is spanked. I can remember times when I would pray in desperation, "Lord, I'm bigger and smarter than my child. Help me find a creative way to bring about the change that is needed!" The Christian parent can freely ask God for direction. *If any of you lack wisdom, let him ask God, who gives it freely to all....*[22] For who knows the heart of the child better than the Heavenly Father? Who knows best how we can bring about the desired change?

Parents are sometimes wrong. It is not easy to confess to a child that we have made a mistake, misunderstanding his intention or his actions. I have never forgotten an incident that occurred when I was only three years old. My grandmother was taking care of me after the death of my mother. I had asked to go down the street to "play with Marietta." Grandma said no. So I walked down the sidewalk only a **little** way, until I came to the crack in the sidewalk that led to the sidewalk in front of Marietta's house. Some men were working with a jackhammer in the street. Delighted with the sound, I sat down to watch. After awhile I got up and returned home.

Grandma met me at the door, said "I told you **not** to go to Marietta's house!" and spanked me. After I was through crying, I explained to Grandma that I hadn't disobeyed, and about the men working in the street. She took me in her arms, set me on her lap and soothed my tears. "I'm so sorry!" she told me. "Grandma was wrong to spank you. Will you please forgive me, Honey?" How her love made me want to please her always! And I still want to, even though she has been with the Lord for a long, long time.

Conflicting expectations

Each infant is a unique individual, with an innate temperament present at the time of birth unlike that of any other person ever born. We often compare babies and children in looks, size, weight and behavior, but this leads to false expectations and is unfair to the child.

Others also make comparisons—brothers, sisters, grandparents, aunts, uncles, church friends. They not only compare our child with others, but many of these people have ideas about how our child should be raised. We can listen to the advice (it might even be good!), but should base our decisions on what we know is best for our child, suitable to his age, temperament and understanding.

This is not always easy to do. One time in church our five year old was wiggling around as usual, standing up, sitting down, leaning against me, in constant motion. I know some people wondered why I didn't take her out and spank her! The reason I didn't was because she was being **very** good. She was sweet natured, loving, obedient, quiet, but it was physically impossible for her to sit still for any length of time. She had been so restless in the womb that it had been difficult to carry her to term. Now as an adult she is still always on the go.

Our three year old son was sitting quietly on the other side of me. Imagine the astonishment of those around me when I picked **him** up, carried him out and spanked him! Although he was sitting still, the naughty, rebellious looks he was giving me were not to be tolerated. I knew many people thought I had spanked the wrong child, but I knew my children and others did not.

Another son when three years old rebelled every Sunday morning at putting on "Sunday" clothes. It was traumatic for him not to be allowed to wear the everyday clothes he was happy in. I finally realized that the issue was unimportant. I didn't want him to grow up hating church simply because he hated the clothes he had to wear! From then on I let him wear his little jeans to church. He was clean, but not "dressed up." People may have looked askance at his clothes (for people still dressed for church in "those days"), but I knew my child's heart. He has grown up loving God, is faithful at church, and is still **very** particular about what he wears! Only now he wants everything he wears to be perfectly coordinated so that he looks "just right." I needn't have worried that he would grow up looking like a slob.

The kind of freedom a child has at home may differ from the freedom he experiences elsewhere, and he has to learn to live with differing expectations. Some parents are more casual than others and will give the child freedom to roam the house, explore, eat anywhere, sleep where he wants. The parents are not bothered by the lack of regular eating and sleeping hours.

But when the child is elsewhere, he may have to make some adjustments. When our grandchildren come to our house, they are to follow "our" rules. Conflict in these matters is not a question of being "right," but of where the child is and with whom he is interacting. At school he is to obey the school's rules. Wise parents will allow their children to work out these problems of behavior with other adults, without leaping to the child's defense unnecessarily. Some grandparents give the children greater freedom than they have at home. When the child protests at home, "But Grandma lets me..." the parent can reply, "Yes. But at home we do it this way."

When the school and teen years come and children wail, "but everyone is doing it!" our response can be, "Maybe so. But in our family we do it this way, and this is the behavior we expect of you."

Confirmation

What a beautiful thing it is to have our children grow up and confirm by their lives that our care of them has been fruitful! Jesus said, *By their fruit you shall know them.*[23] The "fruit" of a family is clearly seen by the outcome in the lives of its grown children.

If we have consecrated ourselves and our children to God, within the framework of the body of believers in Jesus Christ, if we have lovingly affirmed them from birth and applied correction as needed, the years will confirm it. Judgment should not be passed too soon. The prodigal son had the right upbringing, but rebelled and went off, for a time. He **did** return, for God's promise holds true, *Bring a child up in the way he should go, and when he is old he will not turn away from it.*[24]

The prodigal son knew he was still loved. He knew his father would receive him back. He was prepared to humble himself and accept the consequences of his wrong behavior. But did punishment await him? Not at all! His father knew his son had already suffered the consequences of his own actions, and the father expected and believed in his son's eventual return. *His father saw him coming while he was still a long way off, and his heart welled with compassion. And the father ran, and embraced his son and kissed him!*[25]

How much healing that father's loving embrace brought to his son's troubled heart! Our growing and grown children still need the warm hugs of loving parents, and we need theirs. Jesus tells the story of a beggar—a grown man—being comforted in

Abraham's bosom.[26] The Bible says that Jesus, God's Son, is to be found *in the bosom of the Father.*[27] The beloved disciple, John, loved to lean on Jesus' bosom.[28]

All the essence of healing is in the forgiving, accepting, warm embrace of another. Our children need our forgiveness, and we need theirs. We need to embrace each other in healing love, forgiving and being forgiven, *forgetting those things which are behind....*[29] The days of discipline end. The days of loving embraces last a lifetime.

An African Mother's Prayer

Now the children are asleep, my Lord,
I am tired and would spend a half hour in the
   stillness with Thee.
I want to bathe my soul in Thy infinity,
   like the workingmen
Who plunge into the surf to shed the dust and sweat
   of their bodies.
Let my burning heart feel Thy ever-renewing power;
Let my clouded spirit be lost in the crystal clarity
   of Thy wisdom.
Heal my unworthy love in the waters of Thy love
   which is so true, steady and deep.
O Lord, I couldn't stand being a mother one more day,
   if I thought I had to account for all my faults.
I am all sin.
My love walks over my wisdom. But I love my children.
I know that their little, seeing eyes see through me,
   right to my soul; I know that they imitate me.
Help me, O Lord, to be good in the deepest of
   my intentions, good in all my desires.
Make of me what I wish my children to be,
   with a heart that is strong, true, and great.
Help me not to be annoyed by little things.
Give me the large view of things, a sense of proportion
   so that I can truly judge what is important
   and what is not.
Lend me strength to be a real mother to my children,
   knowing how to turn right their souls
     and their imagination,
   knowing how to help them unfold their dreams
     and care for their bodies.

*Guard them against evil and let them grow up
healthy and pure.
This I ask in the name of our Lord, Jesus Christ.*[30]

NOTES
1. Prov. 20:11 Jerusalem Bible. **2.** Prov. 22:6. **3.** Deut. 5:5; 11:18-21 NIV and AV. **4.** 2 Cor. 8:5. **5.** 1 Tim. 1:12. **6.** Ps. 139.5. **7.** Isa. 58:8. **8.** Mt. 6:12. **9.** Lk. 7:8. **10.** Phil. 2:5-13. **11.** Lk. 9:42-52.
12. C.S. Lewis. **The Narnia Tales.** New York. Collier Books. 1970.
13. 1 Cor. 3:3-6. **14.** Walt Whitman, "A Child Went Forth." **15.** Josh. 1:5; Ps. 23:1-4. **16.** Is. 7:16. **17.** Prov. 22:15 NIV. **18.** Prov. 13:24. **19.** Heb. 12:6-8. **20.** Heb. 12:10.
21. James Dobson. **The Strong-Willed Child.** Wheaton, Il. Tyndale House. 1978. Reprinted by permission.
22. James 1:5. **23.** Mt. 7:15. **24.** Prov. 22:6. **25.** Lk. 15:20. **26.** Lk. 16:22, 23. **27.** Jn. 1:18. **28.** Jn. 13:13. **29.** Phil. 3:13.
30. From the Committee on World Literacy and Christian Literature. Translated by Frederick Rex from the French, as it appeared in **Envoi,** No. 1, Nov. 1954, an illustrated monthly published in what was at that time the Belgian Congo.

A Time to Lose

My heart is not proud, O Lord,
  my eyes are not haughty;
I do not concern myself with great matters
  or things too wonderful for me.
But I have stilled and quieted my soul;
  like a weaned child clinging to its mother,
  like a weaned child is my soul within me.[1]

The one unchanging fact of human life is change. We are not as we were yesterday, nor is there permanence in any of our relationships with others. Our lives are constantly moving, changing, interchanging, like the mountain streams rushing downward toward the sea, branching out in many directions, merging again at times and then separating as they spill across the landscape toward the end.

Each separation brings us a sense of loss as we are weaned from one kind of relationship in order to enter into another, different form. The first weaning comes as a child leaves the body of its mother, thrust out of the warm, soft darkness in which everything necessary for its life was provided in the nest of her body. The dry air is sucked into baby's lungs and assaults his skin. The sharp light pierces his eyelids. Empty space meets the thrusting of his arms and legs rather than the safe boundaries of the enfolding womb.

For the mother too, there may be a sense of loss as she touches her empty abdomen with wondering fingers, but this loss is overwhelmed by the joy of welcoming the new baby into her arms, and the welcome end of the pregnancy at its appointed time.

Early weaning

The second weaning is from the breast of the mother. This weaning begins as soon as anything other than breastmilk is put into the baby's mouth. The bottle-fed baby has in effect been weaned from the breast at birth, all biological dependence on the mother severed with the cutting of the umbilical cord. The bottle-fed baby eats from a spoon earlier than the breastfed baby, often drinks from a cup earlier—and may cling to his bottle as a source of comfort long after he is receiving all his nourishment from other sources.

Many of us in the last two or three generations have suffered deprivation of maternal/infant bonding at birth or through insufficient time at the breast. We compensate in inadequate ways such as compulsive nibbling, chewing gum, or smoking cigarettes. Even such seldom noticed habits as compulsively putting one's hands to one's face, stroking the nose or chin or cheeks may be ways of compensating for the loss of sufficient facial skin contact with the breast of the mother. For it is not only inside his mouth that the breastfed baby finds satisfaction. The warmth and smooth softness of the skin of the mother against his lips, nose, cheeks, chin, hands, and body is remembered in his subconscious.

At the present it is estimated that more than half the women in the United States breastfeed at the time they leave the hospital with their babies. But many of these mothers wean the baby to a bottle soon afterward, discouraged because of sore nipples or out of fear that the baby is not getting enough milk. They lack supportive persons or sufficient knowledge about how to adjust the milk supply to the baby's needs. Ironically, the mothers who often feel the greatest sense of loss and/or guilt over weaning are those who wean the baby early. Although the first reaction may be one of relief, later on they become quite defensive about their decision, a sign of subconscious guilt.

Other mothers have had to wean their babies early out of necessity, against their own desire for some difficult reason such as severe illness, family disharmony or other emergency situation. For whatever reason baby was weaned early, such mothers need to allow themselves to grieve! Inner healing comes far more quickly and permanently when they accept the fact that it **is** a loss. This sense of loss helps the mother respond to her infant like a breastfeeding mother in all the other important ways, easing the transition for both herself and the baby.

A breastfed baby needs no food other than the mother's milk

until he is at least six months old. In one sense all weaning is mother-initiated, for she is the one who first introduces the baby to bottle, cup or spoon, thus diminishing the dependence of the baby upon her as his biological lifeline.

Those who choose to wean their baby early (that is, before at least eight or nine months) should do it slowly, for the milk supply must be allowed to decrease gradually to avoid problems of breast engorgement and possible breast infections. Gradual weaning also gives the baby time to adjust to the change. Food from the family table (mashed or strained at first) decreases the baby's appetite for milk, and his increasing activities wean him away from the need for the mother's constant attention. A little sucking first thing in the morning, at bedtime, and a time or two for comfort during the day will gradually diminish the milk supply until baby loses interest.

A well-loved, well-socialized, well-fed baby weaned from the breast early may make a good adjustment, but will still experience a sense of loss, undefined and unexpressed. Life is different for him or her. The wise parent will substitute other pleasures and personal warmth to fill this need.

Toddler weaning

Baby-led weaning is defined as the baby continuing to breastfeed until discontinuing of his or her own accord. A baby who weans himself will do it gradually. A baby who suddenly stops nursing may be reacting to some type of trauma such as a move, a new bed or new room, or a cold which makes it hard to breathe. After a day or two he will probably want to nurse more than ever, if his mother continues gentle encouragement to take the breast. (She may need to hand express some milk in the meantime, to prevent engorgement and maintain the milk supply.)

There are mothers who begin to feel their babies will never want to wean. One mother of a two year old son wept, "Why didn't someone tell me it would be like this? I want **out**!" But eventually her son weaned, and she nursed her next baby happily on into the toddler years, her own expectations having changed and matured.

If the milk supply is adequate and a baby nearing a year old continually refuses the breast, obviously he or she is ready for weaning. In this case the mother may feel a little rejected, unless she is also ready and willing to let her baby wean.

The average time for children around the world to wean

themselves is between two and three years of age. A few children need a little mothering from the breast longer than this, but they are the exception rather than the rule. One five year old said wistfully to her mother, "Mommy, I'm **trying** to stop!"

The more a child clings to the mother, the more he needs the breastfeeding to continue. Others may blame the mother for "keeping" the child dependent, wrongly blaming breastfeeding for the child's clinging behavior. But it works the other way around. A child may be going through a dependent phase, but it is not true that breastfeeding makes him more dependent, nor will weaning make him more grown up and independent. Allowing the child to continue nursing will help satisfy his need for security and provide a stable foundation for his later independence.

The Bible tells of children who nursed far beyond infancy. The Psalmist says, *I have comforted myself like a weaned child.*[2] It is the child—no longer an infant, who is able to comfort himself. Sarah nursed Isaac until he was old enough to be annoyed by the teasing of his older half-brother, Ishmael:

> *And Sarah said, "God has made me laugh, so that all who hear will laugh with me. Who would have said to Abraham that Sarah would give suck to children?" And the child grew, and was weaned.... And Sarah saw the son of Hagar mocking Isaac.*[3]

God answered Hannah's prayer for a son, and she breastfed him until he was old enough not only to live away from his mother, but to assist Eli in the care of the tabernacle. He was probably four or five years of age by this time.

> *Hannah said, "I will not go up to the house of the Lord until the child is weaned, and then I will bring him, so that he may appear before the Lord and stay there permanently. So the woman waited and gave her son suck until she weaned him.*[4]

A still clearer reference to toddler nursing is found in the story of the mother who lost seven sons during the Maccabean period. Just before the last son was killed for refusing to renounce his faith,

> *....she leaned towards him, and flouting the cruel tyrant, she said in their native language: "My son, take pity on me. I carried you nine months in the womb, suckled you three years, reared you and brought you up to your present age....*[5]

Toddler nursing is the norm, and not the exception. If the mother is eating correctly and getting enough rest it is no drain on her body. She can even continue to breastfeed during another pregnancy, and then breastfeed both the new infant and the toddler until the latter loses interest. The older toddler greatly benefits from breastfeeding when he is sick. It helps both to comfort him and to insure that he gets enough fluid. It is a means of soothing a frightened or hurt child. At such times the child enjoys sucking at the breast for a moment even when milk is no longer present. But the day will come when he or she returns to the breast no more and moves on to new interests.

Widening horizons
Mother/child interaction continues in new ways after the child is weaned from the breast. The child who has had a close relationship with the mother through the early months and toddler years may now focus much more attention on the father. Father and child can now do "special things" which do not include the mother. She need not feel rejected as the child develops this special closeness to daddy, for it is good sign of growing maturity and independence. The child's horizons are widening, from the mother's bosom, from the arms and lap of both parents, from the house, from the yard, and ultimately on into his or her own walk through life with the Lord.

Each new experience of separation brings a certain amount of guilt and anxiety to the parents. Mothers do not necessarily experience this separation anxiety more keenly than the fathers, although they may express it more freely. Leaving an infant in the nursery the first time can cause anxiety, sometimes harder on the parents than the child. One mother of a year old baby would leave the church service several times to run down to the nursery and make sure her baby was all right. It was her third child. The women in the nursery were offended. "Doesn't she think we're able to take good care of her baby?" They failed to understand that the mother was suffering separation anxiety. She needed the baby more than he needed her.

Each separation is anticipated with mixed feelings of pride

and regret. Parents must consider not only whether the child is ready, but also whether they themselves are ready for the separation. Loosening the fabric of closeness without tearing the delicate foundation of a child's security needs the wisdom of the Lord. No one else can tell the parents what to do, and their decisions, if wisely made, may vary from child to child even in the same family.

The start of school is another "weaning," with a sharper sense of pride and loss, joy and doubt. Although the mother may be glad the child can go to school, she may be hurt by the child's transference of infallibility from the parents to the teacher. Anything the parent says may be countered with, "But teacher says,..." We need to recognize our own mixed feelings toward the child's teachers. If it is a matter of the wrong teacher, or the wrong school, that is a different matter. It is the parents responsibility to see that the child is in a school which does not crush his spirit or violate the principles he learns in his own home.

Letting go

A child's increasing independence is normal in the transition from home to the larger world. Even teenage rebellion may be a healthy expression of the need to stop leaning on the parents. If we allow our children to differ from us in areas which are less important, giving them more and more responsibility for their own decisions, this defuses their inner need to reject everything the parents stand for.

The lack of physical closeness, eye-to-eye contact and attentiveness to the child's interests during the early years often leads to greater rebellion and rejection of the parents during the high school years. And parents who hold on too tightly, too authoritatively, may produce an explosion that disrupts the household and brings everyone grief.

By the time a son or daughter graduates from high school, any continuing influence we have on their lives comes far more from what we are than from what we say. Whether they go away to work or to college, it is definitely the end of one era and the beginning of another. The homesickness and depression common to college freshmen is an unconscious reaction to the fact that they are now really on their own. The parental home will never again be "home" in the same way as before. They have passed a milestone leading away from home.

The wedding day is another time of separation anxiety, a sad/happy event. Why do we sometimes feel like crying at weddings even when the bride and groom are not our own children? The audience is participating vicariously in this final act of "letting go." Fathers seldom cry at weddings, although it would be all right if they did. But the stiff look on the father's face reveals that letting go is not easy for him either.

The separation is now complete. No matter how close the bond of love between parent and child, the decision-making is no longer in the parents' hands. If the young couple want advice, let them ask for it. Otherwise all well-meaning attempts to advise or help will be looked upon as "meddling."

The circle of love that begins with husband and wife and expands to include a child, and another, and another begins with the parents above and the children beneath. But as the years pass, the circle of love rotates. In time parents and children are equally adults, and as time goes on the children even begin to assume a parenting role. For example, my newly grown son will say, "Now Mother, when you speak in public you have a bad habit of stopping in mid-sentence and starting a new sentence." Or he will say, "Now, Mother, don't get upset. It's not that important." "Now, Mother,. . . ." Our children help us keep in step with the changing times and set bold examples of faith for us. We can thank God for the day when we can begin to look up to them!

I have yet to hear an older parent say, "I regret that I spent so much time with my children." It is true there are days when it seems the child will never grow up, that one will never be free from the chores, the meals, the clutter, the need for one's attention, the financial responsibilities. But the years pass more swiftly than we know and do not return again. Our children are with us such a short time after all, and then are gone.

Where do they go, the days and the decades,
days so filled with goodness—
we lived them like they'd always be—
days that brought such tiredness and hurt
we thought they would not pass
and days when we scarcely knew
whether to laugh or cry because they marked
both beginnings and endings. . . .

How could he have a son of his own
when we just brought him home from the hospital,
and why do we insist on calling the littlest one

> *the baby when he is in third grade?*
> *And how could I be forty-three when I*
> *am just barely thirty?*
> *Where do they go, the days and the decades?*⁶

Grief

We have all known the pain of separation from loved ones, both family and close friends. Jesus said to His disciples, *Now I am going to him who sent me.... And because I have said these things to you, sorrow has filled your hearts. But I tell you the truth. It is best for you that I go away.*⁷ Sorrow and grief are parts of everyone's life, and even Jesus experienced them, for He was *a man of sorrows and acquainted with grief.*⁸

The five normal stages of grief that we experience over any loss have been defined in secular literature as anger, denial (it just can't be!), bargaining (if only, then—), depression, and finally resignation/acceptance. These stages of grief are experienced even if only a part of one's body has been lost through accident or surgery. Recognizing these emotions as normal helps the suffering person to overcome his loss.

Surgery which involves the loss of some sexual function, even though the decision was voluntarily made, often brings emotions and reactions that may not have been anticipated. Vasectomy (male sterilization), tubal ligation (female sterilization), hysterectomy (removal of the uterus), and mastectomy (removal of a breast) bring not only physical loss but may affect the way one feels about himself as a man or a woman.

Miscarriage brings grief. If the loss of the fetus was due to abortion, the woman represses any thought of grief, erasing the brief events of the past weeks from her mind as if they had never been. But whether the loss of the fetus was accidental or deliberate, the fact is that a human life **was** and now is not. The woman's body remembers, and must make the adjustment from the pregnant to the non-pregnant state with its accompanying hormonal changes and emotions. And the subconscious mind remembers.

A woman often experiences little moments of depression after a miscarriage, or a desire to cry sometimes. Condolences like, "You're young yet," do not comfort. Nor does it help to be told that a certain percentage of all pregnancies end in miscarriage and one can always try again. There is self-doubt. What is wrong with my body that I could not keep the growing child? Or was something wrong with the child? If so, could it happen again?

If the miscarriage was in the early weeks of pregnancy, the father probably will not feel the loss as keenly as his wife. But a wise husband will allow his wife to grieve. It is the most normal, healthy way to respond to the loss. It is even all right to fantasize. Would the baby have been a boy or a girl? The young mother can sit in the presence of Jesus and talk with Him about "what might have been," and let her love rise to the spirit of the unborn infant in His bosom.

Death is the final weaning, the final separation. The time comes when it is not an unborn child who is lost, but our father, mother, spouse, or—unthinkable!—our baby or our child. Many of us have attended a funeral which has been like a celebration, a time of victory and even exultation, a time when the presence of the Lord Jesus holds up the bereaved ones with a peace and strength they have seldom experienced before. This is one of the great privileges of God's children.

But then the songs are over. Friends and relatives return to their homes. Condolences pour in for awhile, but only for awhile, and then others forget. The flowers on the grave wilt and turn brown. The bed remains empty. There is silence, where once a loved voice was heard. Regrets.

"God lent him and takes him," you sigh—
—Nay, there let me break with your pain.
God's generous in giving, say I,
And the thing which He gives, I deny
That He can ever take back again.

He's ours and forever. Believe,
O father!—O mother, look back
To the first love's assurance! To give
Means, with God, not to tempt or deceive
With a cup thrust in Benjamin's sack.

He gives what He gives; be content.
He resumes nothing given,—be sure.
God lend?—where the usurers lent
In His temple, indignant he went
And scourged away all those impure.

He lends not, but gives to the end,
As He loves to the end. If it seem
That He draws back a gift, comprehend

> *'Tis to add to it rather,... amend*
> *And finish it up to your dream.*[9]

The Bible does not say we cannot grieve, but only that we are not to grieve like those who have no hope, who do not know the living God:

> *We want you to understand about those who sleep in death, brothers and sisters, so that you are not overcome by grief like those who have no hope. For since we believe that Jesus died and rose again, so we believe that God will bring to life again those who have fallen asleep, in company with Jesus.*[10]

Often we do not allow a person to talk about the one they have lost. But they need to talk! God gave us memories to use, to remind us of all the happy times, the comical times, the hard times—which we can laugh about now, or over which we might shed a few tears. It takes longer to get over the death of a loved one if there is an attempt to keep from grieving. Yet because it is painful for us to be around a grieving person, we stay away. How much better if we accept tears and grief as God's comforting, normal, beautiful gifts, given to us as means of healing and restoration.

Protestants often act as though the dead person never lived at all, and cannot be talked about because they are now *with the Lord.* Catholics seem to have more awareness of the continuity of the lives of their lost ones. I was moved to tears as I stood in a little circle of Catholic friends praying around the altar for their lost ones: "Lord, bless my mother," prayed one, "my father," prayed another, "my sister." "Be with my friend...." Each mentioned a loved one by name who was with the Lord.

"But," some protest, "they don't need our prayers any more, for they are already fully blessed." Perhaps so. But it comforts **us** to speak their names before our Heavenly Father and makes the circle of love seem unbroken, which it really is.

It takes about three years for an individual to recover fully from grief over the death of a loved one. Months may go by in which the thought does not trouble him, and then unexpectedly sadness settles in again for a while.

One mother of a seven year old was told not to grieve, because it was "just his body" that had died and been laid in the grave. "But," she said softly, "it was not only his soul that I loved. I loved his body too. I carried it in my womb, gave birth to it, held, stroked, washed and clothed that little body. I can still feel the firm roundness of his little limbs, see the laughter of his brown eyes and the sun-gold that reflected in the strands of his soft hair...." She grieved, and wisely so.

Little John Philip Lawrence was born on May 2, 1976. He came into the world to be a playmate to his sister Cheryl and brother Timothy and to bring joy to his mommy and daddy. But Johnny didn't stay in this world long enough to become a playmate, and on June 9, 1976 he went home to Jesus. He had been born with a defective heart and underwent corrective heart surgery twice before he was two weeks old. The finest medical staff available fought to save him until he would be old enough for more complete heart surgery. His little body clung tenaciously to life for five weeks.

As I prayed for him and his family I asked the Lord for guidance, and He gave me this passage:

> *The Spirit of the Lord is upon me; because the Lord has anointed me to...* **bind up the brokenhearted,** *to proclaim liberty to the captives, and the* **opening of the prison** *to them that are bound;... to appoint unto them that mourn in Zion beauty for ashes, the oil of joy for mourning, the garment of praise for the spirit of heaviness; that they might be called trees of righteousness, the planting of the Lord, that he might be glorified.*[12]

From this I understood that my prayers for Johnny's healing were more likely to be answered in Life than in this life. My ministry would be to bring comfort to the mourning parents. A few days later I stood with them by Johnny's bed in the intensive care pediatrics ward of the university hospital. The thoughts of my own three weeks' old grandson were in my heart as we watched this little one struggle for life. Several times that day his heart had stopped and been restimulated, but just before ten o'clock in the evening it faltered once more beyond return.

Swiftly the kind nurse detached the medical equipment from the baby and removed the respirator from his mouth. We pulled up a rocking chair for the mother and she was given her baby to hold in his dying moments. As she rocked him, wept over him and kissed him, his daddy stooped beside them to kiss his little head again and again. The nurse and I stood silently beside them, grieving for their grief. The two grandmothers and some of the young aunts and uncles stood just behind us.

Tears were rolling down all our cheeks as little John Philip was committed into the hands of Jesus for all eternity, his spirit released from the suffering prison of the little body in which it had been bound. The painful look on his tiny face changed to one of most beautiful peace, like the face of a little angel. It was one of the most sacred moments of my life.

After returning home, grieving over the pain of the young parents in this loss, the Lord seemed to speak to me again. He said, "Little John Philip is with Me, his presence gracing heaven."

Life is Change

What is life? Back and forth, in and out, up and down, inhale, exhale. Life is like the cool waves of the ocean falling unceasingly upon the shore, only to be sucked back into the mighty abyss. The mind is filled with sparkling knowledge and hard, cold facts, bright gems from the deep mines of the universe, only to be tossed back into the void of ignorance. Food goes in the mouth but soon goes out as energy or waste. Fresh air fills the lungs and then the harmful by-products are sent harmlessly back into space. The sun rises and the sun sets. Men live and then die. Back and forth, in and out, up and down, inhale, exhale. Life is rhythm.

Every snowflake has its design, every small child its own unique delightfulness, every flower its petals, every man his flaws. A blade of grass has billions of orderly molecules, a drop of water is the same in all its many parts. A mountain has its special beauty, a man has his talents. Life is patterns.

The ocean is troubled, always stirring, bubbling, boiling and never the same. A child grows to his maturing and soon withers to an old man. The earth fails to remain in the same place but casts itself uncaring through space. A man is driven by his nature to seek what is new. Life is change.[13]

NOTES
1. Ps. 131:1, 2 NIV & NEB. **2.** Ps. 131:2 **3.** Gen. 21:5-9. **4.** 1 Sam 1:22-28.
5. Maccabees 7:27, 28. This remarkable passage in the Apocrypha shows not only the courage of the mother of the seven sons tortured before her eyes for their faith in God, but also her hope of a resurrection.

"She watched her seven sons all die in the space of a single day, yet she bore it bravely because she put her trust in the Lord. She encouraged each one in turn in her native language. Filled with noble resolution, her woman's thoughts now fired by a man's spirit, she said to them: 'You appeared in my womb, I know not how; it was not I who gave you life and breath and set in order your bodily frames. It is the Creator of the universe who moulds man at his birth and plans the origin of all things. Therefore he, in his mercy, will give you back life and breath again, since now you put his laws above all thought of self.'" Vs. 20-23.

6. Bob Benson. **Come Share the Being.** Nashville. Impact Books. 1974. Pp. 92, 92.

7. Jn. 16:5-7. **8.** Isa. 53:3

9. Elizabeth Barrett Browning. Stanzas, 6, 7, 9 and 10 of her poem, "Only a Curl."

10. 1 Thess. 4:13, 14. **11.** 2 Cor. 5:8.

12. Isa. 61:1-4. While I was writing this chapter, a birth announcement arrived in the mail saying that a healthy baby girl had been born to Johnny's parents, three years after his death.

13. Dan Wessel. Printed by permission.

A Time to Remember

Remember how the Lord your God led you all the way in the desert these forty years, to humble you and to test you in order to know what was in your heart, whether or not you would keep his commands....
Observe the commands of the Lord your God, walking in his ways and revering him. For the Lord your God is bringing you into a good land—a land with streams and pools of water, with springs flowing in the valleys and hills; a land with wheat and barley, vines and fig trees, pomegranites, olive oil and honey, a land where bread will not be scarce and where you will lack nothing....
When you have eaten and are satisfied, praise the Lord your God for the good land he has given you. Be careful that you do not forget the Lord your God.... Otherwise, when you have eaten and are satisfied, when you build fine houses and settle down,... then your heart will become proud and you will forget the Lord your God, who brought you out of Egypt, out of the land of slavery.[1]

All that has been written thus far has presented an ideal of the way things ought to be—the way we want them to be. But in our pilgrimage through this present life many things are not as we had hoped. We have not prayed as we ought, nor sought the Lord's counsel as closely as we should have. We have made mistakes and hurt other people; others have grieved and wounded us. We have suffered onslaughts from Satan, the enemy of our souls. We all remember yesterdays that were not as they might have been.

Remembered hurts

The most recent hurts are the ones we remember the most vividly. They may come from a painful situation that seems unrelieved day after day. But although we remember the last incident most intensely, all the pain of previous wrong accumulates in the memory until the day comes when one tiny hurt is just "the last straw."

What wounds us most deeply is often the pain which comes because we are following God. When we set our hearts to obey the will of God in everything, the initial result is persecution rather than blessing. It comes in the most hurtful form—from those we love most, at church and at home. The Psalmist mourns:

> *It was not an enemy who reproached me, for then I could have borne it. Neither was it someone who hated me who turned against me, or I would have stayed away from him. But it was you! a man my equal, my guide, my dear friend. We had taken sweet counsel with each other, and had walked into the house of God together.*[2]

Jesus also experienced this kind of rejection. The first time he preached in Nazareth after His anointing by the Spirit of God, the members of His home synagogue were so angry they forced Him to the edge of the hill on which the city was built to *throw him down headlong.*[3] Later in His ministry they were still not open to Him:

> *Coming to His own country he taught them in their synagogue, so that they were astonished and asked, "Where did this man get this wisdom and these mighty works? Isn't this the carpenter's son? Is not his mother called Mary? Are not his brothers James and Joseph and Simon and Judas? And are not all his sisters with us? Where then did this man get all this?" And they took offense at Him.*
>
> *But Jesus said to them, "A prophet is not without honor except in his own country and in his own house." And He did not do many mighty works there because of their unbelief.*[4]

Jesus said, *A prophet is not without honor . . . except* **in his own house!** Yet it should not surprise us, for Jesus also said:

> *Do not think that I have come to bring peace on earth. I have not come to bring peace, but a sword. For I have come to set a man against his father, and a daughter against her mother, and a daughter-in-law against her mother-in-law, and a man's foes will be those of his own household.... He who does not take his cross and follow me is not worthy of me.*[5]

When we attempt to bring the things of the Spirit of God into our every day relationships at home, our parents, spouse, in-laws, or children may throw up their hands, accusing us of being so "heavenly-minded" we are "no earthly good." It is not an easy thing to live for God! We can take comfort in the fact that even Jesus knew this pain, for his friends accused him of losing His mind, and his mother and brothers came to remonstrate with Him. He knew what was in their minds and refused to see them. He pointed to those in the room listening to His every word and said, *Here are my mother and my brothers. Whoever does the will of God is my brother, and sister, and mother.*[6]

When division or misunderstandings arise over any of the matters discussed in this book, for example, what is one to do? Peter said, *We ought to obey God rather than men.*[7] But the **manner** in which we obey God may mean the difference between a family restored to harmony or one in which divisions deepen. For Peter also said:

> *Finally, all of you have unity of spirit, sympathy, love of the brethren, a tender heart and a humble mind. Do not return evil for evil or reviling for reviling; but on the contrary bless, for to this you have been called, that you may obtain a blessing....*
> *Now who is there to harm you if you are zealous for what is right? But even if you do suffer for righteousness sake, you will be blessed. Have no fear of them, nor be troubled, but in your hearts reverence Christ as Lord. Always be prepared to make a defense to any one who calls you to account for the hope that is in you, yet do it with gentleness and reverence; and keep your conscience clear, so that, when you are abused, those who revile your good behavior in Christ may be put to shame.*[8]

No power on earth can stand before the loving, forgiving, humble person who serves another in the love of Jesus through

His Spirit, even when there is disagreement. And Paul also says that the wife or husband of an unbelieving (not necessarily "un-Christian") spouse is the means through which the children are made holy.[9] Notice that! **One** spouse walking with the Lord assures that the children will be "holy." So we can never blame our disagreeable marriage partner if our children do not end up following the Lord. The one who has the faith is the one who carries the responsibility before God, and God will answer those prayers.

In the household where husband and wife are not spiritually in harmony, the one with the most maturity is the one responsible to humble himself or herself before the Lord, asking God for a greater work of grace in his or her own heart. As the hurting one begins to walk moment by moment with the Lord, he or she can listen to His advice in each troubling situation and quietly obey what He says. This is not a matter of "memorizing principles" and applying the right one. Rather, it is a matter of listening to the Spirit of Jesus with the inner ear, for He will give wisdom when we ask.[10] This will defuse the immediate crisis, and smooth the way toward eventual reconciliation.

John Wesley once said, "There is nothing like family trouble to make a person spiritual!" More than anything else, this kind of trouble causes us to cast ourselves upon the Lord. He first brings peace to our own heart, and then works through us to bring His victory in the situation in His own time. It may not be a problem with the spouse; it may be with other family members, or with friends, but the solution is the same.

We are not to build a storehouse of memories of the hurts against us, letting each new assault add to the whole. Each rejection is to be treated as an isolated incident. *Love does not brood over injuries.*[11] We can take heart in the example of Jesus' family. The day came when they were all His loyal followers, and His own brother James even became the head of the church in Jerusalem.[12]

Day by day forgiveness, then, is the key to a memory healed of the pain of being sinned against. We need to come before the Lord in prayer, confess to Him those things which have wounded us, and ask His forgiveness to flow through us toward those who caused the hurts, whether in the past or in the present moment.

Remembered failures

The memories of personal failure are like ropes that bind us, so that we are afraid to follow the Lord freely lest we fail again. All of us at times feel overwhelmed by family and other responsibilities, inadequate to carry out our own ideals. If we did not feel this way at the outset, circumstances will prove it so! I knew all the answers to happy married life, before I was married. I knew all the answers to the problems of raising children, before I had any. After our first child was born I thought I was the perfect mother because of her model behavior. However, as other children came along I realized our first daughter was "good" not because I was such a good mother, but because of her own gentle, happy disposition.

The first step in being set free from the bondage of remembered failures is to look into our past and see what *root of bitterness*[13] we may still be harboring against those who have hurt us. Our unforgiveness of others is not only a judgment against them but also leads us right into the trap of self-condemnation. If someone else does something wrong we consider it a "sin." If we do the same thing, we call it a "mistake." Thus do we attempt to justify our own sinfulness! Yet the feeling of guilt remains. For the Bible says, *You have no excuse, whoever you are, when you judge someone else: for in passing judgment on him you condemn yourself, because you, the judge, are doing the very same things.*[14]

We need to look into our memories and make sure that we have forgiven our parents, our brothers and sisters, our teachers, our former classmates, our spouses, doctors, nurses, friends, or any others who have hurt us, whether it was intentional or not. Only then are we able to freely forgive ourselves for our "mistakes."

Jesus said we are not only to forgive, but He also said to *love your neighbor **as yourself**.*[15] We cannot love our sinning neighbor as we ought until we forgive ourselves. Sometimes we are like the unforgiving servant whom the master forgave an uncountable debt, who then turned around and grabbed a fellow servant, demanding that he pay every red cent. And who is that "servant" whom we grab, choke, and from whom we demand accountability? Is it not often our own selves? We demand such a high standard of perfection from ourselves that we either live under continual self-justification or self-condemnation.

The ability to love and forgive ourselves comes when we admit that in ourselves there is not enough wisdom, piety, love or goodness to be the kind of spouse or parent that we ought, or to do anything right. Only then are we able to grasp the truth that the *grace of Jesus **is** enough for all our weaknesses.*[16] We need to see ourselves as the sons and daughters of God, able to draw from Him moment by moment all the grace we need. This grace covers past sins and failures with forgiveness and present difficulties with wisdom.

Hidden memories

Some of our unhappy memories go so far back that we cannot recall them in our conscious minds. Or they may have been repressed, buried in the subconscious as too painful to think about. Agnes Sanford first taught about "the healing of the memories" during the 1950's. Then in 1966 she wrote about it in her beautiful book, **The Healing Gifts of the Spirit.**[17]

When I read Mrs. Sanford's book shortly after it was published I decided to take a faith walk with Jesus back through the years of my own life as she suggested, to see what hidden hurts or unforgiveness might be festering there. I began with my conception and moved on through my birth.

Each day during prayer I centered my attention on the next little period of my life, lifting myself first as a little babe and then as a little child into the light of God's presence, waiting for Him to lift a forgotten grief to the surface. Often I could not remember what the difficulty was, but the remembered **feeling** was still there. As it surfaced, sometimes I would weep as if my heart would break! I would allow the grief to be expressed in the presence of Jesus, until peace came. The next day I would do the same again, bringing to Him the next little section of my life.

Once the Lord brought to my attention an incident that had ocurred when I was seven years old. It was a small, childish thing, but to my astonishment I found myself crying inconsolably as if still a small child! Finally the peace came, and I moved on in my memory walk with Jesus.

Through the weeks in which I pursued this memory walk such peace filled my heart that I began to pray in this way for each of my loved ones—my father, stepmother, husband, children, friends, one by one. They knew nothing of it because I told no one. Since there was no way I could know many of their most painful memories, I simply prayed *in the Spirit,* pausing over each portion of each life until a peace came to me, and then moving on until my spirit bumped into a "grief," interceding then for that grief to be soothed and healed, and for any hindrance in my relationship with them to be removed.

I undertook praying in this way for a missionary friend in Indonesia. To my astonishment, as I prayed for her day after day *in the Spirit,* nothing but peace ever came! Finally I wrote and told her that I had been praying for the healing of all her memories, but that the Lord had not lifted a single burden to my heart. Praying over the years of her life had been like praying over a smooth, peacefully moving stream. She wrote back thanking me, and explained why I had found no burdens for her in this deep level of prayer. Agnes Sanford had already prayed for her for the healing of her memories! This amazing experience conviced me more than ever of the value and effectiveness of this kind of prayer.

When we pray for each other in this unselfish way, the broken unity over which we have grieved is healed first at a deep level of the spirit. By entering into another's pain in the spirit, our own unforgiveness and judgmental attitudes melt away in the love of Jesus. Paul says in Romans that we can be the avenue through which the Holy Spirit *prays in griefs too deep for words.*[18] The Father hears, answering with His perfect peace in those for whom we pray.

The unspeakable memory

We live in a violent world in which incest, rape, sodomy, adultery and assault abound. Many people carry memories so shocking they cannot be shared. The memories are pushed back into the closet of the mind, but like menacing ghosts hover just below the surface, subconsciously influencing many of our attitudes toward ourselves, our families and others.

The victims of such sins often carry a deep sense of shame even though they were in no way at fault. Women especially have uncounted shameful memories of being sexually abused. It may be from a pinch on the "fanny" by a stranger on a bus, or a lustful look that makes one feel undressed. It may be memories of male relatives and family friends who were always harassing little girls with "naughty" comments or roving fingers. If wives are cold and unresponsive, it may be some buried childhood memory that brought a sense of shame. These may seem small offenses compared to incest and rape, but they also deeply wound the spirit, the dignity of one's personhood even as a little girl.

When we pray alone for the healing of memories, the gentle Holy Spirit will never allow a memory to come to our attention that we cannot handle in prayer by ourselves. He is so sensitive to our vulnerability that He only brings up "safe" things. Even then, He only exposes one unpleasant memory at a time for healing, for we could never successfully pray over a whole mountain of grief all at once. Jesus says to us, *I have many things to tell you, but you cannot bear them now.*[19]

We need a trusted, godly, mature Christian man or woman to face these shocking, shameful things with us in prayer. I say "mature" because only those who have lived long enough to have experienced many sorrows will have the compassion to bring God's healing without **any** condemnation. In the presence of a loving, wise man or woman of God we can walk, together with Jesus, down into the dark basement of the memory where these terrifying things lie.

A great deal of harm has been done by some counselors who have attempted to bring inner healing by following a program of "steps," including confession and asking forgiveness. This is totally different from a Spirit-led experience of inner healing. There must be no probing, but a quiet waiting, in an atmosphere of prayer, for anything the suffering one might want to share. There must be no "rape of the soul," no drawing out of experiences whose exposure will add to the person's pain. The healing is done by the Spirit of Jesus in the inner man, not in the intellect through following a prescribed plan.

When the distressing memory surfaces, time must be allowed for grief, for something precious **was** lost. And then the Spirit of God begins to heal the grief, *making all things new.*[20] As God continues His healing work deep in our hearts, we may even be able to thank Him for those awful experiences. For now we will be far better able to comfort other sufferers,[21] assuring them that God indeed gives *beauty for ashes,*[22] causing a garden to blossom in our hearts out of the ashes of our pain.

Childbirth practices in our culture are a common cause of shock and shame. The assaults on the sensibilities of some women has had an impact similar to rape. When one mentions the possibility of unhappy childbirth memories, a common first reaction is denial. Yet when the repressed memories begin to surface, what pain and griefs often emerge!

One young woman said her childbirth experience was fine, just fine, no problem. Weeks later she said, "Why did you ask that? The more I recall, the worse I realize it was!" When she looked at the experience realistically, without repressing any part of it, she found many unhealed griefs. God's inner healing came only as she accepted the catharsis of working through her disappointments honestly.

Sometimes the unspeakable memory is not something done

against our person or our dignity, but shameful sins which we ourselves committed, perhaps even after we had received Jesus as our Savior. Others may have thought we were models of virtue, and only we know the truth. These may be sexual sins such as repeated masturbation, heavy petting and "almost" coitus during the teen years, coitus outside marriage or even with other partners after marriage. Such sins need to be repented of and turned from. But many times a sense of guilt and shame remains. If so, it is wise to seek out a mature, older Christian, confess our wrong and hear from their lips the words of our Lord's forgiveness.

It may be that God will bring to our attention some restitution that needs to be made for our wrong doing. Other times no restitution is possible. One time in praying with a young Christian mother for the healing of memories a measure of peace came to her, but something still troubled her. Try as she would, she could not recall what it might be. We prayed again, but still she was not completely free. We waited to see if the Holy Spirit would reveal her trouble. Suddenly a look of anguish came over her face and she cried out, "My baby! I killed my baby! Oh! I killed my baby!" She buried her face in her hands and wept bitterly. Early in one of her pregnancies she had had an abortion. She had been counselled at the time that it was the wise thing to do and had agreed with the decision. She had pushed the memory down past recall, but now the gentle Spirit of God brought it to light so that she might experience His forgiveness and peace.

Confess your sins to one another, and pray for one another, so that you may be healed.[23] This does not mean that we are to be dumping every little wrong on each other. But in these deep areas of shame and grief we not only need the assurance of God's forgiveness in His Word. We also may need to hear the spoken words of forgiveness from one of His servants to feel truly free. "The Lord has forgiven you. You are now as pure in His eyes as the day you were born.[24] Go your way in the peace and joy of the Lord."

Remembered joys

Our memories serve not only as storehouses of sorrows until God heals them. They also serve the marvelous function of filling our minds with remembered joys. We need to remember all the good things God has done for us, all the many answers to prayer that we so quickly forget in the urgency of our new petitions.

Over and over the Bible reminds us to **remember** *the lovingkindness of the Lord.*[25]

> *Remember all the way which the Lord your God led you.... You shall remember the Lord your God, for it is He who gives you power to get wealth....*[26]

> *Bless the Lord, O my soul, and do not forget all his benefits, who forgives all your iniquities, who heals all your diseases, who crowns you with lovingkindness and tender mercies....*[27]

> *I consider the days of old. I remember the years long ago. I commune with my heart in the night. I meditate and search my spirit.... I will call to mind the deeds of the Lord. I will remember the wonders of old. I will meditate on all thy works, and muse on thy mighty deeds.*[28]

It is also good to think of all the experiences of joy and scenes of loveliness with which God has filled our lives, for which we did not even ask. These blessings are far more numerous than our sorrows. I remember the happiness of our fifth grade daughter who became jump rope champion of our city of 70,000, and her excitement at the opportunity to demonstrate her skill on television. I remember how often our back yard looked like the bicycle brigade as her active friends—mostly boys—came over to play.

Children's voices filled our house during the day, a friend or two for each of our several children. I remember young voices on the front step filling the early evening air with the cries of "Moonlight, starlight!" games, and the sounds of running feet and laughter.

In times of stress when tempers flare and relationships are strained, it is wise to pause and be reminded of the happy times. A young wife was struggling with difficulties between her husband and herself. A wise counselor suggested, "Try to remember some area in which you and your husband used to be in tune."

She thought a moment and then replied, "I can't remember any!" But later on the happy memories began to surface. Her impulse was to push them back down and nurse her anger. She didn't **want** to remember the happy times! But as she allowed these memories to rise, remembered blessings began to strengthen her to face the trials of the moment as passing events that God could heal.

Pictures and mementoes help bring back happy memories, though each item is a vain attempt to catch the moment and hold onto it. Although we cannot keep the moment, we can long be reminded of its happiness.

> *Grandmother asked to have the boxes down*
> *From the high shelves where they had gathered dust,*
> *Unopened. Now space was needed and she must*
> *Sort out the trash to burn. Her son, man-grown,*
> *Piled them beside her chair, with basket near*
> *To catch the discard. Thin fingers broke the strings*
> *And let the musty smell of shut-up things*
> *Creep out: A christening robe, full, long and sheer,*
> *"Award of Merit" for fourth-grade proficiency*
> *In spelling; letters, War One, from overseas;*
> *A dried corsage; a bottle of colored sand....*
> *She lifted them out, then put them back with care*
> *And firmly said, "There was no rubbish there."*[29]

Building memories

Memory is one of the finest gifts of our Creator. It is through the integration of memories that our personalities develop. Although our ideas change and grow and our bodies continually change from youth to age, yet each of us is the same "I" looking out on the world that we were "back then."

I am three years old, sitting on a tiny red chair in a country Sunday school singing "Jesus loves me, this I know." I am a school girl, hurrying to class across the train-yard, with the snow-capped peaks of the Sierra Nevada mountains filling the horizon of my vision. I am the bride walking down the aisle on my father's arm toward my groom. I am the lonely granddaughter by the casket of my godly grandmother. I am in labor.... I am a grandmother hurrying to the hospital with my husband for our first peek at a new grandchild. I am myself, then, now, and through eternity.

Since happy memories are so important, parents need to plan ways in which to build them in their children. It is impossible for us to know what little things they may recall, good and bad, but we can deliberately plan some customs and events they may never forget. For our family it was cross-country trips in the summer time with a station-wagon loaded with children, sleeping bags and suitcases, the tent tied on top of the car. And birthdays were always a special event. Christmas traditions developed over the years. Each Christmas Eve we had a "program" which the children planned and performed themselves. One year we made a tape of their program, and it has become a tradition to replay it every year, laughing and wiping our eyes and remembering together. Christmas morning was the "birthday cake" for Jesus (coffee cake with a big candle) before opening gifts. And so on. Each family builds its own traditions.

But the traditions that are most easily remembered are like those of our Jewish friends, whose Sabbath family celebration has been little changed through long centuries. The synagogue is not the key to the survival of Judaism; it is the weekly Jewish tradition in the home that welds the bonds of love in memories that stretch back through time.

At the close of the Old Testament it says that *those who feared the Lord spoke often to one another. And the Lord listened, and heard it, and a book of memories was written before him for those who feared the Lord, and who thought upon his name.*[30]

If a Memory Book is being prepared for us in heaven by the Lord, should we not build a storehouse of happy memories for our children here? If God remembers how we talk about Him to each other, should we not fill our children's lives with experiences of His goodness and the joys of this present life? Then when we are gone, they will be able to draw out of the storehouse of their hearts happy memories to encourage each other in the Lord, like the householder of whom Jesus spoke, *who brings forth out of his treasury things new and old.*[31] Our children will then be able to say to us, "Thanks for the memory!"

NOTES
1. Deut. 8 NIV. 2. Ps. 55:12-14. 3. Lk. 4:16-30. 4. Mt. 13:53-58. 5. Mt. 10:34-37 RSV. 6. Mk. 3:21-35. 7. Acts 5:29. 8. 1 Pet. 3:8-17. 9. 1 Cor. 7:14. 10. Jas. 1:2-5. 11. 1 Cor. 13:4 NIV.
12. Acts 21:18. James, the brother of John, had been martyred by this time. (Acts 12:2).

13. Heb. 12:15. **14.** Rom. 2:1. **15.** Mt. 19:19. **16.** 2 Cor. 12:8-10.
17. Agnes Sanford. **The Healing Gifts of the Spirit.** New York. Lippincott. 1966. Trumpet edition, 1976. See also **Behold Your God.** St. Paul, MN. Macalaster Park Publishing. 1958.
18. Rom. 8:26-30 NEB. **19.** Jn. 16:12. **20.** 2 Cor. 5:17; Rev. 21:5. **21.** 2 Cor. 1:3, 4. **22.** Isa. 61:3. **23.** Jas. 5:16. **24.** 1 Thess. 5:23, 24. **25.** Ps. 48:9. **26.** Deut. 8:2, 18. **27.** Ps. 103:2-5. **28.** Ps. 77:5-7, 11, 12.
29. Nellie Burget Miller. **30.** Mal. 3:16. **31.** Mt. 13:52.

The Family of God

They devoted themselves to the apostles' teaching and to the fellowship and to prayer. Everyone was filled with awe, and many wonders and miraculous signs were done by the apostles. All the believers were together and had everything in common. Selling their possessions and goods, they gave to anyone as he had need. Every day they continued to meet together in the temple courts. They broke bread, praising God and enjoying the favor of all the people. And the Lord added to their number daily those who were being saved.[1]

But now in Christ Jesus you who once were far away have been brought near through the blood of Christ.... For through him we both have access to the Father by one Spirit. Consequently, you are no longer foreigners and aliens, but fellow citizens with God's people and members of God's household, built on the foundation of the apostles and prophets, with Christ Jesus himself as the chief cornerstone. In him the whole building is joined together and rises to become a holy temple in the Lord. And in him you too are being built together to become a dwelling in which God lives by his Spirit.
... For this reason I kneel before the Father, from whom his whole family in heaven and on earth derives its name.[2]

The church is the family of God, the members of God's household, the sons and daughters of the heavenly Father.[3] God's family of believers includes people of all ages from every nation and from every generation. The local church is the visible symbol of this larger family of God. This local body of believers is not meant to be like a country club with only adult members, but a "home" for all ages, without partiality. The prophet Joel sounds the summons:

> *Call a solemn assembly;*
>   *gather the people.*
> *Consecrate the congregation;*
>   *assemble the old people.*
> *Gather the children,*
>   *even those that suck the breast.*
> *Let the bridegroom leave his room,*
>   *and the bride her chamber....*
> *I will pour out my Spirit on all flesh:*
>   *your sons and your daughters shall prophesy;*
> *Your old men shall dream dreams,*
>   *and your young men shall see visions.*
> *I will pour out my Spirit even upon*
>   *the servants and the servant girls.*[4]

The covenant

When an infant is born to a couple in the local church, the parents enter into a covenant relationship with the congregation. Even if there is no formal service of consecration, there is the tacit understanding that the whole assembly shares responsibility for the faith of the children of its members.

A formal ceremony of dedication or christening is a public acknowledgment of this covenant. The child is consecrated to God. The parents are consecrated in their role of bringing their child up to love and serve God. The assembled congregation witnessing the ceremony is a part of this consecration and may even be asked to give a verbal commitment. In this way the new parents with their infant acknowledge their dependence upon the loving supervision of the local church. They are to be uplifted by the prayers and cooperation of the larger family of the church in guiding the child to personal faith in Jesus Christ.

But in how many churches is this responsibility carried out? How many churches provide resources for young parents, helping them cope with their new spiritual responsibilities before God? Some churches have discussion groups for mothers of small children. But has anyone ever heard of groups formed to guide fathers of young children in their new responsibility as priests of their households?

Christian parents who want to raise their children by following the biblical examples of such things as closeness, touching, breastfeeding, co-family sleeping, and loving discipline face numerous obstacles. It may be difficult for them to move against the cultural trend in their own congregation, which reflects Western culture more than biblical cultures. They may not find the affirmation and support that was implicit in the consecration ceremony.

For example, where in the church can a mother breastfeed her baby? There is no reason why a tiny baby cannot be breastfed right in the church service. If the parents sit near the back, the mother can nurse the baby quietly, a little blanket thrown over her shoulder for modesty, and no one will be the wiser. Mama and daddy can sit together. Baby can stay with mama, nursing quietly when hungry, and worship can be a family joy. What a blessing it is when this is possible without the risk of offending the members of the congregation!

Some church nurseries will not accept a baby if he or she will not take a bottle, or they may not allow parents into the room. Even if the mother is allowed into the nursery to nurse her baby, what would she do about her breastfeeding toddler? The mother breastfeeding a one, two or three year old child needs a comfortable, private place to which she can go. It can be a women's lounge (if the other women are not scandalized by the Old Testament custom of nursing young children). Privacy is needed for modesty's sake, for the toddler pulls the blanket away, tries to unbutton mama's dress or thrusts his hands into her bosom. Some will not allow her to cover her breasts in any way. (Older toddlers can be taught to cooperate. Nurslings older than 2 or 3 can learn to wait until they are home to "have mama.")

The church "family"

The function of the local church is not only to propagate doctrine, but also to serve the needs of **all** its people. A church "family" consists of everyone from the infant to the elderly. If the church is truly "my Father's house," then those who participate are my brothers and sisters, aunts and uncles, nieces and nephews.

Western culture is one of unbiblical isolation in which individuals are alienated from one another. The relatives of newly married couples often live long distances away from them so that the couple has no extended family support. At birth the newborn is taken from the mother, placed in an "isolette," fed from a bottle, and cared for much of the time by baby sitters and preschool teachers until old enough for school. The direction of his growth is away from the family until his own marriage. By then his middle-aged parents may be on their way to a retirement village where no children are allowed, and later on be placed in nursing homes for the elderly.

Our churches and Sunday schools have not escaped this cultural pattern of alienation. The baby is locked into age segregation from his first Sunday in church. Every age has its own program from nursery through college, to young marrieds' classes, to classes for the elderly which are often sex segregated as well. One elderly lady complained, "I don't care to be with other old ladies **all** the time!"

This age segregation extends through most church activities. How many children learn that prayer meetings are too "boring" for children, by always being in their own clubs rather than in a place of prayer? Children sing in their own choirs, have their own parties, and too often grow up and go their own way without ever having been drawn into the heart and life of the church family.

Jesus said, ***Let the children come to me,***[5] when mothers brought tiny infants and children into the teaching circle of His disciples. What better way is there for children to learn the ways of the Lord than to be present at least sometimes in the assembly, participating in the praise and prayer and singing? (Don't we all smile when a little voice sings out at the end of a phrase when everyone else has stopped?) Children need to hear the testimonies and the laughter, see the tears, witness the Lord at work in the altar calls. And whatever happened to families sitting together in church? Even parents need to feel that they "belong," with the pleasure of growing children and teenagers worshipping beside them rather than with their peers in the balcony.

A recent study of children's ministries demonstrates that churches which segregate children and adults during worship are the ones whose memberships most often ultimately decline. The same study revealed that churches which encouraged all ages to take part in worship were enjoying growth. Churches were warned that "unless young children are made welcome in worship services, babies and toddlers included, they will never see themselves as part of the whole congregation."[6]

One creative church had bean bag chairs made. Little children had the choice of sitting up in front on the bean bags or with their parents, whichever they preferred. These children had "the best seats in the house" from which to view what the Lord was doing.

Small groups which meet for Bible study or prayer often assume that everyone will leave their small children with baby sitters. But why can provision not be made for the children to play quietly in a room near by? Those present could take turns caring for the children or could hire a neighbor girl or boy to babysit (teenage boys make fine babysitters). The children should be free to come in to their parents at any time they feel the need to be close to mommy and daddy, as long as they are quiet.

In New Testament times churches often began as the members of a single household.[7] In some parts of the world today church growth is most rapid where "house churches" are again being established. At first it might be only one household which accepts the Lord. As other families accept Jesus as Savior, they continue to meet in homes like the early church, whose members *broke bread together from house to house.*[8]

The Lord has prospered some of our churches until they are ministering to hundreds and even thousands of people. But this hugeness needs to be balanced by provision for every believer to be a part of some home fellowship group, some "family" of all ages within the larger church structure. This church family of several households will learn to know the needs, joys and concerns of everyone among them, functioning as an extended family.

"Singles" groups are springing up in churches across the United States. Although there are some advantages in this provision for single people, at the same time it is a sad commentary on current church life. We are brothers and sisters in the Lord, whether married or not. Men and women ought to have the opportunity to experience family love even if they are not married. This will also help keep childless adults, whether married or single, from becoming disgusted with the presence of little children. The modern grandparent who gladly lives in an "adult only" community would then be unheard of. We often think about the dependence of children on adults, but it is equally true that adults, including unmarried adults, need interaction with young children.

The single parent, whether unmarried, widowed or divorced,

faces still harder problems. James reminds us that *religion which is pure and without fault is this: to visit the fatherless and the widows in their affliction.*[9] This implies not only practical help, but also loving relationships which draw these people into the church family. Jesus promises to be *husband of the widow,*[10] and *father of the fatherless.*[11] He is also mother of the motherless and gives strength and wisdom to the single father.

My mother died when I was two years and my brother six weeks old. In the dark of night my father went out to a deserted park near the river and threw himself weeping on the ground. He pleaded with the Lord for guidance in being both father and mother to his motherless babes. His prayer has been abundantly answered!

I was probably the first (and perhaps only) three year old girl to have been a regular member of YMCA camps in the mountains, where Dad was a camp counselor. He took me along wherever he could. As teenagers my brother and I went with him every Sunday that he was invited to preach in churches in the area (he taught high school during the week). I thought he was the best preacher in the world! Churches, conferences—we were included as part of the activities wherever he went, even though we did not "fit" the age or sex categories.

The handicapped, the retarded, the elderly, also need a rightful place within a small circle of the larger church "family." They need to feel they belong and are dearly loved by people who care about them. God *places the solitary ones in families.*[12]

> *If a brother or sister is ill-clad and in lack of daily food, and one of you says, "Go in peace, be warmed and filled," without giving them the things needed for the body, what good is that?*[13]

> *Do not rebuke an older man but exhort him as you would a father. Treat younger men like brothers, older women like mothers, younger women like sisters, in all purity.*[14]

The Eucharist

> *The cup of blessing which we bless, is it not the communion of the blood of Christ? The bread which we break, is it not the communion of the body of Christ?*
>
> *For we being many are one bread, and one body: for we all partake of that one bread.*[15]

Jesus gave His body and poured out His life's blood to make us one. When we share in the bread and cup of Communion, we are participating in an act of "oneness." When we share meals together, each meal can be a Eucharist, uniting us to one another and our living Lord as one body.

> *And as they were eating Jesus took the bread, and blessed it, and broke it and gave it to them saying, "Take, eat. This is my body. And he took the cup, and when he had given thanks **(eucharisteo)**, he gave it to them and they all drank of it. And he said to them "This is the blood of the new testament, which is shed for many."*[16]

In quoting these words of the Lord Jesus, Paul adds that many of the problems in the local community of believers, including sickness, is the result of their lack of unity. He rebukes them for divisions, contentions, and even heresies, and concludes by saying that *anyone who eats and drinks without recognizing the body of the Lord eats and drinks judgment on himself. That is why many among you are weak and sick, and a number of you have fallen asleep.*[17] Earlier in the same epistle he had written, *I plead with you, brothers and sisters, that you be perfectly united in mind and thought.*[18]

What Paul is requesting is humanly impossible. Not only is Christ's church on earth fragmented and divided, but there is friction in every family, every small fellowship of believers, every church. The body of Christ, His bride, is full of *spots, wrinkles, blemishes.*[19] But hidden in the word **eucharisteo,** which we have come to associate with holy communion, is God's provision for our living together: **charis,** grace.

No earthly utopia is possible. But the grace of God not only brings us salvation, it also makes it possible for us to get along with each other. Without the active presence of God's grace the local believers are simply a collection of individuals, not a community of believers. Without God's grace "community life is little more than a superficial juxtaposition of individual lives!"[20]

> *For by grace **(charis)** are you saved through faith; and that not of yourselves. It is the gift of God; not of works; lest any one should boast. For you are God's workmanship....*[21]

The Greek word ***charisma*** (plural: ***charismata)*** is also translated as grace: *For the wages of sin is death, but the free grace **(charisma)** of God is eternal life in Jesus Christ our Lord.*[22] The grace of God is *manifold,*[23] that is, many-faceted, like a prism in the sunlight, and takes many varied forms. The graces, the charisms of the Holy Spirit, transform our personalities, fill us with love, joy, peace, gentleness.[24] His grace makes it possible for us to live together in peace. He graces us with the ability to bless one another through a word of wisdom, a word of knowledge, or through the graces of healing.[25] These charisms of the Spirit are graces which He is causing to blossom in our lives.

*For I long to see you, that I may impart some spiritual grace **(charisma)** to strengthen you.*[26]

*For the graces **(charismata)** and the call of God are irrevocable.*[27]

*Having then graces **(charismata)** according to the grace **(charis)** given to us, let us use them....*[28]

*Now there are diversities of graces **(charismata),** but the same Lord.... There should be no discord in the body, but the members should have the same concern for one another.... For you are the body of Christ.*[29]

Thus Christians are by definition "charismatic," graced by God in many ways. And together we give thanks *(eucharisteo)* around the table of our Lord, who makes us one body. He even makes the words that come out of our mouths full of grace, like those of Jesus:

*There was a general stir of admiration; they were surprised that words of such grace **(charis)** should fall from his lips. "Is this not Joseph's son?" they asked....*[30]

You are the fairest of men; grace is poured upon your lips.[31]

The charisms of the Spirit of God make it possible for us to live, work, worship and serve together as families, as local fellowships, as members of Christ's body on earth. How we need these graces in our lives! We need family grace, loving grace, healing grace, Divine gentleness and power.

In South Africa, there used to be an old lady who visited our home once in a while. She was one of the sweetest, most blessed creatures I ever met. My, when she came into my office and sat down for five minutes, she brought the consciousness of God, a restfulness and a peace of mind. From her whole person there seemed to radiate that blessedness that can be described only as the grace of God, and the very atmosphere would become pregnant with it. I would make excuses to take her through the house. I wanted her to leave that beautiful emanation all over the place. Because when she was gone, it seemed the house settled down, the noisy children ceased to influence, and all invisible unrest disappeared. It was the Grace of God.[32]

Notice how often in Paul's opening words in his letters he says, *Grace and peace to you.*[33] The grace comes first, and brings peace, peace in our hearts, peace among each other. Even little babies respond. One pastor sometimes blesses a crying baby by placing his hand on its head and saying firmly, "The **peace** of Jesus to you!" Our culture would say "this works like a charm." But we say, "The charism works!"

Grace and healing go hand in hand. The disunity in our homes and churches leads to much unnecessary illness,[34] but the opposite is also true. The gracious Holy Spirit brings oneness among us, and also restores body, soul and spirit to harmony. A loving hand placed on a sleeping child who is restless or ill ministers to its troubled spirit. "The peace of Jesus to you, my child. In His name, be whole."

It is often easier to show grace to those who are "down and out," than to those closest to us. The closer we live to each other, the more grace we need in order to be able to get along! But what do we do about those "thorns in the church,"[35] those people who stir up trouble, will not listen to the others, and are always causing us grief? Richard Baxter suggests an answer:

This is the time for crowning with thorns.... We can now scarce pray in our families, or sing praises to God, but our voice is a vexation to them.... You, brethren, who can now attempt no work of God without losing the love of the world, consider, you shall have none in heaven but will

*further your work, and join heart and voice with you in
your everlasting joy and praise. Till then, "possess ye
your souls in patience" (Luke 21:19). Bind all reproaches
as a crown to your heads. Esteem them greater than the
world's treasures.... We shall then rest from all our sad
divisions, and unchristian quarrels with one another. How
lovingly do thousands live together in heaven, who lived at
variance on earth!*[36]

The **eucharisteo,** the body and blood of Christ Jesus, should
not only heal the differences in our homes, our small fellowships,
but bring healing to the whole body of Christ. Juan Carlos Ortiz
says our difficulty in getting along with Christians of other
denominations and persuasions is because we are still children,
and it is natural for children to quarrel. Paul says, *I cannot speak
to you as spiritual men, but as to babes in Christ,... for there is
jealousy and strife among you.*[37]

*We are called to renew our spirits. When we meet
somebody, we try to determine if he is renewed. If he is not
renewed, we think,* **Poor man!** *So then we have the
"renewed" and the "not renewed," those who have the vision and those who don't.
So the groupist spirit among Christians is a real problem. The way in which we have divided ourselves is
childish.... When we were in the world, we fought for
politics or sports—the Giants or the Dodgers. Now we fight
for doctrine. We have a holy fight.... How the Spirit of
God grieves!*[38]

But when we allow the warmth of God's grace to work among
us it is a witness to the world. Jesus said, *Everyone will know
you are my disciples by the love which you show each other.*[39] This
love does not end with our human family or church family, for
we are also to *love our neighbors as ourselves.*[40] It does not matter if they are agnostics, secularists, materialists, humanists,
atheists, communists, spiritists, pagans—we are to love them
with the love of Christ. Our little fellowship is not to be a ghetto
in which we close ourselves off from the crying needs of the
family of mankind. By God's grace, we can love them as he
loved us.

> *God's love has been poured into our hearts by the Holy Spirit which has been given to us.... God's love for us was proven by the fact that while we were still sinners, He died for us.*[41]

The wilderness

There is another word of which **eucharisteo** reminds us. It is the word **chara,** joy! The joy that Jesus gives cannot be taken from us, no matter how hard the circumstances. *I have said these things to you so that my joy **(chara)** might be in you, and that your joy might be complete.*[42] After promising us joy, Jesus goes on to say that *in the world you will have tribulation. But be of good cheer. I have overcome the world!*[43]

The apostle Peter warns God's children to stay closely united, in order to protect each one. *Be sober. Be watchful. Your adversary the devil prowls around like a roaring lion, seeking whom he may devour.*[44] The hurting, lonely one we allow to wander off, unnoticed, may become a prey to the evil one. Like the children of Israel, our journey through the wilderness of life is not to be an individual one, but is to be a communal experience in which each member of every household is accounted for. We are all in this together, facing possible days of hard times and persecution. There have been more Christian martyrs in this century than in all the centuries since Jesus first came.

But there is a bright side to persecution. "O happy days of persecution, which drove us together in love!"[45] Baxter wrote. Christians who have been imprisoned under totalitarian regimes tell us what joy it is to discover a brother or sister in the Lord.

All over the world Jesus is drawing His people together in households, in communities, or in closer bonds of small fellowships in our big churches. These are preparations for possible hard days ahead. When another war comes—and we know from Scripture that there will be wars until the Lord returns—once again we may of necessity be *breaking bread from house to house, holding all possessions in common.*[46] Persecution drove the first Christians together, so that they were *in every house teaching and preaching Jesus Christ, ... rejoicing to be counted worthy to suffer for His name.*[47]

If such times come to the Western churches as they already have to some of the Eastern and third world churches, we will need all the graces, the charisms of the Holy Spirit to sustain us, even for some of us the grace to accept martyrdom for Jesus. In such times, how blessed are those small Christian fellowships whose members know how to deliver their own babies, breastfeed their infants and toddlers, and pray for the healing of their sick! Together they will share miracles of protection, provision and wholeness, as have the little house churches in China, now hesitantly emerging after a generation of purges.

There are a number of practical steps to take to be prepared for possible famine, war, financial collapse or persecution. One is to throw away our charge cards and obey Scripture which says, *Owe no man anything but to love each other.*[48] In times of national distress, those in debt will be at the mercy of their creditors. Jesus wants us free. We can learn to share with each other now, rather than spending beyond our means.

It might become necessary to set aside emergency supplies of food, water, medicine and fuel (for heat and light).[49] Money is worthless if there is nothing to buy! If we are sensitive to the prompting of the Holy Spirit, He will guide each family and each little fellowship group in setting aside the right amounts of the right supplies, at the right time, with enough to share with others also. When darkness fell over the land of Egypt, all God's children had light in their homes.[50]

Any hard days that may lie ahead may not yet be *the end of the world.*[51] Numerous times during the last two thousand years God's people thought it might be so, but then times of blessing returned. The promise is still true that *the wilderness will blossom as a rose.*[52] Nevertheless, we are advancing together through the wilderness of this present life against the gates of hell,[53] as sons and daughters of another Realm, *looking for a city whose builder and maker is God.*[54]

And you shall be betrayed both by parents, and brothers, and relatives, and friends; and some of you shall they cause to be put to death. And you shall be hated of all men for my name's sake.... And when these things begin to come to pass, then look up, and lift up your heads; for your redemption is drawing near.[55]

The consummation

Jesus says an amazing thing to His disciples before His crucifixion: *Some of you shall be put to death.... but not a hair of your head shall perish!*[56] This seeming contradiction is an affirmation of the resurrection of the body. This earthly body returns to dust *(adamah),* yet not a hair is lost! Although we are spirit, as God is Spirit, yet our spirits are clothed in flesh and shall one day be clothed in new **flesh.**

How often our picture of heaven is of disembodied, sexless, invisible spirits (ghosts) floating around in the ether! But that is not what the Bible says:

> *So also is the resurrection of the dead. It is buried in corruption. It is raised in incorruption. It is sown a natural body. It is raised a spiritual **body**.*[57]

After Jesus rose from the dead He said to His disciples, *A spirit does not have flesh and bones as you see that I have. Handle me, and see!*[58] And we shall be like Him. [59]

Every special joy of this earthly life will blossom into a greater joy. We shall be eating and drinking as Jesus did after His resurrection,[60] walking and leaping and praising God, and even soaring through the air.[61] We will retain our individuality. We will know each other.[62] There will be diversity in our unity, for we will not be blended together like vegetables through a sieve into the soup. Our unity will not be a blending with earth, air, fire and water in which all personal distinctiveness is lost as some religions teach.

Rather, it will be a **com**-unity among believers patterned after *the plural unity of God himself. At one time our theology so stressed the oneness of God that we ran the risk of looking upon him as uni-personal.... We cannot minimize either the unity or the trinity of God, there is unity in trinity and trinity in unity.*[63]

Our unity will be so great that the word "family" can no longer describe its closeness. We will be closer to each other than that. The joys and ecstasy of sexuality will not be lost, even though we will *not marry nor be given in marriage.*[64] The deepest expression of human love between man and wife will be sublimated in as deep a love for everyone. It is impossible for God to describe heaven to us in terms which we can understand. It is more difficult than for us to describe the principle of aerodynamics to a two year old. God describes heaven in terms of a marriage:

> *In loving one person and one's children, a human being can better understand God's love and care for all. Promise, commitment, concern, spring from love. But there is also a foretaste of bliss in the gift of sexual pleasure. The*

delights and joys of sexual orgasms may be a preparation for heaven. Fallen man needs a training in joy, among other things. Sexual ecstasy can confirm a message of the beauty of the world....

There would be no marriage of two-in-one flesh in heaven, because in an all-in-one-flesh community all would be married to all. The coming of the kingdom is even described as the "marriage of the Lamb," a wedding of joy. With space and time overcome, love for one another could be expressed transcendently in all the ways of expressing love. In a transfigured person all the individual's faculties and capacities would be unified, and full communion with others would be possible. With sexual identity transcended, the ecstasy of male-female coupling could be expanded to all human relationships....[65]

Jesus never married in His earthly life because He was already promised in marriage to a bride, the new Eve. If He had married a woman in the flesh it would have broken His commitment to the rest of us! His virginity was not a denial of sexuality, but a symbol of a still deeper unity to come. It is a mystery how God can love every one of us totally all at the same time, without detracting one iota from His personal love and attention for each of us! We shall be able to love like that.

Now we have only a dim idea of the bliss this union will be. As members of the bride of Jesus—now so full of spots and wrinkles and soiled garments—we shall be clothed in dazzling wedding clothes for the consummation of our marriage to Him!

Listen! My Lover!
　Look! Here he comes,
Leaping across the mountains,
　bounding over the hills....
My lover spoke and said to me,
　"Arise, my darling,
　my beautiful one, and come with me.
See! The winter is past;
　the rains are over and gone.
Flowers appear on the earth;
　the season of singing has come....
Arise, come, my darling;
　my beautiful one, come with me.[66]

In that day when the new Eve, the Church, is wedded to the new Adam, Christ Jesus, we can walk together along the banks of the river of life among the trees of the Garden, whose leaves are for the healing of the nations. We can freely eat of the Tree of Life.[67]

The way is still open for anyone who has not yet received Jesus as Savior. *The Spirit and the bride say, Come. And let anyone who is thirsty, come. And whoever will, let him take of the water of life freely. He who gives witness to these things says, "I assure you, I am coming soon!"*

Amen. Come, Lord Jesus!

*The grace **(charis)** of our Lord Jesus Christ be with you all.*
Amen.[68]

NOTES
1. Acts 2:42-46 NIV. **2.** Eph. 2:13, 17-22; 3:14, 15 NIV. **3.** 1 Cor. 6:16-18. **4.** Joel 2:16, 28, 29. **5.** Lk. 18:15-18.
6. A report by Rev. Stan Stewart to a United Methodist Conference on Ministries with Children. Quoted in **Eternity,** December, 1979. P. 51.

Family Crusade Projects have been held in Latin America since 1976 by Overseas Crusades Ministries, Inc. (3033 Scott Blvd., Santa Clara, CA 92052). Evangelistic ministries are adapted to family needs, and hundreds of broken families have been healed. Before the Family Crusades a retreat is held for pastors **and their wives,** where attention is directed to their own family relationships. They are also trained to teach healthy family living to the people of their congregation.

7. Rom. 16:5; 1 Cor. 16:19; Col. 4:15; Philemon 2. **8.** Acts 2:46. **9.** Jas. 1:27. **10.** Isa. 54:4, 5. **11.** Ps. 68:5. **12.** Ps. 68:6. **13.** Jas. 2:15. **14.** 1 Tim. 5:1, 2 RSV. **15.** 1 Cor. 10:16, 17.
16. *Eucharisteo* is also found in Mt. 26:27; Lk. 22:17-19 and 1 Cor. 11:23-30.
17. 1 Cor. 11:18, 19. **18.** 1 Cor. 1:9-13. **19.** Eph. 5:27.
20. Leon Joseph Cardinal Suenens. **A New Pentecost?** New York. Seabury Press. 1974. P. 103.
21. Eph. 2:8, 9. **22.** Rom. 6:23. **23.** 1 Pet. 4:10; Eph. 2:7. **24.** Gal. 5:22, 23. **25.** 1 Cor. 12:1, 7-11. **26.** Rom. 1:11. **27.** Rom. 11:29. **28.** Rom. 12:6. **29.** 1 Cor. 12:4, 7, 25, 27a. See also 1 Cor. 1:7; 7:7; 12:9, 28, 30, 32; 2 Cor. 1:11; 1 Tim. 4:14; 2 Tim. 1:6; 1 Pet. 4:10.
30. Lk. 4:22 NEB. **31.** Ps. 45:2 RSV
32. The John G. Lake Sermons. Ed. by Gordon Lindsay. Dallas, TX. Christ for the Nations. 1949, 1978. Pp. 97, 98.
33. Rom. 1:7; 1 Cor. 1:3; 2 Cor. 1:2; Gal. 1:3, etc.

34. 1 Cor. 11:18-34. Medical science also attests to the close relationship between mind and body. Disorders in one disturb the harmony of the other. All discord creates emotional tensions, with their negative physical results including lowered resistance to disease. In the realm of the spirit, discord blocks the gracious moving of the Holy Spirit and quenches the power of His presence.

35. Hos. 9:5, 8 KJV. *What will ye do in the solemn day, and in the day of the feast of the Lord?... nettles shall possess them: thorns shall be in their tabernacles;... the prophet is a snare of a fowler in all his ways, and hatred in the house of his God.* See also Num. 33:55; Josh. 23:13; Prov. 15:19; 2 Cor. 10:10; 12:7-10; 2 Tim. 4:14.

36. Richard Baxter. **The Saints' Everlasting Rest.** Ed. by Glenn Hinson. New York. Doubleday. 1978. Pp. 51, 52.

37. 1 Cor. 3:1, 3.

38. Juan Carlos Ortiz, **Cry of the Human Heart.** Carol Stream, IL. Creation House. 1977. Pp. 31-33. Reprinted by permission.

39. Jn. 13:35. **40.** Mt. 22:37-40. **41.** Rom. 5:5, 8; Jn. 3:16, 17. **42.** Jn. 15:11. **43.** Jn. 15:32. **44.** 1 Pet. 1:8.

45. Baxter, **op. cit.** P. 52. **46.** Acts 2:44-46. **47.** Acts 5:41, 42. **48.** Rom. 13:8. See also Luke 3:14; 1 Tim. 6:8; Heb. 13:5; Phil. 4:11-13 NIV.

49. Maria Hirschman. **Are You Prepared?** Hansi Ministries, Inc. P.O. Box 552. Huntington Beach, CA 92648.

50. Ex. 10:23. **51.** Mt. 13:39, 40. **52.** Isa. 35:1, 2. **53.** Mt. 16:18. **54.** Heb. 11:13-16. **55.** Lk. 21:16-18. **56.** Lk. 21:16, 17. **57.** 1 Cor. 15:42-55; 2 Cor. 5:1-4. **58.** Lk. 24:39. **59.** 1 Jn. 3:1, 2. **60.** Lk. 24:34-43. **61.** 1 Thess. 4:17. **62.** Mt. 22: 29, 30.

63. Suenens, **op. cit.** Pp. 192, 193. **64.** Mt. 22:30.

65. Sidney Cornelia Callahan. **Beyond Birth Control: The Christian Experience of Sex.** New York. Sheed & Wood. 1968. P. 50.

66. S. of S. 2:8-13 NIV. **67.** Rev. 21:9; 22:1-5. **68.** Rev. 22:17-21. **69.** 2 Cor. 6:16, 18.

The Family of God

And God said, I will dwell with them....
  and they shall be my people;...
  and ye shall be my sons and daughters.[69]

I'm so glad I'm a part of the family of God—
  I've been washed in the fountain,
    cleansed by His blood!
Joint heirs with Jesus as we travel this sod,
  For I'm part of the family,
    the family of God.

You will notice we say "brother and sister"
  around here—
It's because we're a family and these folks
  are so near;
When one has a heartache we all share the tears,
And rejoice in each victory
  In this family so dear.

From the door of an orphanage to the house of the King—
  No longer an outcast,
    A new song I sing;
From rags unto riches,
  from the weak to the strong,
I'm not worthy to be here,
  But, praise God, I belong!

I'm so glad I'm a part of the family of God—
  I've been washed in the fountain,
    cleansed by His blood!
Joint heirs with Jesus as we travel this sod,
  For I'm part of the family,
    the family of God.

"The Family of God." Words by William J. & Gloria Gaither and music by William J. Gaither. © Copyright 1970 by William J. Gaither. All rights reserved. Reprinted by permission.

Appendix

Acknowledgments

I am deeply indebted to my husband of over 36 years, Walter W. Wessel, Ph.D., biblical scholar, translator and professor, for his continuing encouragement of my independent research.

Thanks also go to our sons and daughters and grandsons and granddaughters, who have taught me so much. This book is not theory, but has been tested and tempered through raising a family of six children, each of whom has widely differing interests and temperaments. Without them this book could not have been written.

Special thanks go to Kathy and Deryl Nesper who urged me to write this book so that they could begin a teaching series on natural childbirth in the churches of Fresno, California. Not willing to wait for the book to be written, they began using the rough draft for their first series. The comments of the many couples they have since guided through the series have helped to refine the final draft.

My thanks also go to others who unexpectedly called or wrote urging me to write a sequel to **The Joy of Natural Childbirth** which could be the basis for a teaching series in churches. In each case I could assure them that I had already started writing! Clearly, God's time had come.

Our daughter Sharyl Adams burned the midnight oil for months as she skillfully edited the book and gave valuable insights from her own experiences. Our daughter Margaret Wilke also had many helpful insights to offer. Both of them are experienced La Leche League leaders. I am deeply indebted to them both.

It would be impossible to mention all those who read the manuscript and offered suggestions, but I would especially like to thank the following:

Rev. G. L. Johnson, pastor of Peoples Church, Fresno, whose support encouraged us to begin the project;

Ed Wheat, M.D., a Christian family physician who is also a certified sex therapist, for his help with the chapters on marital sex;

Marielle Lapointe, M.D., one of the medical consultants to Serena Canada (a family planning and counseling service) for her invaluable advice for the chapter on fertility and conception prevention;

Gregory White, M.D., medical consultant to La Leche League International and one of the founders of the American College of Home Obstetrics, for his encouraging comments.

And above all, thanks are due to our wonderful God and Savior, who is teaching us how to enjoy more fully the marvelous world He has made.

Permission Credits

Richard Baxter. **The Saints Everlasting Rest.** Ed. by Glenn Hinson. New York. Doubleday. Copyright © 1978.

Constance A. Bean. **Labor and Delivery: An Observer's Diary.** New York. Doubleday. Copyright © 1977 by Constance A. Bean.

Bob Benson. **Come Share the Being.** Nashville. The Benson Company. Copyright © 1974 by Impact Books.

Robert A. Bradley, M.D. **Husband-Coached Childbirth.** New York. Harper & Row. Copyright © 1965, 1974.

Sidney Cornelia Callahan. **Beyond Birth Control: The Christian Experience of Sex.** New York. Sheed & Ward. Copyright © 1968.

Chambers, Oswald. **My Utmost for His Highest.** New York. Dodd, Mead & Co. Copyright © 1935 by Dodd, Mead & Company.

Glenn Clark. **I Will Lift Up Mine Eyes.** New York. Harper & Row. Copyright © 1937.

Eldridge Cleaver. **Soul On Fire.** Waco, TX. Word Books. Copyright © 1978.

James C. Dobson, M.D. **The Strong-Willed Child.** Wheaton, IL. Tyndale House. Copyright © 1978.

Catherine de Hueck Doherty. **The Gospel Without Compromise.** Notre Dame. Ave Maria Press. Copyright © 1976.

_____ **Poustinia.** Notre Dame. Ave Maria Press. Copyright © 1975.

Geraldine Lux Flanagan. **The First Nine Months of Life.** New York. Simon & Schuster. Copyright © 1962.

William J. & Gloria Gaither. "The Family of God." Alexandria, IN. Gaither Music Company. Copyright © 1970 by William J. Gaither.

William H. Hodges, M.D. "International Milk Companies and Breast Feeding." Published in "Insight: A Special Report." Valley Forge. PA. International Ministries: American Baptist Churches in the U.S.A.

John & Sheila Kippley. **The Art of Natural Family Planning.** Cincinnati, OH. The Couple to Couple League. Copyright © 1975, 1979.

Frank Lake, M.D. "A Revolution in Understanding." Published in "Report from the Research Department." 1979. See also **Studies in Constrictive Confusion** Available from Clinical Theology Association, Lingdale, Weston Avenue, Nottingham NG7 4BA, England.

John G. Lake. **The John G. Lake Sermons.** Ed. Gordon Lindsay. Dallas TX. Christ for the Nations. Copyright © 1949, 1978.

C.S. Lewis. **A Grief Observed.** New York. The Seabury Press. Copyright © 1961 by N. W. Clerk.

Francis MacNutt. **The Power to Heal.** Notre Dame. Ave Maria Press. Copyright © 1977.

Marilyn A. Moran. **Birth and the Dialogue of Love.** Leawood, KS. New Nativity Press. Copyright © 1981.

Watchman Nee. **A Table in the Wilderness.** Fort Washington, PA. Christian Literature Crusade. Copyright © 1965. Kingsway Publications LTD, East Sussex, England.

Juan Carlos Ortiz. **Cry of the Human Heart.** Carol Stream, IL. Creation House. Copyright © 1977.

Carl C. Pfeiffer, M.D., Ph.D. **Zinc and Other Micro-Nutrients.** New Canaan, CT. Keats Publishing, Inc. Copyright © 1978 by Carl C. Pfeiffer.

Marion Sousa. **Childbirth at Home.** Englewood Cliffs, NJ. Prentice-Hall. Copyright © 1976 by Marion Sousa.

Leon Joseph Cardinal Suenens. **Your God?** New York. The Seabury Press. Copyright © 1978 by Leon Joseph Cardinal Suenens.

_____ **A New Pentecost.** New York. Seabury Press. Copyright © 1974.

Deborah Tanzer, Ph.D. **Why Natural Childbirth?** Garden City, NY. Doubleday. Copyright © 1972.

Ed Wheat, M.D. and Gaye Wheat. **Intended for Pleasure.** Old Tappan, NJ. Fleming H. Revell Company. Copyright © 1977 by Fleming H. Revell Company.

I would also like to thank the following for permission to quote portions of letters or comments: The Birthplace Newsletter, Gainesville, FL, courtesy of Judith Levy, Ph.D.; Charles and Norma Cushing, Larry and Sharon Douglas, Connie Seekins and Muriel Strand.

Resources

American Academy of Husband-Coached Childbirth. Box 5224, Shermon Oaks, CA 91413.

An organization that certifies teachers in the Bradley method of natural childbirth.

American College of Home Obstetrics. 644 No. Michigan Ave., Suite 610, Chicago, IL 60611.

ACHO collects and publishes data on the safety and advantages of home births, gathering data from member physicians for publication, and helping to overcome the isolation of many home obstetricians.

American College of Nurse-Midwifery. 1000 Vermont Ave. NW, Washington, D.C. 20005.

ACNM is an interdisciplinary health discipline focusing on the childbearing family with respect for human dignity and worth, while emphasizing excellence in preparation for its practitioners and expecting their professional behavior to be in keeping with the high standards of the organization.

Apple Tree Family Life Teaching Series. Box 9883, Fresno, CA 93795.

Dedicated to fostering education in and through local churches on personhood, marriage, sexuality, natural family planning, natural childbirth, breastfeeding, weaning, child nurture and Christian family lifestyles.

Birthing. Box 415, Winona Lake, IN 46590.

A monthly newsletter about childbirth, providing information and books and materials in order to further childbirth goals.

Christian Marriage Encounter. Box 1297, Colorado Springs, CO 80901.

A ministry to married couples and families with week-end retreats and continuing support in couple communication.

Clinical Theology Association. c/o Dr. Frank Lake, Director. Lingdale, Weston Ave., Nottingham, NG7 4BA, England.

A Christian professional organization which sponsors workshops in Basic Personal Growth and Primal Integration. Its growing collection of data on the relevance of the Maternal-Foetal Distress Syndrome offers new dimensions to psychotherapy and pastoral counselling.

Couple to Couple League. Box 11084, Cincinnati, OH 45211.

An interfaith organization offering married couples help with the successful practice of natural family planning, it teaches ecological breastfeeding and the full sympto-thermal method in member groups in many localities.

Family Life Mission, North America. 5733 East 25th St., Tulsa, OK 74114.

A marriage counselling service founded by Walter and Ingrid Trobisch while missionaries in Africa, FLM now sponsors Marriage Seminars throughout the world.

The Federal Monitor, ed. Ann Gray, Drawer 1, McLean, VA 22101.

Published by Maternal and Child Health Legislative Alert

(MCHLA), this organization keeps its members informed about state and federal governmental activities affecting the health of women and children, with a special emphasis on childbearing.

Home Oriented Maternity Experience. 511 New York Ave., Takoma Park, WA, D.C. 20012.

A national organization to support and assist couples who wish to give birth at home, with emphasis on safety.

The Human Life Center. St. John's University, Collegeville, MN 56321.

An international center which helps people of all faiths with programs for marriage preparation, marriage enrichment, birthright counseling, parent effectiveness training, child abuse, death and dying, care of the aged and infirm, sexuality and natural family planning.

Imprints. Box 70625, Seattle, WA 98107.

The review newsletter/catalog of the Birth and Life Bookstore. Lynn Moen, President, was formerly manager of the ICEA bookstore for many years.

International Childbirth Education Association. Box 20048, Minneapolis, MN 55420.

A valuable resource agency for all those who want information concerning childbirth education, the ICEA is a federation of independent childbirth education groups worldwide, sponsoring numerous regional conferences and a biennial convention.

La Leche League International. 9616 Minneapolis Ave., Franklin Park, IL 60131.

Women who want help in breastfeeding will find valuable counsel through the literature and staff of LLLI, which has thousands of local chapters across the United States and in other countries.

Napsac International. Box 267, Marble Hill, MO 63764.

Napsac (InterNational Association of Parents and Professionals for Safe Alternatives in Childbirth) is dedicated to implementing family-centered childbirth programs that meet the needs of families as well as provide the safe aspects of medical science.

The People's Doctor, ed. Dr. Robert Mendelsohn, 664 No. Michigan Ave., Suite 720, Chicago, IL 69611.

A newsletter on medical issues to keep laymen as well as physicians aware of trends in health care.

Read Natural Childbirth Foundation, Inc. 1300 So. Eliseo Drive, Suite 102, Greenbrae, CA 94904.

A non-profit educational organization founded to promote the philosophies and techniques of Dr. Grantly Dick-Read, and to preserve his life work as it relates to childbirth.

Scriptural Counsel, Inc. 130 No. Spring St., Springdale, AR 72764.

Dr. Ed Wheat, Bible-believing family physician and marriage counselor, has developed a unique counseling series on cassette for couples needing information on sex techniques and sex problems in marriage.

Serena. 55 Parkdale, Ottawa, Ontario K1Y 1E5, Canada.

For over 20 years Serena (Service for the Regulation of Natality) has perfected and disseminated natural methods of birth regulation, especially the sympto-thermal method, as a resource for couples in controlling their fertility while deepening their relationship.

Spun, 17 No. Wabash Ave., Suite 603, Chicago, IL, 60602.

The Society for the Protection of the Unborn through Nutrition, founded by Dr. Tom Brewer, demonstrates that restrictive prenatal diets can lead to irreversible brain damage, hyperactivity, learning disorders, premature births and low birth-weight babies, as well as toxemia in the pregnant woman.

The Pennypress, 110023rd Ave. East, Seattle, WA 98112.

Edited by Penny Simkin, The Pennypress has many excellent leaflets, pamphlets and small books on childbirth and related subjects. It is a valuable resource.

Recommended Reading

ALTERNATIVES FOR BIRTH

Brennan, Barbara, CNM and Joan Rattner Heilman. **The Complete Book of Midwifery.** New York: E.P. Dutton, 1977.

This book explains Nurse-Midwifery, and includes a directory of Nurse-Midwifery services in the United States.

Edwards, Margot and Penny Simkin. **Obstetric Tests and Technology. A Consumer's Guide.** Seattle: The Pennypress, 1980.

Pamphlet with invaluable information for childbearing women.

Family-Centered Maternity/Newborn Care in Hospitals. Interprofessional Task Force Secretariat, American College of Obstetrics and Gynecologists, One East Wacker Dr., Suite 2700, Chicago, IL 60601, 1978.

An interdisciplinary position statement which endorses family/centered maternity care and gives specific recommendations. Give a copy to your local hospital.

Fitzgerald, Hermon, Long, Schildroth & Ventra. **Home Oriented Maternity Experience.** Published by H.O.M.E., 511 New York Ave., Takoma Park.

A manual for home birth.

Haire, Doris, **The Pregnant Patient's Bill of Rights—The Pregnant Patient's Responsibilities.** ICEA, Box 20048, Minneapolis 55420.

A pamphlet giving the ACOG statement in support of informed consent and listing a woman's rights and responsibilities in maternity care.

Hathaway, Marjie and Jay Hathaway. **Children at Birth.** New York: Academy, 1978.

A positive report on children's presence at the birth of their siblings, illustrated with over 125 photos.

Hazell, Lester. **Birth Goes Home.** Seattle: Catalyst Publishing, 1974.

A positive report on the increasing demand for home births by intelligent, aware young couples of today, establishing a strong trend.

_____. **Commonsense Childbirth.** New York: Berkeley Publishing Co., 1976.

A complete guide to family-centered natural birth, this book explains how to surround the experience of childbirth with kindness, dignity and joy.

Kitzinger, Sheila. **The Complete Book of Pregnancy & Childbirth.** New York: Alfred Knopf & Random House of Canada Unlimited, Toronto, 1980.

Answers nearly every question an expectant couple might have. Photos, drawings and diagrams are on almost every page. Stresses the importance of gentle birth for the baby as well as the mother.

_____. **The Experience of Childbirth,** 3rd ed. Baltimore: Penguin Books, 1972.

A psychosexual approach to childbirth, with numerous examples from the natural childbirth approach which the author helped develop in England.

Moran, Marilyn. **Birth and the Dialogue of Love.** The New Nativity Press, Box 6223, Leawood, KS 66206, 1980.

An indepth study of childbirth and its role in bringing genuine fulfillment to husband and wife. The conclusion is that birth belongs in the bedroom. Many helpful suggestions for preparing for home birth.

Phillips, Celeste and Joseph Anzalone, M.D. **Fathering: Participation in Labor and Birth.** St. Louis: C.V. Mosby, 1976.

The father's place in labor and delivery, physicians' opinions on the subject and helpful definitions. More than 25 revealing interviews with fathers in Part II.

Simkin, Penny. **Directory of Alternative Birth Services and Consumer Guide.** Published by Napsac, Box 267, Marble Hill, Mo., 1978.

This helpful book provides a list of alternatives birth services across the United States (updated periodically), and offers guidelines on how to judge the quality of the service and its ability to meet the couple's needs.

Sousa, Marion. **Childbirth at Home.** Englewood Cliffs, NJ: Prentice-Hall, 1976.

Issues of home birth and management of complications.

Stewart, David and Lee Stewart. **Compulsory Hospitalization or Freedom of Choice in Childbirth?** Napsac, Box 267, Marble Hill, MO 63764, 1979.

Three volumes, winner of the 1979 Books of the Year Award from the American Journal of Nursing and the American Nurses Association.

_____. **The Five Standards for Safe Childbirth.** Napsac, Box 267, Marble Hill, MO 63764, 1981.

Documents safe childbearing basics: good nutrition, skillful midwifery, natural childbirth, birth at home and breastfeeding.

_____. **Safe Alternatives in Childbirth.** Napsac, Box 267, Marble Hill, MO 63764, 3rd ed. 1978.

Demonstrates that hospitals have never been proven to be the safest place for most mothers to give birth—existing evidence strongly suggests the opposite to be true. Winner of the 1976 Books of the Year Award, American Journal of Nursing.

_____. **21st Century Obstetrics Now!** Napsac, Box 267, Marble Hill, MO 63764, 2nd ed., 1978, 2 vols.

Family-centered hospitals, birthing centers, home birth programs working together

Tanzer, Deborah. **Why Natural Childbirth?** Garden City, NY: Doubleday, 1972.

A psychologist's report on the benefits of natural childbirth to mothers, fathers and babies.

Wallerstein, Edward. **Circumcision: An American Health Fallacy.** New York: Springer, 1980.

Fully documented, it challenges the practice of routine, nonreligious circumcision as not only unnecesary but also potentially harmful.

Walton, Vicki E. **Have it Your Way.** New York: Bantam, 1976.

An overview of pregnancy, labor and postpartum, including alternatives available in the hospital childbirth experience. Excellent diagrams and photos.

White, Gregory. **Emergency Chilbirth.** Police Training Foundation, Franklin Park, IL, 1969.

Basic explanation of procedures for nonhospital deliveries, especially in emergency situations. Simply and clearly presented. An important item if one is planning a home birth.

Young, Diony and Charles Mahan. **Unnecessary Cesareans—Ways to Avoid Them.** ICEA Publications, Box 20048, Minnieapolis, MN 55420.

How to minimize the possibility of a cesarean delivery and increase the potential for optimal outcome should a cesarean become necessary. Fully documented.

BIRTH EDUCATION

Beals, Peg. **Parents' Guide to the Childbearing Year.** ICEA, Box 20048, Minneapolis, MN 55420.

A childbirth education manual for couples and teachers.

Bean, Constance. **Labor and Delivery: An Observer's Diary.** New York: Doubleday, 1977.

Candid reports of births in a variety of settings by an experienced childbirth educator.

Bing, Elisabeth. **Six Practical Lessons for an Easier Childbirth.** New York: Grosset & Dunlap, 1967.

An exposition of the principles and techniques of the Lamaze method of childbirth by a renowned teacher of this method in the United States.

Bradley, Robert, M.D. **Husband-Coached Childbirth.** New York: Harper & Row, 1965, 1974.

A wealth of information for the husband who wants to help his wife adjust comfortably and happily to pregnancy and birth.

Dick-Read, Grantly, M.D. **Childbirth Without Fear,** 4th ed. Revised by Helen Wessel and Harlan Ellis, M.D. New York: Harper and Row, 1972.

This famous classic by the founder of the natural childbirth movement around the world includes the best of his writings from 1933 on, an extensive autobiographical section and 70 photographs from Dr. Ellis' practice. An invaluable addition to every childbirth education library.

_____. **The Practice of Natural Childbirth.** New York: Harper & Row, 1972.

The preparation for childbirth section of **Childbirth Without Fear,** 4th ed.

Gamper, Margaret. **Preparation for the Heir Minded.** Midwest Parentcraft Center, 627 Beaver Rd., Glenview, IL 60025.

A helpful manual based on 25 years as a childbirth educator.

Hartman, Rhondda. **Exercises for True Natural Childbirth.** New York: Harper & Row, 1975.

Simple directions for childbirth preparation from a childbirth educator and mother of five naturally born children.

Noble, Elizabeth. **Essential Exercises for the Childbearing Year.** Boston: Houghton-Mifflin, 1976.

Highly recommended!

Wessel, Helen. **Natural Childbirth and the Family.** Paper edition under the title **The Joy of Natural Childbirth.** Harper & Row, 1963, 1973.

A rare and special blend of Christian faith and medical wisdom.

Young, Joy. **Christian Home Birth.** P.O. Box 33512, Detroit, MI 48232.

Indispensable Scriptural preparation as well as practical natural knowledge for a home birth.

BREASTFEEDING

Applebaum, Richard, M.D. **Abreast of the Times.** New York: Harper & Row, 1973.

Techniques of breastfeeding written in a conversational style by a pedicatrician.

Brewster, Dorothy Patricia. **You Can Breastfeed Your Baby—even in special situations.** Emmaus, PA: Rodale Press, 1979.

Reassuring, specific advice on breastfeeding twins, siblings, premature babies, babies with jaundice, allergies, cleft palate, etc.

Bumgamer, Norma Jane. **Mothering Your Nursing Toddler.** P.O. Box 5064, Norman, OK 73070.

Reassurance and practical help for the mother who breastfeeds her older baby.

Cradeur, Jennifer. **Blessings of the Breasts.** P.O. Box 206, Branch, LA 70516.

Based on Gen. 29:25, this is a Christian viewpoint on breastfeeding.

Hormann, Elizabeth. **Relactation: A Guide to Breastfeeding the Adopted Baby.** 1 Merrill Ave., Belmont, Mass., 1971.

A guide to breastfeeding the adopted baby, or to reestablishing a milk supply.

Jelliffe, D.B. and E.F.P. Jelliffe. **Human Milk in the Modern World. Psychological, Nutritional & Economic Significance.** Fair Lawn, NJ: Oxford University Press, 1978.

Comprehensive account of the psychosocial, nutritional and economic significance of human milk.

Kippley, Sheila. **Breastfeeding and Natural Child Spacing: The Ecology of Natural Mothering.** Baltimore: Penguin Books, 1975.

Covers an extensive survey on the effectiveness of breastfeeding as a means of conception control, as well as the requirement to make it effective for this purpose.

La Leche League. **The Womanly Art of Breastfeeding.** Franklin Park: La Leche League, 1963.

A practical manual by the acknowledged international authorities on breastfeeding.

Lawrence, Ruth A. **Breast-Feeding: A Guide for the Medical Profession.** St. Louis: C. V. Mosby, 1979.

Written by a physician and mother of nine breastfed children, this definitive work is a great asset for the medical profession.

Pryor, Karen. **Nursing Your Baby.** New York: Pocket Books, 1973.

Informative and stimulating, with discussion of how the breasts function and a week-by-week guide.

Raphael, Dana. **The Tender Gift: Breastfeeding.** New York: Schocken Books 1976.

The subtitle, "Mothering the mother—the way to successful breastfeeding" is the theme of this beautiful book, which documents the fact that a mother flourishes when she has supportive care and attention.

FAMILY LIFE

Brazelton, T. Berry, M.D. **On Becoming a Family.** New York: Delacorte (Dell), 1981.

Stresses the importance of interaction with newborns and infants in the early weeks through touch, eye-contact, vocalizing, with the father as well as the mother.

Briggs, Dorothy. **Your Child's Self-Esteem.** Garden City, NY: Doubleday, 1975.

Shows what can be done specifically to build a child's feelings of worth, making it clear that the most effective discipline is not adversary in nature, but constructive and cooperative.

Campbell, Ross, M.D. **How to Really Love Your Child.** Wheaton, IL: Victor Books, 1977.

Dr. Campbell shows how to express love through touch, eye contact, focused attention and loving discipline. Biblical references to support his ideas occur frequently throughout the book.

Dobson, James, M.D. **Dare to Discipline.** Wheaton, IL: Tyndale, 1972.

A Christian psychologist offers urgent advice to parents and teachers.

_____. **Hide or Seek.** Old Tappan, NJ: Fleming H. Revell, 1978.

How to create self-esteem in children and also helping them understand themselves. The idea of "letting a child cry" in some situations is in some disagreement with the theme of the Apple Tree series.

Fraiberg, Selma. **Every Child's Birthright: In Defense of Mothering.** New York: Bantam, 1977.

Especially helpful in evaluating day care standards.

Gresh, Sean. **Becoming a Father: A Handbook for Expectant Fathers.**

Conveys the many options for involvement and shares from his own experience as an expectant and new father.

Hymes, James L., Jr. **The Child Under Six.** Englewood Cliffs, NJ: Prentice-Hall, 1963.

Helps parents see things from the child's perspective. Christians will want to be alert to humanist philosophy as a basis for some of the author's recommendations and make their own decisions from the Christian perspective.

Iatesta, Robert. **Fathers: A Fresh Start for the Christian Family.** Ann Arbor: Servant Books, 1980.

Things will change when the father hears God's call and responds with decision and action. A blend of practical and spiritual advice. Robert Iatesta is the father of six children.

Ilg, Frances L. and Louise B. Ames. **Child Behavior.** Cranberry, NJ: Barnes and Noble, 1972.

Covers child behavior from birth to age 10. Useful guide to child development if norms are not taken too literally.

Johnson, Lois. **Gift in My Arms.** Minneapolis: Augsburg, 1977.

Twenty essays on various problems and feelings faced by a new mother. Deeply rooted in the biblical perspective on these situations.

Klaus, Marshall and John H. Kennell. **Maternal-Infant Bonding. The Impact of Early Separation or Loss on Family Development.** St. Louis: C. V. Mosby, 1976.

This valuable book explores the earliest physical and sensory relationship an infant develops with his parents, and the factors that enhance or inhibit this relationship.

LaShan, Eda J. **The Conspiracy Against Childhood.** New York: Atheneum, 1967.
   Deals with the efforts of some to educate very young children beyond their emotional capacity. Valuable for parents contemplating preschool education for their child.

Newton, Niles. **The Family Book of Child Care.** New York: Harper & Row, 1957.
   This book on baby and child care from pregnancy on contains the soundest findings of modern medicine with the good-humored wisdom of an experienced parent.

Noble, Elizabeth **Having Twins, A Parent's Guide to Pregnancy, Birth and Early Parenthood.** Boston: Houghton-Mifflin, 1980.
   Prenatal care, parenting tips, and fascinating facts dealing with multiple birth.

Ribble, Margaret. **The Rights of Infants.** New York: New American Library, 1973.
   First published in 1945, this readable classic shows the vital part that mothering plays in a baby's normal development.

Stewart, David. **Fathering and a Career.** Napsac, Box 267, Marble Hill, MO 64764.
   Gives perspective on the demands of career advancement and the fathering role.

Szasz, Suzanne, **The Unspoken Language of Children.** New York: Norton, 1980.
   A photo-essay on the feelings of children.

Thevenin, Tine. **The Family Bed: An age-old concept in child rearing.** Box 16004, Minneapolis, MN 55416.
   Advocates co-family sleeping (either children with their parents or with other siblings) as a way to solve bed and night time problems with young children, create a closer bond within the family, and give children a greater sense of security.

Young, Diony. **Bonding: How Parents Become Attached to their Baby.** ICEA, Box 20048, Minneapolis, MN 55420, 1978.
   Explanation of bonding behavior, factors influencing bonding, role of the father and siblings.

FERTILITY

Billings, John. **Natural Family Planning: The Ovulation Method.** Collegeville, MN: The Liturgical Press, 1973.
   Describes the mucus only approach to fertility awareness.

Halverson, Kaye with Karen Hess. **The Wedded Unmother.** Minneapolis: Augsburg, 1980.
   The personal story of a woman who struggles to understand and accept infertility.

Kippley, John and Sheila Kippley. **The Art of Natural Family Planning,** 2nd ed. Couple to Couple League, Box 11084, Columbus, OH 45211, 1979.

The most complete text available on natural family planning. The first part of the book explains "why," the second part the "how" of the sympto-thermal method of natural family planning.

Kippley, John. **Birth Control and the Marriage Covenant.** Collegeville, MN: The Liturgical Press, 1976.

One of the very few books written in the immediate post-Humanae Vitae years which supports the encyclical from a theological point of view, it develops the concept that marital coitus is meant to be a renewal of the marriage covenant.

Kippley, Sheila. **Breastfeeding and Natural Child Spacing: The Ecology of Natural Mothering.** New York: Harper & Row, 1975.

Covers an extensive survey on the effectiveness of breastfeeding as a means of conception control, as well as the requirements to make it effective.

Menning, Barbara Eck. **Infertility, A Guide for the Childless Couple.** Englewood Cliffs, NJ: Prentice-Hall, 1977.

Covering both the medical and psychosocial aspects of this problem, it is particularly sensitive to the emotional impact of infertility.

Parenteau-Carreau, Suzanne, M.D. **Love and Life. Fertility and Conception Prevention,** 2nd ed. Serena Canada, 55 Parkdale, Ottawa, Ontario K1Y 1E5, 1975.

Written by a medical consultant to Serena Canada since 1962, this pamphlet provides a clear, fully illustrated description of the processes governing fertility, to enable couples to make wise choices.

Pharand-Lapointe, Marielle, M.D. & F. Kavanagh-Jazrawy. **Planning Your Family the S-T Way,** 2nd ed. Serena Canada, 55 Parkdale, Ottawa, Ontario K1y 1E5, 1981.

An introduction to the sympto-thermal method of natural family planning, providing an overview of the method and its advantages, and sample charting procedures.

Roetzer, Elizabeth. **Family Planning the Natural Way.** Old Tappan, NJ: Revell, 1981.

A most helpful book on natural family planning with specific, easy to understand instructions.

Suenens, Cardinal Leo Joseph. **Love and Control.** Westminster, MD: The Newman Press, 1967.

Explains the teachings of the Catholic church on marriage, sexuality, regulations of births and periodic abstinence.

Trobisch, Ingrid. **An Experience of Love: Understanding Natural Family Planning.** Old Tappan, NJ: Revell, 1981.

The well-loved author of **The Joy of Being a Woman** and other Trobisch books expands on the philosophy of natural family planning.

HEALTH AND NUTRITION

Apgar, Virginia, M.D. and Joan Beck. **Is My Baby All Right?** New York: Trident Press, 1972.

The famous Apgar score for newborns is used in almost all hospitals for assessing his or her state at birth on a scale of 1 to 10. The Apgar score is a prime indicator of the baby's future development.

Brewer, Thomas H., M.D. **Metabolic Toxemia of Late Pregnancy: A Disease of Malnutrition.** Springfield, IL: Charles C. Thomas, 1966.

A medical treatise on metabolic toxemia with a history of cases and treatment in a long-range study of clinical patients.

Brewer, Gail Sforza with Thomas Brewer, M.D. **What Every Pregnant Woman Should Know: The Truth about Diets and Drugs in Pregnancy.** New York: Random House, 1977.

Importance of good nutrition during pregnancy. Relation of toxemia and birth defects to malnutrition.

Gazella, Jaqueline Gibson. **Nutrition for the Childbearing Year.** Wayzata, MN: Woodland, 1979.

Reasons for a good prenatal diet and the importance of breastfeeding, includes a helpful chapter on the selection and preparation of foods.

Goldbeck, Nikki and David Goldbeck. **Supermarket Handbook: Access to Whole Foods.** New York: Signet, 1973.

A guide to good nutrition for the whole family.

Howell, Mary, M.D. **Healing at Home.** Boston: Beacon, 1979.

A pediatrician's guide to more health and less doctoring for your children.

Jacobson, Edmund, M.D. **You Must Relax.** New York: McGraw Hill, 1937, 1962.

This priceless book offers advice for those with heart ailments, high blood pressure, stomach distresses, and gives specific methods for relieving tension and relaxing the mind without drugs, medicines, hypnosis or any other form of "mind" manipulation. Invaluable as an aid to learning relaxation for childbirth and breastfeeding.

Johnson, Roberta, ed. **Mother's in the Kitchen.** Franklin Park, IL: La Leche League, 1971.

Collection of recipes stressing good nutrition, economy and ease of preparation.

Macnutt, Francis. **Healing.** New York: Bantam, 1974.

A Scripturally sound, balanced approach to prayer for healing, this is one of the finest books on the subject by a gifted Christian scholar.

_____. **The Power to Heal.** Notre Dame: Ave Maria Press, 1977. Sequel to **Healing.** Excellent insights into supernatural healing.

Mendelsohn, Robert, M.D. **Confessions of a Medical Heretic.** Chicago: Contemporary Books, 1979.

A critique of many established medical practices by a famous physician.

Pfeiffer, Carl, M.D. **Zinc and Other Micro-Nutrients.** New Canaan, CT: Keats Publishing, 1978.

A helpful explanation of the need for minerals in the diet, and sound advice for balanced nutrition.

INNER HEALTH

Clark, Glenn. **I Will Lift Up Mine Eyes.** New York: Harper & Row, 1937.

This creative, inspiring little classic should be in the hands of every person who wants to achieve his or her high goals.

Daily, Starr. **Well-Springs of Immortality.** St. Paul: Macalaster Park, 1941.

Seven meditations which lead to a conviction of immortality and give a meditational experience of eternal life, by a saintly Christian.

Doherty, Catherine de Hueck. **The Gospel Without Compromise.** Notre Dame: Ave Maria Press, 1976.

Living for others as Jesus commanded is the key to joy.

_____. **Poustinia.** Notre Dame: Ave Maria Press, 1974.

Reveals new ways of growing in the Christian life by one who has the gift of a great and joyous faith and of making life an adventure, a pilgrimage of love.

Frankl, Victor. **Man's Search for Meaning.** New York: Washington Square Press, 1963.

A survivor of the concentration camps of World War II shows how suffering can help in the discovery of the meaning of life.

Fromm, Eric. **The Art of Loving.** New York: Harper & Row, 1956.

A classic in the literature, demonstrates that love is a commitment revealed in actions, and does not vacilate with circumstances as emotional attachments may.

Lake, Frank, M.D. **Clinical Theology.** London: Dartman, Longman & Todd, Ltd., 1966.

A masterful study of the importance of theology and psychology working together for emotional health. As a Christian, Dr. Lake brings his profound spiritual insights into his practice as a psychiatrist.

Missildine, W. Hugh. **Your Inner Child of the Past.** New York: Simon & Schuster, 1963.

Describes how childhood experiences affect one's adult responses, an insight that helps cope with situations in more mature and creative ways.

Montagu, Ashley. **Touching, the Human Significance of the Skin.** New York: Columbia University, 1971.

An invaluable study of the physical and psychological importance of the skin. Touching deprivation can lead to both physical and emotional disorders.

Moseley, J. Rufus. **Perfect Everything,** rev. ed. St. Paul: Macalaster Park, 1949, 1952.

Reveals that Jesus is "Perfect Everything," perfect light, perfect birth, perfect baptism, perfect love, perfect health and healing, perfect triumph. A masterpiece!

Ortiz, Carlos, **The Cry of the Human Heart.** Carol Stream, IL: Creation House, 1977.

This innovative pastor from South America stresses the need to apply the command of Jesus to "love one another." The cry of every human heart is to be loved.

Sanford, Agnes. **Behold Your God.** St. Paul: Macalaster Park, 1958.

A masterful study of how to pray effectively and to increase one's faith in order to help and heal the sick and troubled, and bring our Lord's kingdom on earth.

_____. **The Healing Gifts of the Spirit.** New York: Trumpet/J.B. Lippincott, 1966, 1976.

Mrs. Sanford coined the phrase "inner healing" and has taught thousands of clergy and others how to apply it, from her own personal experiences since the early 1950's. This is still the best book on the subject.

Tournier, Paul, M.D. **The Person Reborn.** New York: Harper & Row, 1966.

One of the best of Dr. Tournier's numerous books which integrate modern psychology and biblical faith, the many case histories in this remarkable book show how it is possible for each person to find happiness and fulfillment, to be, in the biblical sense, truly reborn.

IN UTERO

Flanagan, Geraldine Lux. **The First Nine Months of Life.** New York: Simon & Schuster, 1962.

Beautifully illustrated book on the baby's development from conception to birth.

Gots, Ronald and Barbara Gots. **Caring for Your Unborn Child.** New York: Bantam, 1979.

Effect of nutrition, drugs, infections and environment on the unborn child.

Hanes, Mari. **The Child Within.** Wheaton, IL: Tyndale, 1979.

This is a "workbook" for the pregnant woman, providing much spiritual insight and growth for the woman who puts forth the effort to complete it.

Lake, Frank, M.D. **Studies in Constrictive Confusion.** Published by CTA, Lingdale, Weston Ave., Nottingham NG7 4BA, England, 1980.

An invaluable, pioneering study of the influence of maternal emotions on the fetus, with extensive illustrations and diagrams of the occurrence of "Umbilical Affect," positive and negative, its manifestations and fetal reactions.

Macaulay, Susan Schaeffer. **Something Beautiful from God.** Westchester, IL: Cornerstone Books, 1981.

The miracle of life before birth simply and beautifully told in words and full color in-the-womb photos. Ideal as a read-aloud book for children.

Miles, Judith. **Journey from an Obscure Place.** Minneapolis: Dimension Books, 1978.

Written as if by an unborn child, this book contains fascinating insights into the physiological development of the baby and convincing arguments against abortion.

Montague, Ashley. **Life Before Birth.** New York: New American Library, 1964, rev. 1977.

Ways a mother can affect the physical and emotional development of her child before birth.

Nilsson, Lennart. **A Child is Born: The Drama of Life Before Birth.** New York: Dell, rev. ed. 1977.

Human reproduction from conception to birth with outstanding photographs. It is not necessary to read the text to enjoy the book—the pictures and captions alone are worthwhile.

LONELINESS AND LOSS

Bowlby, John, M.D. **Attachment and Loss.** 2 vols. New York: Basic Books, 1969, 1973.

One of the first physicians to use the phrase "maternal deprivation," Dr. Bowlby documents the importance of mother/infant closeness and breastfeeding.

Conway, Sally. **You and Your Husband's Mid-Life Crisis.** Elgin, IL: David C. Cook, 1980.

A Christian wife tells how wives can effectively cope with the tremendous upheaval that sometimes occurs when their husbands reach midlife.

Conway, Tim. **Men in Mid-Life Crisis.** Elgin, IL: David C. Cook, 1978.

It is common knowledge that women may have difficulties in midlife, but the fact that men also often suffer a midlife crisis has been kept in a dark closet. At last the problem can be faced openly, with perspectives helpful not only to the man suffering the crisis, but to all those around him who are affected by it.

Decker, Beatrice. **After the Flowers Have Gone.** Grand Rapids: Zondervan, 1973.

Tells how God led her through her own grief to found the fellowship called THEOS.

Dunker, Marilee Pierce. **Man of Vision—Woman of Prayer.** Nashville: Thomas Nelson, 1980.

The daughter of Bob Pierce, founder of World Vision and his wife Lorraine, Mrs. Dunker not only relates the tremendous achievements of her famous father but candidly discusses the often traumatic relationship of her parents.

Esses, Betty Lee. **If I Can, You Can.** Monroeville, PA: Whitaker House, 1974.

The wife of a famous evangelist tells of their trying marriage before Jesus saved her husband and the marriage. She also shares how God helped them overcome the tragic loss of their two year old.

Gauchat, Dorothy. **All God's Children.** New York: Hawthorn, 1972.

This compassionate book about exceptional children and their many problems is an affirmation of all human life.

Haggai, John Edmund. **My Son Johnny.** Wheaton, IL: Tyndale, 1978.

Story of a terribly brain-damaged baby whose mother poured her life into caring for him until his death at age 25, John Haggai is convinced that from the prison of an inadequate body, his son interceded powerfully for his ministry.

Kaufman, Barry Neil. **Son Rise.** New York: Harper & Row, 1976.

Moving story of the persistence of a dedicated couple in reaching out to their autistic child, heedless of the negative advice given by medical authorities.

Klaus, Marshall H. and John H. Kennell. **Maternal-Infant Bonding: The Impact of Early Separation or Loss on Family Development.** St. Louis: C.V. Mosby, 1976.

Demonstrates the importance of early infant-parent interaction. Also suggests loving care of parents of sick, premature, malformed infants or of infants who die.

Lewis, C.S. **A Grief Observed.** New York: Seabury Press, 1961.

A moving personal journal written after the death of his wife from cancer.

Marshall, Catherine. **To Live Again.** Old Tappan, NJ: Revell, 1972.

The grief experienced over the death of her husband Peter Marshall opened up a whole new dimension of life for Catherine Marshall, who became a famous author.

Phillips, Carolyn. **Michelle.** Ventura, CA: Regal Books, 1980.

Story of an eight year old whose leg was amputated due to a malignant tumor, who faced the reality of death and accepted the loss of her leg and eighteen months of chemotherapy with awesome courage.

Pizer, Hank & Christine O'Brien Palisnki. **Coping With A Miscarriage.** New York: Houghton-Mifflin, 1981.

Clear, reassuring explanation of the causes, process and treatment of miscarriage, with guidelines for choosing a doctor and assessing proposed methods of treatment.

Richards, Larry and Paul Johnson, M.D. **Death and the Caring Community: Ministering to the Terminally Ill.** Portland. Multnomah Press, 1980.

Richard's unique skill as an educator combines with Johnson's background both as physician and cancer patient to teach us how to minister effectively to life-threatened individuals and their families.

Sarnoff-Schiff, Harriet. **The Bereaved Parent.** New York: Penguin, 1977.

A practical and reassuring book on how to cope with the death of a child and how to rebuild the lives of the survivors.

Smith, Harriet Whitall. **God of All Comfort.** Chicago, Moody Press.

This little book, along with **The Christian's Secret of a Happy Life,** has survived for a century because of its timely solutions to any trouble.

Timmons, Tim. **Loneliness is Not a Disease.** Eugene, OR: Harvest House, 1981.

An experienced family life counsellor and pastor opens the way for the healing of hurts and relationships. Written with honesty and humor.

Van Auken, Sheldon. **A Severe Mercy.** New York: Harper & Row, 1977.

The story of his courtship, marriage and subsequent death of his wife to cancer, and how her faith brought him to Christ.

MARRIAGE

Demarest, Donald. **Marriage Encounter.** St. Paul, MN: Carillon Books, 1977.

Explains the step-by-step methods used in marriage encounter groups to foster effective communication between husband and wife.

Dobson, James, M.D. **What Wives Wish Their Husbands Knew About Women.** Wheaton, IL: Tyndale, 1975.

Includes an important section on hormonal changes during menopause.

Gallagher, Charles, S.J. **The Marriage Encounter.** New York: Doubleday, 1975, Bantam, 1978.

A priest-counsellor in numerous marriage encounter weekends offers valuable insights into the effectiveness of the program.

Landorf, Joyce. **Tough and Tender.** Old Tappan, NJ. Fleming H. Revell, 1976.

A sensitive portrayal of the husband and wife roles in marriage.

Small, Dwight. **Marriage an Equal Partnership.** Grand Rapids: Baker Book House, 1980.

Equal partnership in marriage is affirmed in the context of mutual servanthood in obedience to Ephesians 5:21-23.

Suenens, Cardinal Leo Joseph. **Love and Control.** Westminster, MD: The Newman Press, 1967.

Explains the teachings of the Catholic church on marriage, sexuality regulation of births and periodic abstinence.

Timmons, Tim. **Maximum Marriage.** Old Tappan, NJ: Revel, 1976.

Practical advice in resolving conflict and establishing desirable attitudes.

Trobisch, Walter. **I Married You.** New York: Harper & Row, 1971.

Profound insights on the husband/wife relationship by the founder of Family Life Mission, he includes experiences he and his wife Ingrid have shared in maturing together.

PERSONHOOD

Booth, Catherine. **Female Ministry: Women's Right to Preach the Gospel.** New York: Salvation Army, 1975.

First published in 1859, shows that Paul's major theme is unity in Christ which destroys all barriers between Christians. Wife is subject to husband by divine order but this is no barrier to public ministry.

Bushnell, Katherine. **God's Word to Women.** Privately reprinted by Ray B. Munson, Box 53, No. Collins, NY 14111.

A definite study of women's role from Genesis to Revelation in a step-by-step exposition by a Greek scholar in the last century. Most exhaustive study ever published.

Cardozo, Arlene Rossen. **Woman at Home.** New York: Jove Publications, 1976.

Contains a good discussion on why it is all right to be a homemaker, offering many suggestions on ways to make staying at home challenging and fulfilling.

Clark, Stephen B. **Man and Woman in Christ.** Ann Arbor: Servant Publications, 1980.

The roles of men and women in the light of Scripture and the social sciences, Clark maintains that both opponents and advocates of change in the roles of men and women seldom understand the usefulness social roles have been in human society.

Derstine, Gerald. **Woman's Place in the Church.** Gospel Publications, Bradenton, TX 33505, 1977.

This Mennonite preacher shows that Scripture teaches no limit to the public ministry of any woman led of the Holy Spirit who is living in divine order (i.e., in harmony with) her husband and the leaders of her congregation.

Gundry, Patricia. **Woman Be Free.** Grand Rapids: Zondervan, 1977.

Scholarly research from New Testament times through the early church fathers to the present time yields some surprises, showing how the position of women has fallen in the course of history since the early church.

Mollenkott, Virginia. **Women, Men and the Bible.** Nashville: Abingdon, 1977.

A theologically oriented study of the roles of men and women, with conclusions documented from Scripture.

Penn-Lewis, Jessie. **The Magna Charta of Women.** Minneapolis: Bethany Fellowship, 1975.

First published in 1919, this is a summary of Katherine Bushnell's earlier massive collection of Bible study essays on women in Scripture.

Scanzoni, Letha & Nancy Hardesty. **All We're Meant to Be.** Waco, TX: Word, 1974.

Theological skill is combined with knowledge of the social sciences to broaden contemporary discussion of women's roles.

Troutt, Margaret. **The General Was a Lady.** Nashville: Holman, 1980.

The story of Evangeline Booth, whose father founded the Salvation Army. Evangeline was the seventh child, becoming one of the most dynamic and effective leaders the Salvation Army has ever known.

Williams, Don. **The Apostle Paul and Women in the Church.** Ventura: Gospel Light, 1977.

Summarizes the content and argument of each of the Pauline epistles, and within that established context concludes that Paul's real view of women emerges apart from contemporary polemical considerations.

Yoder, Elizabeth and Perry Yoder. **New Men, New Roles.** Newton Campus: Faith & Life Press, 1977.

Men and women are urged to be mutually submissive, teachable and servants of one another. The questions and exercises make this a fine book for small groups.

SEXUALITY

Callahan, Sidney Cornelia. **Beyond Birth Control: The Christian Experience of Sex.** New York: Sheed & Ward, 1968.

Emphasizes the beauty of the marriage relationships in all its aspects, as a symbol of the love and unity of the body of Christ.

Hollender, Marc H. "Women's Wish to be Held: Sexual and Nonsexual Aspects," **Medical Aspects of Human Sexuality,** Oct. 1971.

Demonstrates that in some women the desire to be held and cuddled is the major sexual aim and not just foreplay.

Newton, Niles. **Maternal Emotions.** New York: Hoeber Medical Division, Harper & Row, 1955.

A classic study of women's feelings toward aspects of their sexuality, and their reactions to medical intervention.

Scully, Diana. **Men Who Control Women's Health: The Miseducation of Obstetrical-Gynecologists.** Boston: Houghton-Mifflin, 1980.

The author, a sociologist, spent three years scrutinizing two hospital training programs specializing in obstetrics and gynecology. She questions the methodology of the resident's training, which largely ignores education of surgical skills, sexuality and psychology but stresses the acquiring of surgical skills, not always in the woman's best interests.

Trobisch, Ingrid. **The Joy of Being a Woman, and What a Man Can Do.** New York: Harper & Row, 1975.

Discusses the major realms of a woman's experience, sexual response, fertility and conception control, pregnancy, birth, breastfeeding, menopause and maturity written from a Christian viewpoint.

Trobisch, Walter, **I Loved a Girl.** New York: Harper & Row, 1963.

What began as a correspondence between an African young man and his pastor (Walter Trobisch) has become a classic, translated into numerous languages.

Wallerstein, Edward. **Circumcision: An American Health Fallacy.** New York: Springer Pub., 1980.

Fully documented, challenges the practice of routine, non-religious circumcision as not only unnecessary but also potentially harmful.

Wheat, Ed. M.D. and Gaye Wheat. **Intended for Pleasure.** Old Tappan, NJ: Revell, 1977.

An illustrated book on sex technique and sexual fulfillment in marriage written by a Christian family physician and his wife.

Wheat, Ed. M.D. **Love-Life for Every Married Couple.** Grand Rapids: Zondervan, 1980.

Sequel to **Intended for Pleasure.**

Index

Abel, 100
Abraham, 3, 19, 39, 41, 100, 106, 144, 206
Abortion, abortifacients, 84, 85, 93, 94, 95, 265
Abstinence, 85, 92, 93
Adam, 9, 11, 12, 13, 14, 28, 43, 48, 67, 100, 284
Adam, adamah, 7, 13, 100, 206, 281
Adams, Sharyl, 289
Adelphos, 24
Adrenalin, 164
Androgen, 10
African parable, 69
Aner, 48, 113
Anesthesia (see Medications)
Angels, 8, 18, 158, 218,
fallen, 109
Anna, 27
Apple Tree, ix, x, 50, 66
Astrology, 176-7
Augustine, St., 23
Bed, co-family sleeping, 204, 212, 224, 272
Billings method, 91
Birth centers, birthing rooms, 173 ff.
Bonding, 59, 172, 215ff.
Bradley, Robert A., 65, 143, 294
Brain-waves, 136
Braxton-Hicks, 148, 156
Breastfeeding, 206ff, 224
Breast milk, 209
Breath, 8, 119
during labor, 120-124, 149, 163
during birth, 124, 158
and spiritism, 180
Breech, 170, 194
Brephos, 107
Brewer, Tom, 126
Bride, 11, 12, 39, 52, 250
of Christ, 11-14, 25, 29, 40, 43, 284

Brother, 23, 141, 240, 275
God as, 5
Browning, Elizabeth Barrett, 256
Caesar, Julius, 176
Cain, 99, 111
Catholic, 47, 94, 253
Cervix
identifying, 53
changes during fertility, 84, 90
during childbirth, 150, 157
Cesarean delivery, 9, 162, 164, 168-170, 179
Charis, charisma, 276ff
Childbirth, 111, 131, 143, 178
Children
at birth, 189
of Israel, 3
Christ (Messiah, Anointed One), 11, 26, 28, 33, 100, 284
Chul, 6
Church, 11, 13, 14, 25, 41, 62, 139, 209, 271ff., 284
Clark, Glen, 29
Coitus, 52, 58-60, 131, 157, 169, 224
Colostrum, 206
Community of believers, 33, 276ff., 282
Conception, 50, 83, 104
Conceptus *(see also* fetus), 104, 106, 140ff.
Condom, 87, 94
Contraception, 84-87
Creator, 6, 9, 12, 17, 128, 147, 267
Cross, 13, 102, 175, 276
Curse of Eve, 100
Daniel, 28
David, 20, 71
Daughter, 6, 25, 270
Death, 8, 13, 252ff.
Demons, 109, 175, 181
Derstine, Gerald, 29
Diaphragm, 87, 94

Dick-Read, Grantly, 122, 127, 135, 194, 294
Diethylstilbestrol (DES), 94
Discipline, 229ff., 233
Distraction, 154, 165-6
Doherty, Catherine, 48, 143
Dostoevsky, 217
Dragon, 100, 176, 181
Earth, 6, 115, 282
Eden, ix, 68, 284
Ejaculation, 56ff.
Elohim, 5, 6, 7
Enema, 171
Energy field, energy blocks, 176
Episiotomy, 158, 168-9, 179, 190, 224
Estrogen, 10, 87
Eternal life, 13, 282ff.
Etzev, 112
Eucharist, 175ff.
Eve, 11-14, 21, 28, 48, 67, 99, 111-113, 283-4
Exercises for childbirth, 128ff.
Eye-to-eye contact, 10, 60, 81, 201, 226, 235, 249
Ezer, 9, 15
Fallopean tubes, 83, 85
Family, 5, 9, 19, 20, 214, 240, 282
Father, 4, 108, 215
  God as, 5, 8, 14, 16, 111, 191, 270
Fertility cycle, 89-91
Fetus (embryo), 110-112, 140-142
Flanagan, Geraldine, 143
Fornication, 35
Frogs, 176
Garden, x, 8, 14, 68, 114, 284
Genes, 140, 141
Grace, 33, 45, 47, 276ff.
Grandparent, 42, 104, 107, 239, 241, 267, 274
Grief, 251ff.
Gune, 48, 113
Halloween, 181
Havah (chavah), 13, 21

Healing, 60, 102
  of memories, 110, 258-265
Heaven, 100, 282
Holistic,, 176
Holy Spirit (*see* Spirit)
Home birth, vii, x, 174, 182ff., 190, 196
Homosexuality, 35, 48
Hormones, 157, 225
  androgen, 10
  estrogen, 10, 87
  oxytocin, 157, 187
  progesterone, 89
Huldah, 27
Hupotasso, 49
Husband, 33, 37, 40, 60, 113, 128, 220
  and childbirth, 151, 157, 186-7
  God as, 5, 73, 151
Husbandman, 8, 43, 186
Hymen, 52, 53
Hypnotism, 166, 175, 179
Hyperventilation, 124
Iatrogenic, 164
Induction of labor, 157
Infertility, 87, 111, 118
Intrauterine device, 84, 85
Ish, isshah 10
Israel (see Jews, Jewish)
Jacobson, Edmund, 135, 143
Jehovah, 3, 4, 5, 14, 24, 27, 110, 112
Jesus, 3, 8, 13, 14, 18, 21, 206, 227, 258, 284
Jerusalem, 24, 25, 39, 40
Jews, Jewish, 24, 94, 100, 112, 150, 157, 268
Johnson, G.L., 289
Joseph, 28, 108, 199, 218
Judah, 144, 194
Karate, 180
Karma, 176
Kegel, Arnold, 54, 130
Kippley, John and Sheila, 95ff.
Labor, 16, 144, 148, 151, 157, 168

Lake, Frank, 112
Lapointe (Pharand-Lapointe), Marielle, 290
Lay midwives, 174
Let-down reflex, 151, 188
Lewis, C.S., 37
Life-line, 48, 106, 231
Lilith, 181
Mantra, 180
Marriage, 18, 33, 36, 62, 66, 79, 283
Martin, Francis, 14
Mary, 13, 14, 101, 107, 108, 112, 153, 199, 218, 258
Medication for birth, 91, 156, 165, 168, 171, 178
Memory, 75, 145, 156, 169, 177 258ff.
Messiah, 13, 100, 107
Midwifery, 180ff.
Miscarriage, 104, 111, 118, 251-2
Monitor (fetal), 168, 172
Montagu, Ashley, 65
Moran, Marilyn, 143
Morbidity and mortality, 195
Moses, 46, 102, 216
Mother, 11, 24, 221ff.
  Church as, 11
  God as, 5, 8, 211-2
  Israel as, 24
Mucus sign, 89-91, 146
Naming, 205ff.
Natural family planning, 88, 103
Nee, Watchman, 15
Nesper, Kathy, 289
Nirvana, 176
Noble, Elizabeth, 158
Nurse-midwifery, 173, 180
Nutrition, 115ff.
Occult, 177, 181
Orgasm,
  female, 55, 58
  male, 56, 57
  birth orgasm, 157, 187
Ovaries, 84
Ovum, 83, 141

Ovulation, 85, 87, 102
Owls, 176, 181
Oxygen, 120, 151, 168
Oxytocin (the "love" hormone), 58, 157, 187
Pain, 161
  and labor, 151, 162-164, 178
Paradise lost, 67
Paul, 11, 18, 28, 30, 31, 107
Pelvic rock, 129ff.
Penis, 50, 52, 56
Perineum, 53, 155, 158
Person, God as, 3, 11, 12
Personhood, 42, 47, 222
Peter, 17, 46, 259
Pfeiffer, Carl, 123, 126, 143
Pettit, Hermon, 32, 76
Philadelphia, 24
Pill: birth control, 84-5, 87-8
Pitocin, 171
Placenta, 202
Pleura, 11
Posterior, 178, 192
Priest/father, 108, 200, 219
Priest/husband, 11, 12
Priscilla, 27
Privacy, 62, 188-9
Progesterone, 89
Protestants, 94, 253
Psychic experiences, 175
Pubococcygeus muscle, 54
Read, *see* Dick-Read
Rebecca, 39, 51, 94, 111
Reincarnation, 126, 176
Relaxation, 126, 134ff.
Religion, false, 174
Sanford, Agnes, 262, 269
Sapphira, 46
Sarah, 24, 39, 41, 106, 144, 206, 213
Satan, 13, 46, 100-102, 174-5
Savior, 12, 13, 17, 21, 43, 100, 283
Semen, 51, 90
Serpent, 13, 99-101, 176
Septuagint, 11- 51

"Singles," 274-5
Sister, 24, 141, 275
  God as, 5
Shaving, 168, 171
Skin-to-skin (*see* Touching)
Soma, 62, 63
Snakes, 176
Spermatozoa, 83, 141, 142
Spirit, 8, 11, 18, 103-105
Spirit, Holy, 4, 6, 8, 11, 16, 18, 25, 27, 29, 108, 109, 138, 139, 176, 192, 212, 227, 259, 270
Spiritism, spiritualism, 175-177, 184
Suenens, Cardinal, 14
Tanzer, Deborah, 186, 196
Taurine, 210
Tension, 134ff.
Toddler Nursing, 246-8, 272
Toffler, Alvin, 223-228
Timothy, 107
Touch, 59, 157, 188, 200 208, 215, 241-2
Transcendental meditation, 180
Transition, 153-158
Trinity, 5, 12, 13, 14, 33
Trobisch, Ingrid 79

Tsela, 9, 11
Unity, 5, 33, 43, 259, 281
Uterus, 54, 57, 183, *(see also* Womb)
Vagina, 50, 94, 155
Vasectomy, 86, 94
Vegetarian, 126, 176
Vulva, 53
Weaning, 244ff.
Wessel, Walter, ix, 289
Wheat, Ed, 56, 65, 290
Whiskey nipple, 172
White, Gregory, 290
Wholistic, 176
Wife, 33, 37, 42, 43, 61, 113, 128,
  God as, 5, 27
Wilke, Margaret, 289,
Williams, Don, 29
Witches, 175, 181,
Working mothers, 219, 221, 223
Womb, 6, 54, 47, 99, 103, 104, 140, 150, 183, 199
Yalad, 6
Zinc, 126, 132, 143
Zion, 25, 39,

About the Author

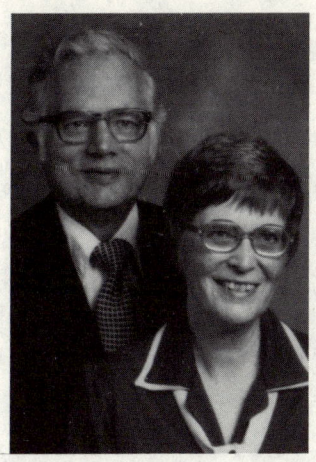

The author and her husband

Helen Wessel is the mother of six children and an ever increasing number of grandchildren. She married Walter Wessel, Ph.D., in 1945, a New Testament scholar who is currently teaching at Bethel Seminary West in San Diego.

A graduate of Sioux Falls College with a major in English literature, she also studied Greek and Hebrew in Bible school and seminary, as well as sociology and psychology in the graduate school of the University of Minnesota.

Mrs. Wessel has been actively involved in natural childbirth education since the publication of her first book in 1963, **Natural Childbirth and the Christian Family.** She is past president of the International Childbirth Education Association and one of the founders of the La Leche League and CEA of Minneapolis/St. Paul.

She is founder and president of Bookmates International, Inc., a non-profit organization dedicated to stimulating the circulation of Christian and family life books to the disadvantaged people of the world.

Childbirth in Emergency

Before birth

1. Stay calm and pray.

   Ask the God of all creation to help you know instinctively what to do.

2. Wash your hands.

   If there is time, wash your hands in soap and water thoroughly and dry on a clean towel.

3. Lean against cushions or a wall, in a semisitting position on clean towels or newspapers.

   Do not lie down on your back!

4. Bear down **gently**.

   If there is a strong urge to push, grasp your knees, lean forward and bear down gently, keeping your mouth open and breathing as normally as possible without holding your breath.

5. **Stop pushing** when baby's head causes a burning, stretching sensation.

   Let baby's head and shoulders be born by uterine contraction alone, to help keep your perineum from tearing.

During birth

6. Support baby's head in your hands as he is born.

   Also support his body as the shoulders emerge. Baby will rotate as he is born so that he will be facing you. Draw him up toward you over the pubic bone as he emerges.

7. Remove the membranes at once from the baby's face.

   Break the bag of waters immediately if it has not yet broken (tear it open with your fingertips), so baby can breathe.

8. Lay baby over your abdomen, head slightly lower than body.

   This position helps any mucus drain from his nose and throat.

9. Wipe away any mucus from the baby's nose and mouth, and cover baby.

10. Put baby to breast if the cord is long enough. **Never pull on it!**

After birth

11. Cough gently with each contraction to help expel the afterbirth.

    This may take from five minutes to an hour. **Do not pull on the cord** to hasten the afterbirth.

12. Do not cut the cord. Wrap afterbirth up with the baby.

    The cord may be cut as soon as sterile supplies are available, first tying it in two places six inches from the navel before cutting. The afterbirth must be saved for examination.

13. Massage the uterus and let baby nuzzle the breast.

    Keep the uterus contracted by periodic gentle massage. Baby nuzzling at the breast also helps keep the uterus contracted, even if he won't nurse. There is less bleeding when the uterus keeps contracting.

14. You may get up and walk around whenever you wish.

    You will need to put on sanitary pads. Be careful not to touch the perineum at any time.

Know these rules by heart from the fifth month on!

If others are present, let them call for emergency help, and assist the mother—but only as **she** wishes. They **must not touch the perineum!**

If baby doesn't breathe at once (they usually do), keep his head slightly lowered and tap gently on his feet. If he still doesn't breathe, cover his nose and mouth with your mouth (through a clean handkerchief if there is one) and breath **gently** and rhythmically into baby's lungs as long as necessary.

Additional books written or edited by Helen Wessel:

Apple Tree Family Life Teaching Manual
(with Kathy Nesper)

Natural Childbirth and the Family

The Joy of Natural Childbirth
(paperback edition of Natural Childbirth and the Family)

Childbirth Without Fear, 4th ed., by Grantly Dick-Read
(revised with Harlan Ellis, M.D.)

The Autobiography of Charles G. Finney

Jubilee: The Autobiography of Hermon Pettit

Hebrews: Handbook for World Revival
(with Hermon Pettit)